# NURSING SCHOOL ENTRANCE EXAM

## Your Guide to Passing the Test

## Third Edition

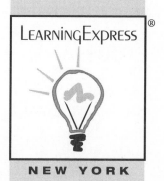

LearningExpress®

NEW YORK

**Library of Congress Cataloging-in-Publication Data**
Nursing school entrance exam.—3rd ed.
    p. ; cm.
    Includes bibliographical references and index.
    ISBN 978-1-57685-902-5
    I. LearningExpress (Organization)
[DNLM:    1.  Nursing—Examination Questions.    WY  18.2]
LC classification not assigned
610.73076—dc23

                                    2011045556

Printed in the United States of America

9 8 7 6 5 4 3 2 1

3rd Edition

ISBN 13: 978-1-57685-902-5

For more information or to place an order, contact LearningExpress at:
    2 Rector Street
    26th Floor
    New York, NY 10006

Or visit us at:
    www.learningexpressllc.com

# CONTENTS

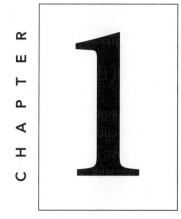

CHAPTER

1

# NURSING SCHOOL ENTRANCE EXAM PLANNER

### CHAPTER SUMMARY

In this chapter, you will learn about career opportunities in nursing and what to expect on the job, as well as essential information about choosing and getting into the nursing school of your choice. You will also find out about the types of entrance tests that nursing schools use to select students.

f you enjoy caring for others and interacting with a wide range of people, and if you cope well when confronted with challenges, nursing is a great career choice. Nursing is also a secure profession with excellent starting salaries and very good job prospects. Job opportunities in nursing abound—registered nurses fill more than 2.6 million jobs, making up the largest healthcare occupation in the nation. And the need for nurses is likely to continue to soar—many of today's nurses are beginning to retire, leaving thousands of job openings. The U.S. population as a whole is also aging, and because older people require more nursing care, the demand for skilled nurses willing to work on the front lines of patient care will also increase. Technological advances in medical care, which allow more medical conditions to be treated, and an emphasis on preventive care also create a greater demand for nurses. As you consider your future in nursing, think about these facts:

- More new jobs are likely to be created for registered nurses than for any other occupation.
- Employers in some areas of the country report a nursing shortage, spurring efforts to attract and keep nurses on staff.
- Hospital outpatient facilities—like same-day surgery centers or rehabilitation centers—offer the most rapid growth in nursing jobs.

To become a nurse, you need to pursue one of three educational routes—a bachelor's degree, an associate's degree, or a hospital diploma. You may also consider becoming a licensed practical nurse (LPN), which requires only one year of training in a vocational or technical school and can be a stepping stone to becoming a registered nurse. Most nursing programs require that you take an entrance test, and that's where this book comes in. *Nursing School Entrance Exam* was designed from real tests, including the admissions test you will face to get into the program of your choice. By tailoring your study plan and using the information in this book, you can achieve your best score and begin the path of your desired career—training to become a nurse.

## Career Opportunities in Nursing

Registered nurses (RNs) provide direct patient care and serve as health educators in the effort to promote wellness and prevent disease. In giving care, they monitor and record a patient's symptoms and progress, give medications, assist in rehabilitation, and teach patients and families about proper care practices. They assist physicians in everything from routine exams and treatments to surgery. There are limits to what a nurse does—state regulations determine the scope of tasks a nurse can perform. But the factor that most influences a nurse's daily workload is the type of healthcare facility in which he or she works. Nurses work in a range of settings: hospitals, doctor's offices, outpatient surgical centers, nursing homes, schools, or work sites. Home health nurses even work in patients' homes. The following is an overview of what you can expect on the job, depending on your work setting.

- *Hospital nurses* make up the largest group of nurses. They provide bedside care for hospitalized patients, observe and record symptoms, and administer treatments and medications. They often work in a specific department of a hospital, such as pediatrics, emergency care, or oncology.
- *Office nurses* work in doctor's offices, clinics, outpatient surgical centers, and emergency medicine clinics. Their job tasks include assisting with exams, giving medications, dressing wounds, and assisting in minor surgeries. They may also do office work and maintain patient records.
- *Nursing facility nurses* provide care for residents in nursing homes or long-term rehabilitation centers. They monitor residents' progress, develop treatment plans, and oversee nursing aides and licensed practical nurses.
- *Home health nurses* work in the patients' own homes. They give medications, check the patient's condition and environment, and instruct patients and caregivers about care and treatment. They may supervise home health aides.
- *Public health nurses* work on the community level in schools, government agencies, retirement communities, or other settings. They educate the public about health promotion and disease prevention strategies in areas like nutrition, smoking cessation, or childcare.
- *Occupational health nurses* provide care to employees at work locations, giving emergency treatments, providing health counseling, or identifying potential health problems in the work environment.

Most RNs earn between $47,000 and $68,000 annually, with the highest paid receiving more than $80,000 annually. Nurses who earned the highest average salaries worked in employment services, followed by hospitals, home healthcare services, physicians' offices, and nursing care facilities.

Licensed practical nurses (LPNs) care for patients under the supervision of a physician or registered nurse. They provide routine bedside care, such as taking vital signs, preparing injections, applying dressings, or collecting testing samples. They also aid patients with feeding, dressing, and bathing. In nursing facilities, LPNs may evaluate the needs of residents and oversee nursing aides. In private offices or clinics, they may be responsible for some administrative work, such as making appointments or maintaining records. The average yearly salary for LPNs is between $28,000 and $50,000. The highest paying LPN positions were found in employment services, followed by home healthcare services, nursing care facilities, hospitals, and physicians' offices.

Working conditions for nurses depend on the type of healthcare facility. For example, work hours vary according to work setting. In nursing homes or long-term rehabilitation centers where residents need around-the-clock care, nurses may work night or weekend shifts. Public health nurses and nurses who work in offices or on industrial work sites follow schedules during regular business hours.

Risks for nurses in hospitals and clinics include coming in contact with patients who have infectious diseases. Nurses must follow a standard set of precautions to reduce their risk for disease or other kinds of danger, like radiation or chemical exposure. Nurses are also susceptible to back injury from moving patients.

## Which Nursing Program Is Right for You?

You may need to consider many factors in deciding the nursing program that is right for you. If your financial situation is tight, you might choose to earn a two-year associate's degree, land a job as a nurse, and then use tuition benefits that come with your employment to take additional courses and work toward a bachelor's degree. Whether you are entering the workforce from high school or making a mid-career change may be another consideration.

Of the programs described in the following list, the bachelor's degree of science in nursing (BSN) offers the most job opportunities. Nurses with bachelor-level education can more easily advance in their jobs, and some positions—like administrative work or those requiring a clinical specialty—may require a bachelor's degree or even an advanced degree.

Nursing programs combine hands-on, supervised clinical experience at a healthcare facility with traditional coursework. In addition to general education requirements, students fulfill courses in

## CHECK YOUR BASIC SKILLS

Nursing requires a range of skills and abilities to perform the job well. Nurses face many challenges on the job—from heavy workloads to long hours on their feet. Review this checklist to see if you fit these job characteristics. Nurses must:

- show caring and sympathy
- look for ways to help others
- demonstrate emotional stability in stressful situations
- have good observational skills
- have physical stamina
- communicate effectively—talking and listening
- be able to direct and supervise (RNs)
- be able to follow orders (LPNs)
- use judgment and make decisions
- know how to problem solve

anatomy, physiology, microbiology, chemistry, nutrition, psychology, and nursing. After completing a nursing program, students must pass a licensing exam to become a nurse. Here is an overview of the degree programs that prepare students for entry-level nurse positions:

- **Diploma Programs** are run by hospitals and usually take three years to complete. These programs are few and their numbers are declining. To broaden their job opportunities, nurses from diploma programs may later opt to earn a bachelor's degree by completing coursework in an RN-to-BSN program. Staff nurse positions often offer tuition reimbursement programs to help allay the cost of additional education.
- **Associate's Degree in Nursing (ADN)** programs are offered by community colleges and last from two to three years. There are about 700 associate-level nursing programs throughout the country. ADN-schooled nurses may also later choose to earn a bachelor's degree to increase their job choices.
- A **Bachelor's of Science Degree in Nursing (BSN)** takes four years to complete at a college or university. More than 670 programs offer this degree. For people who have earned a bachelor's degree in another field and are interested in becoming a nurse, accelerated BSN programs are available; they grant credit for the liberal arts requirements you have already completed. They take from one year to 18 months to complete.

To become a licensed practical nurse (LPN), you must complete a state-approved, one-year training program at a technical or vocational school, community college, or high school. You must also pass a licensing exam. If you want to become an LPN first, but wish to continue your education to become an RN, you can enroll in an LPN-to-RN program. These programs give you credit for your LPN coursework, so you can build upon your training to become an RN.

On the other end of the educational spectrum is a master of science in nursing (MSN). These two-year programs give nurses the opportunity to specialize in clinical training or research. People seeking this degree typically have a BSN or an RN license.

## Selecting a Program That Meets Your Needs

Some considerations for finding a nursing program are obvious. For example, most applicants limit their search by geographic area. Some people need to find a school within driving distance; others are willing to relocate to attend school. An Internet search or a published listing of nursing schools will help locate schools in the area of your choice.

Tuition is another factor in choosing a nursing school—cost can vary depending on whether the institution is private or public, or whether you qualify as an in-state student. Financial aid availability also differs by institution. When you research schools, collect as much information as possible considering these and the factors listed here.

- **Is it approved by the state?** Each state determines the standards for nursing schools and approves them. Your school must be state-approved. However, state approval does not mean that the institution is accredited—for more about accreditation, see the following paragraph.
- **Is it accredited?** Accreditation means that a national accrediting organization, such as the National League for Nursing Accrediting Commission (NLNAC) or the Commission on Collegiate Nursing Education (CCNE), has determined that the nursing school has met certain educational criteria. Earning your degree from an accredited school can give you an edge in the job market—when employers review your educational background, they know you were trained according to an established set of standards. Attending an accredited school also allows you to

continue your education at a graduate-level accredited school. To find out if your preferred school is accredited, contact a school representative or go to the NLNAC's website at www.nlnac.org/home.htm.

- **Pass rate.** What percentage of the school's students passed the nursing licensing exam after graduating? Ask a school representative for information about pass rates from the last five years.
- **What is its focus?** Consider what kind of nursing program interests you (for example, are you interested in a particular clinical specialty?) before you begin your school search. After you choose what kind of program interests you, look for the institution that meets your needs.
- **School size and class size.** Do you want the close-knit community of a small school or the wider mix of students you will find at a large school? Make sure to research the student-to-teacher ratios at prospective schools. Smaller class sizes often mean more attention from faculty.
- **Clinical experience.** What kind of clinical placements does the school offer? How much time does it allot for clinical experience? You can find this information by talking to current students.

## Financing Your Nursing Education

Planning how you are going to pay for your nursing education is essential to your preparation process. The cost of nursing education can be considerable—a four-year program at a state university can be $14,000 a year, and private schools can be more than twice as much. Fortunately, many resources offer financial assistance to nursing students. Financial aid may be awarded based on financial need or on merit and comes in three basic forms—scholarships, loans, or student employment. Be sure to fill out a financial aid form when you apply to nursing school—this form helps schools determine your financial need. Plan on visiting the financial aid office at the school of your

choice or searching the Internet for funding possibilities from a variety of sources, such as the following:

- *Government*: The U.S. Department of Education offers a range of loans and scholarships. The U.S. military also offers financial aid for service people. State governments often provide aid for students attending school in their home state.
- *Your prospective school*: Check with the school of your choice about its scholarships. In addition to aid based on your financial need, you may qualify for a merit-based grant, scholarship, or fellowship.
- *Your employer*: Find out if your employer offers scholarships or tuition reimbursement benefits for education.
- *Nursing associations*: State nursing associations and national professional organizations are other possible sources for financial aid.

## How This Book Can Help You

*Nursing School Entrance Exam* will help you maximize your chances of scoring high on your upcoming exam. Preparing for this important admissions test does not have to be overwhelming—this book will help you organize your preparation process and break it down into manageable steps. Not only does it include hundreds of practice questions and answers, it explains study strategies, so that you can better utilize your time and better learn the key concepts that will appear on your exam. It also offers test-taking tips, a study planner, and practice tests designed from actual entrance exams used by nursing schools today. The explanatory answers that follow the simulated tests are a study guide of their own—helping you understand and review essential ideas and terms. The following is an overview of what you can expect in every chapter.

In Chapter 2, you will learn important test-taking strategies, such as how to pace yourself during the exam, when to guess, and how to combat test anxiety. This chapter presents specific study techniques, giving

## WEB RESOURCES

For more information about funding sources, check out these Web resources:

**U.S. Department of Education**
www.ed.gov
This website has an online financial aid form and offers federal scholarship information.

**National Health Service Corps (NHSC)**
http://nhsc.bhpr.hrsa.gov/
A division of U.S. Department of Health and Human Services, the NHSC offers scholarships and loans for students who agree to practice in a medically underserved area.

**FedMoney.org**
www.fedmoney.org
This is an online guide to all U.S. federal government financial aid programs.

**American Association of Colleges of Nursing (AACN)**
www.aacn.nche.edu
In addition to giving information about scholarships offered by the AACN, this website has links to other government funding sources as well as to other nursing organizations that offer scholarships.

**National Student Nurses' Association (NSNA)**
www.nsna.org
The NSNA offers a scholarship program for nursing students at a range of degree levels.

you several study methods that will aid you in increasing your understanding and retention of material. Varying your study methods will help you avoid boredom in your study sessions and make it easier to learn complicated or difficult topics. You will also learn how to avoid last-minute studying. Be sure to review the helpful strategies in this chapter before you take the practice tests and begin the self-evaluation process described later on in this chapter.

Chapter 3 contains the first of three practice exams. Use the first practice exam as a self-evaluation. Once you complete this practice test and score yourself, you can diagnose your strengths and weaknesses—those areas in which you need more preparation. You can greatly increase the effectiveness of your preparation by targeting your weakest subjects and allotting your study time accordingly.

Chapters 4–9 cover the subject areas found on most nursing school entrance exams: "Verbal Ability," "Reading Comprehension," "Math," "Biology," "Chemistry," and "General Science." Each chapter breaks down and organizes each review topic, highlighting

important terminology and concepts that you need to know for your exam. The biology, chemistry, and general science chapters present material in a clear, concise outline form, so you can easily peruse each subtopic and focus your attention where you need it most. At the conclusion of each chapter, you will find a list of additional resources to help you review topics comprehensively.

Each of these chapters also provides an overview of the kinds of questions you will encounter on the exam and how to tackle them. In addition, you will find practice questions throughout, so you can hone your test-taking skills while you review each topic.

Chapters 10 and 11 contain the last two practice tests. These sample exams use multiple-choice questions just like the ones you will encounter on exam day. By taking these simulated tests and reviewing the answer explanations, you will familiarize yourself with the question types, test format, and subject matter so that you'll feel more prepared and confident on testing day. Read on for more about developing your own study plan, with suggestions about when to take the practice tests so that you can check your scores and still have enough time to focus on the areas in which you need to improve.

## Test Overview

To begin preparing for the test, you need an overview of the type of exam you are facing, and some tips on how to use this book to achieve your best test score. Schools have different requirements for admission, depending on the institution, your choice of study, and whether you are applying for a one-year LPN degree, a two-year RN degree, a four-year BSN degree, a hospital diploma program, or a graduate program. Many accredited nursing schools ask candidates to pass the Registered Nursing School Aptitude Exam (RNSAE), or the Nurses Entrance Test (NET), or the Evolve Reach Admission Assessment Exam (HESI A2), or the Test of Essential Academic Skills (TEAS). Community college LPN programs may require applicants to take the Aptitude for Practical Nursing Exam (APNE). However, even if the school of your choice uses another exam, you will most likely need to demonstrate the essential skills covered in this book. You must show that you can communicate effectively, read and understand college-level materials, and utilize basic math skills. You may also be asked to demonstrate that you have fundamental knowledge about biology, chemistry, natural science, anatomy, and physiology.

Contact the school of your choice immediately to learn about its admissions requirements and test dates and sites in your area. The dates when the test is offered in your area may determine when you take the exam. However, if you have a choice of test dates and have not already applied to take the exam, do not apply until you have conducted the self-evaluation outlined in this chapter. The results of that self-evaluation can help you decide when to take the exam.

The following provides contact information for and an overview of the common nursing aptitude

tests—the NET, RNSAE, and APNE. If you know you will need to take one of these tests, contact the testing agencies in each section for more information about registration, testing locations, and dates.

### Registered Nursing School Aptitude Exam (RNSAE)

Nursing programs that offer degrees ranging from the bachelor's level to a master's degree may require that applicants take the RNSAE. Developed by the Psychological Services Bureau, Inc., this exam consists of five parts and takes about two and a half hours to complete. The first section is divided into three subsections.

- Part 1: Academic Aptitude
    Verbal, 30 questions
    Math, 30 questions
    Nonverbal, 30 questions
- Part 2: Spelling, 50 questions
- Part 3: Reading Comprehension, 40 questions
- Part 4: Natural Sciences (Chemistry, Biology, Health), 90 questions
- Part 5: Vocational Adjustment, 90 questions

### Aptitude for Practical Nursing Exam (APNE)

The Psychological Services Bureau test for practical nursing varies somewhat from the exam for registered nursing. Many community colleges with practical nursing programs use the APNE.

- Part 1: Academic Aptitude
    Verbal, 30 questions
    Math, 30 questions
    Nonverbal, 30 questions
- Part 2: Spelling, 50 questions
- Part 3: Natural Sciences (Chemistry, Biology, Health), 90 questions
- Part 4: Judgment and Comprehension in Practical Nursing Situations, 50 questions
- Part 5: Vocational Adjustment, 90 questions

To register for the RNSAE or the APNE, or to learn about testing sites, contact the school of your choice, or:

Psychological Services Bureau, Inc.
Health Careers Aptitude Tests
977 Seminole Trail
PMB 317
Charlottesville, VA 22901
434-293-5865
www.psbtests.com
Email: info@psbtests.com

### Nurse Entrance Test (NET)

Many RN and LPN nursing programs use the NET as a pre-admissions test. This approximately two-and-a-half-hour test measures your ability in two general academic areas: your critical reading ability and your knowledge of basic math. The test includes two academic sections:

- Mathematics, 60 questions
- Reading Comprehension, 33 questions

Some schools require a different version of this test that includes a written expression section. Find out from the training program of your choice whether this is required. If it is, you will have an additional hour to complete this section.

In addition to reading comprehension and math questions, the basic NET includes questions that evaluate your learning style, stress, and social skills. These nonacademic sections include the following: Test-Taking Skills (30 questions); Stress Level (45 questions); Social Interaction Profile (30 questions); and Learning Style (50 questions). These sections are *not* used to determine whether you will be accepted into a nursing school. The purpose of these sections is to help learning institutions *after* a student has been accepted to their program—it aids the school in considering how a student will best learn—and to increase the likelihood that a student will complete the program successfully.

If you know you need to take the NET, contact the school you are applying to or the testing agency for more information about the test:

Educational Resources, Inc.
7500 West 160th Street
Stilwell, KS 66085
800-667-7531
www.eriworld.com

### Evolve Reach Admission Assessment Exam (HESI A2)

The HESI A2 test is often required as an entrance examination to an accredited nursing program. Each school requires the specific sections it would like its applicants to complete. This guide will help you prep for the basic skills portions of the HESI, along with the biology, chemistry, and anatomy and physiology content.

The academic portion of the HESI A2 exam consists of the following:

- Mathematics, 50 questions
- Reading Comprehension, 47 questions
- Vocabulary and General Knowledge, 50 questions
- Grammar, 50 questions
- Chemistry, 50 questions
- Anatomy and Physiology, 25 questions
- Biology, 25 questions
- Physics, 25 questions

### Test of Essential Academic Skills (TEAS)

Nursing schools sometimes require that students take the TEAS, which can predict whether or not students have the skills required for nursing school and NCLEX-RN or PN success. Developed by ATI Nursing Education, this exam is a multiple-choice assessment of basic academic knowledge in reading, mathematics, science, and English.

The TEAS consists of a total of 170 questions:

- The Math subtest, 45 questions
- The Science subtest, 30 questions
- The English subtest, 55 questions
- The Reading subtest, 40 questions

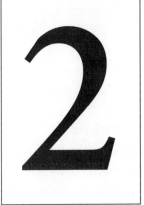

CHAPTER

2 ▶ THE
LEARNINGEXPRESS
TEST PREPARATION
SYSTEM

### CHAPTER SUMMARY

Taking a nursing school entrance exam can be tough, and your career in nursing depends on your passing the exam. The LearningExpress Test Preparation System, developed exclusively for LearningExpress by leading test experts, gives you the discipline and attitude you need to succeed.

**F**irst, the bad news: Taking the nursing school entrance exam is no picnic, and neither is getting ready for it. Your future career depends on passing the test, but there are all sorts of pitfalls that can keep you from doing your best on this all-important exam. Here are some of the obstacles that can stand in the way of your success:

- Being unfamiliar with the format of the exam
- Being paralyzed by test anxiety
- Leaving your preparation to the last minute
- Not preparing at all!
- Not knowing vital test-taking skills: how to pace yourself through the exam, how to use the process of elimination, and when to guess
- Not being in tip-top mental and physical shape
- Arriving late at the test site, having to work on an empty stomach, or shivering through the exam because the room is cold

What's the common denominator in all these test-taking pitfalls? One word: control. Who's in control: you or the exam?

Now the good news: The LearningExpress Test Preparation System puts *you* in control. In just nine easy-to-follow steps, you will learn everything you need to know to make sure that you are in charge of your preparation and your performance on the exam. Other test takers may let the test get the better of them; other test takers may be unprepared or out of shape—but not you. You will have taken all the steps you need to take to get a high score on the nursing school entrance exam.

Here's how the LearningExpress Test Preparation System works: Nine easy steps lead you through everything you need to know and do to master your exam. Each of the steps listed below includes both reading about the step and one or more activities. It is important that you do the activities along with the reading, or you won't be getting the full benefit of the system.

Step 1. Get Information
Step 2. Conquer Test Anxiety
Step 3. Make a Plan
Step 4. Learn to Manage Your Time
Step 5. Learn to Use the Process of Elimination
Step 6. Know When to Guess
Step 7. Reach Your Peak Performance Zone
Step 8. Get Your Act Together
Step 9. Do It!

If you have several hours, you can work through the whole LearningExpress Test Preparation System in one sitting. Otherwise, you can break it up and do just one or two steps a day for the next several days. It is up to you—remember, you are in control.

# Step 1: Get Information

**Activities: Read Chapter 1, "Nursing School Entrance Exam Planner," and use the suggestions there to find out about your requirements.**

Knowledge is power. Therefore, first, you have to find out everything you can about the nursing school entrance exam. Once you have your information, the next steps will show you what to do about it.

## *Part A: Straight Talk about the Nursing School Entrance Exam*

Why do you have to take this exam, anyway? Because an increasing number of people need the kind of care that only a nurse can provide. And, since more and more people need these services, there is growing concern about the quality of care the patients receive. One way to try to ensure quality of care is to test the people who give that care to find out if they have been well trained. And that's why your state or the agency you want to work for may require you to take a written exam.

It is important for you to remember that your score on the written exam does not determine how smart you are or even whether you will make a good nurse. There are all kinds of things a written exam like this can't test: whether you are likely to show up late or call in sick a lot, whether you can be patient with a trying client, or whether you can be trusted with confidential information about people's health. Those kinds of things are hard to evaluate on a written exam. However, it is easy to evaluate whether you can correctly answer questions about your job duties.

This is not to say that correctly answering the questions on the written exam is not important! The knowledge tested on the exam is knowledge you will need to do your job, and your ability to enter the profession for which you have trained depends on your passing this exam. And that's why you are here—to achieve control over the exam.

### Part B: What's on the Test

If you haven't already done so, stop here and read Chapter 1 of this book, which gives you an overview of the written exam. Later, you will have the opportunity to take the sample practice exams in Chapters 3, 10, and 11.

## Step 2: Conquer Test Anxiety

**Activity: Take the Test Anxiety Quiz on page 12.**
Having complete information about the exam is the first step in getting control of the exam. Next, you have to overcome one of the biggest obstacles to test success: test anxiety. Test anxiety can not only impair your performance on the exam itself; it can even keep you from preparing! In this step, you will learn stress management techniques that will help you succeed on your exam. Learn these strategies now, and practice them as you complete the exams in this book so that they will be second nature to you by exam day.

### Combating Test Anxiety

The first thing you need to know is that a little test anxiety is a good thing. Everyone gets nervous before a big exam—and if that nervousness motivates you to prepare thoroughly, so much the better. Many well-known people throughout history have experienced anxiety or nervousness—from performers such as actor Sir Laurence Olivier and singer Aretha Franklin to writers such as Charlotte Brontë and Alfred Lord Tennyson. In fact, anxiety probably gave them a little extra edge—just the kind of edge you need to do well, whether on a stage or in an examination room.

Stop here and complete the *Test Anxiety Quiz* on the next page to find out whether your level of test anxiety is something you should worry about.

### Stress Management Before the Test

If you feel your level of anxiety getting the best of you in the weeks before the test, here is what you need to do to bring the level down again:

- **Get prepared.** There's nothing like knowing what to expect and being prepared for it to put you in control of test anxiety. That's why you are reading this book. Use it faithfully, and remind yourself that you are better prepared than most of the people taking the test.
- **Practice self-confidence.** A positive attitude is a great way to combat test anxiety. This is no time to be humble or shy. Stand in front of the mirror and say to your reflection, "I'm prepared. I'm full of self-confidence. I'm going to ace this test. I know I can do it." If you hear it often enough, you will come to believe it.
- **Fight negative messages.** Every time someone starts telling you how hard the exam is or how it is almost impossible to get a high score, start telling them your self-confidence messages above. If the someone with the negative messages is you telling yourself you don't do well on exams or you just can't do this, don't listen.
- **Visualize.** Imagine yourself reporting for duty on your first day as a nurse. Think of yourself helping patients and making them more comfortable. Imagine coming home with your first paycheck. Visualizing success can help make it happen—and it reminds you of why you are working so hard to pass the exam.
- **Exercise.** Physical activity helps calm down your body and focus your mind. Besides, being in good physical shape can actually help you do well on the exam. Go for a run, lift weights, or go swimming—and do it regularly.

You need to worry about test anxiety only if it is extreme enough to impair your performance. The following questionnaire will provide a diagnosis of your level of test anxiety. In the blank before each statement, write the number that most accurately describes your experience.

0 = Never
1 = Once or twice
2 = Sometimes
3 = Often

____ I have gotten so nervous before an exam that I simply put down the books and didn't study for it.

____ I have experienced disabling physical symptoms, such as vomiting and severe headaches, because I was nervous about an exam.

____ I have simply not showed up for an exam because I was scared to take it.

____ I have experienced dizziness and disorientation while taking an exam.

____ I have had trouble filling in the little circles because my hands were shaking.

____ I have failed an exam because I was too nervous to complete it.

____ **Total:** Add up the numbers in the blanks above.

## Your Test Anxiety Score

Here are the steps you should take, depending on your score. If you scored:

- **Below 3**, your level of test anxiety is nothing to worry about; it is probably just enough to give you that little extra edge.

- **Between 3 and 6**, your test anxiety may be enough to impair your performance, and you should practice the stress management techniques listed in this section to try to bring your test anxiety down to manageable levels.

- **Above 6**, your level of test anxiety is a serious concern. In addition to practicing the stress management techniques listed in this section, you may want to seek additional, personal help. Call your local high school or community college and ask for the academic counselor. Tell the counselor that you have a level of test anxiety that sometimes keeps you from being able to take an exam. The counselor may be willing to help you or may suggest someone else with whom you should talk.

### Stress Management on Test Day

There are several ways you can bring down your level of test anxiety on test day. They will work best if you practice them in the weeks before the test, so that you know which ones work best for you.

- **Deep breathing**. Take a deep breath while you count to five. Hold it for a count of one, then let it out for a count of five. Repeat several times.
- **Move your body**. Try rolling your head in a circle. Rotate your shoulders. Shake your hands from the wrist. Many people find these movements very relaxing.
- **Visualize again**. Think of the place where you are most relaxed: lying on the beach in the sun, walking through the park, or whatever makes you feel good. Now close your eyes and imagine you are actually there. If you practice in advance, you will find that you only need a few seconds of this exercise to experience a significant increase in your sense of well-being.

When anxiety threatens to overwhelm you right there during the exam, there are still things you can do to manage the stress level.

- **Repeat your self-confidence messages**. You should have them memorized by now. Say them quietly to yourself and believe them!
- **Visualize one more time**. This time, visualize yourself moving smoothly and quickly through the test, answering every question correctly, and finishing just before time is up. Like most visualization techniques, this one works best if you have practiced it ahead of time.
- **Find an easy question**. Skim over the test until you find an easy question, and answer it. Getting even one circle filled in gets you into the test-taking groove.
- **Take a mental break**. Everyone loses concentration once in a while during a long test. It is normal, so you shouldn't worry about it. Instead, accept what has happened. Say to yourself, "Hey, I lost it there for a minute. My brain is taking a break." Put down your pencil, close your eyes, and do some deep breathing for a few seconds. Then you will be ready to go back to work.

Try these techniques ahead of time, and see if they don't work for you!

## Step 3: Make a Plan

**Activity: Construct a study plan.**

Maybe the most important thing you can do to get control of yourself and your exam is to make a study plan. Too many people fail to prepare simply because they fail to plan. Spending hours poring over sample test questions the day before the exam not only raises your level of test anxiety, but also will not replace careful preparation and practice over time.

Don't fall into the cram trap. Take control of your preparation time by mapping out a study schedule. On the following pages are two sample schedules based on the amount of time you have before you take the written exam. If you are the kind of person who needs deadlines and assignments to motivate you for a project, here they are. If you are the kind of person who doesn't like to follow other people's plans, you can use the suggested schedules here to construct your own.

Even more important than making a plan is making a commitment. You can't review everything you learned in your nursing courses in one night. You need to set aside some time every day for study and practice. Divide your test preparation into sessions of at least 20 minutes a day. Small, manageable, daily sessions over the course of several weeks will do you much more good than two hours of cramming on Saturday. In addition, making study notes, creating visual aids, and memorizing can be quite useful as you prepare. Each time you begin to study, quickly review your last lesson. This act will help you retain all you have learned and help you assess if you are studying effectively. You may realize you are not remembering some of the material you studied earlier. Approximately one week before your exam, try to determine the areas that are still most difficult for you.

Don't put off your study until the day before the exam. Start now. A few minutes a day, with half an hour or more on weekends, can make a big difference in your score.

## Self-Evaluation

One way to find out how to focus your study time is to conduct a self-evaluation. Begin by taking the practice test in Chapter 3 to highlight areas in which you are strongest and those in which you need more work. You do not have to time yourself—just make sure you have allotted enough time to complete the test in one sitting. When you have finished, score your exam using the answer key at the end of that chapter. Then, match your percentages on each section with the analysis below.

Most people do better on some sections of the exam than on others, but most also find that the varia-

tion is within a certain range; that is, it is rare to score under 50% in one section and over 90% in another. If you are one of those rare types, don't worry; it just shows you where most of your preparation time should go.

But if you are more typical, where your section scores tend to cluster on the following chart should tell you something about when you should take the exam, if you have a choice, and how much time you will have to put in to prepare. If your score in a section clusters in the "under 25%" category, you should really consider postponing taking the exam until you have had some time for serious study. If your score is in the middle ranges, then you can go ahead and take the exam, but you should plan to put aside a fair amount of time to study between now and exam day. Finally, if your score is in the "over 75%" category, you can still benefit from the practice tests and review chapters in this book—your study time will most likely ensure a high score on the entrance exam.

| SECTION SCORE | ANALYSIS |
|---|---|
| under 25% | You need concentrated work in this area. Your best bet is to take an additional course. If that is not possible, contact your school's guidance or academic counseling office to arrange for a tutor. Turn to the chapter of this book pertaining to this section of the test only after you have taken that course or spent at least two months in tutoring; at that point, you will be ready to get maximum benefit from the tips and practice questions in the chapter. |
| 51–74% | This area may not be your strong suit, which is why you should not only work through the relevant chapter, but also use the additional resources listed at the end of that chapter. You might want to find a tutor or form a study group with other students preparing for a nursing school entrance exam. |
| over 75% | Congratulations! You do not need a lot of work in this area. Turn to the relevant chapter of this book to pick up vital tips and practice that can give you extra points in this area. |

## Planning for Success

Based on the amount of time you have before the exam, four customized schedules follow. If you are the kind of person who needs deadlines and assignments to motivate you for a project, here they are. If you prefer to design your own study timeline, use the suggested schedules to help you create an effective plan.

Be sure to research the content of the specific entrance test you will be taking in order to adapt the given schedules for your exam. For example, if you are taking the NET, you may plan to spend less time on the science-related chapters, realizing that this topic is not covered with as much depth as the RNSAE or APNE. (However, because the reading comprehension section of the NET focuses on science material, do not skip these chapters altogether!)

In constructing your plan, you should take into account how much work you need to do. If your scores on the first practice exam were not what you hoped, you should take some of the steps from Schedule A and work them into Schedule D somehow, even if you have only two weeks before the exam. Similarly, your scores on the practice exam should help determine how much time you have to spend preparing each week. If you scored low, you might need to devote several hours a day to test preparation. If you scored high, a few hours a week will probably be enough.

Even more important than making a plan is making a commitment. You cannot get ready overnight for a nursing school entrance exam. Set aside some time every day—or every other day, if your scores were high and you have months until the exam—for study and practice. An hour every day or every other day will do you much more good than a day or two of cramming right before the exam.

## Learning Styles

Each of us absorbs information differently. The way that works best for you is called your dominant learning method. If you were to help a friend assemble a bookcase that arrived in many pieces, how would you begin? Do you need to read the directions and see the diagram?

Would you rather hear your friend read the directions to you and tell you which part connects to another? Or do you draw your own diagram?

The three main learning methods are visual, auditory, and kinesthetic. Determining which type of learner you are will help you create tools for studying.

1. **Visual Learners** need to see the information in the form of maps, pictures, text, words, or math examples. Outlining notes and important points in colorful highlighters and taking note of diagrams and pictures may be key in helping you study.
2. **Auditory Learners** retain information when they can hear directions, the spelling of a word, a math theorem, or poem. Repeating information aloud or listening to your notes on a tape recorder may help. Many auditory learners also find working in study groups or having someone quiz them beneficial.
3. **Kinesthetic Learners** must *do*! They need to draw diagrams, write directions, etc. Rewriting notes on index cards or making margin notes in their textbooks also helps kinesthetic learners to retain information.

## Mnemonics

Mnemonics are memory tricks that help you remember what you need to know. The three basic principles in the use of mnemonics are imagination, association, and location. Acronyms (words created from the first letters in a series of words) are common mnemonics. One acronym you may already know is **HOMES**, for the names of the Great Lakes (**H**uron, **O**ntario, **M**ichigan, **E**rie, and **S**uperior). **ROY G. BIV** reminds people of the colors in the visible light spectrum (**R**ed, **O**range, **Y**ellow, **G**reen, **B**lue, **I**ndigo, and **V**iolet). Depending on the type of learner you are, mnemonics can also be colorful or vivid images, stories, word associations, or catchy rhymes that you create yourself. Any type of learner, whether visual, auditory, or kinesthetic, can use mnemonics to help the brain store and interpret information.

## Schedule A: Six Months to Exam

You have taken the first practice test in Chapter 3 and know that you have at least six months in which to build on your strengths and improve in areas where you are weak. Do not put off your preparation. In six months of five hours a week, you can make a significant difference in your score.

| TIME | PREPARATION |
|------|-------------|
| Exam minus 6 months | Pick the one section in which your percentage score on the practice exam was lowest to concentrate on this month. Read the relevant chapters from among Chapters 4–9 and work through the exercises. Use the additional resources listed in that chapter. When you get to that chapter in the plan below, review it. |
| Exam minus 5 months | Read Chapter 5, "Reading Comprehension," and work through the exercises. Practice reading textbooks and professional journal articles about healthcare, and quiz yourself on each chapter or article you read. Read Chapter 9, "General Science Review," using your reading comprehension skills. Find other people who are preparing for the exam and form a study group. |
| Exam minus 4 months | Read Chapter 7, "Biology Review," and work through the sample questions. Use the resources listed at the end of the chapter for a comprehensive review. Doing all this reading is a good way to practice your reading comprehension skills, too. |
| Exam minus 3 months | Read Chapter 8, "Chemistry Review," and work through the exercises. Use the resources listed at the end of the chapter, or your old textbooks, to review topics you are shaky on. |
| Exam minus 2 months | Read Chapter 6, "Math Review," and work through the exercises. Give yourself additional practice by making up your own test questions in the areas that give you the most trouble. |
| Exam minus 4 weeks | Read Chapter 4, "Verbal Ability," and work through the exercises. Use at least one additional resource listed here. |
| Exam minus 2 weeks | Take the practice test in Chapter 10. Use your scores to help you decide your focus for this week. Go back to the relevant chapters and get the help of a teacher or your study group. |
| Exam minus 1 week | Review the first two sample tests, especially the answer explanations. Then, take the practice exam in Chapter 11 for extra practice. As you study this week, concentrate on your strongest areas and decide not to let any areas where you still feel uncertain bother you. Go to bed early every night this week so you can be at your best by test time. |
| Exam minus 1 day | Relax. Do something unrelated to your nursing school entrance exam. Eat a good meal and go to bed at your new early bedtime. |

## Schedule B: Three to Six Months to Exam

If you have three to six months until the exam, you have just enough time to prepare, as long as you put in at least seven or eight hours a week. This schedule assumes you have four months; stretch it out or compress it if you have more or less time.

| TIME | PREPARATION |
|------|-------------|
| Exam minus 4 months | Read Chapter 5, "Reading Comprehension," and work through the exercises. Practice your reading comprehension skills as you work through Chapter 9, "General Science Review," and the resources listed at the end of that chapter. Find other people who are preparing for the exam and form a study group. |
| Exam minus 3 months | Read Chapters 7 and 8, "Biology Review" and "Chemistry Review," and work through the exercises. Use the resources listed at the end of the chapter, or your old textbooks, to review topics you're shaky on. |
| Exam minus 2 months | Read Chapter 6, "Math Review," and work through the exercises. Give yourself additional practice by making up your own test questions in the areas that give you the most trouble. |
| Exam minus 4 weeks | Read Chapter 4, "Verbal Ability," and work through the exercises. Use at least one of the additional resources listed there. |
| Exam minus 2 weeks | Take the practice test in Chapter 10. Use your scores to help you decide where to concentrate your efforts this week. Go back to the relevant chapters and get help from a teacher or your study group. |
| Exam minus 1 week | Review the first two sample tests, especially the answer explanations. Read over the test-taking strategies in Chapter 2. Then, take the sample test in Chapter 11 for extra practice. Choose the one area in which your scores are lowest to review this week. Go to bed early every night this week so you can be at your peak by test time. |
| Exam minus 1 day | Relax. Do something unrelated to your nursing school entrance exam. Eat a good meal and go to bed at your new early bedtime. |

## Schedule C: One to Three Months to Exam

If you have one to three months until the exam, you still have time to get ready, but you should plan to put in ten hours a week. This schedule is built around a two-month time frame. If you have only one month, spend a couple of extra hours a week so you can get all the steps in. If you have three months, include some of the steps from Schedule B.

| TIME | PREPARATION |
|------|-------------|
| Exam minus 8 weeks | Read Chapter 5, "Reading Comprehension," and work through the exercises. Use your reading comprehension skills as you review Chapter 9, "General Science Review." |
| Exam minus 6 weeks | Read Chapters 7 and 8, "Biology Review" and "Chemistry Review," and work through the exercises. Use the resources listed at the end of the chapters, or your old textbooks, to review topics you're shaky on. |
| Exam minus 4 weeks | Read Chapter 6, "Math Review," and work through the exercises. |
| Exam minus 2 weeks | Read Chapter 4, "Verbal Ability," and work through the exercises. |
| Exam minus 1 week | Take the practice test in Chapter 10. Use your scores to help you decide where to concentrate your efforts this week. Go back to the relevant chapters, and get the help of a teacher or friend. Go to bed early every night this week so you can be at your peak by test time. |
| Exam minus 4 days | Take the practice exam in Chapter 11 for extra practice. |
| Exam minus 1 day | Relax. Do something unrelated to your nursing school entrance exam. Eat a good meal and go to bed at your new early bedtime. |

### Schedule D: Two to Four Weeks to Exam

If you have just two to four weeks until the exam, you really have your work cut out for you. Carve two hours out of your day, every day, for study. This schedule shows you how to make the most of your time if you have just two weeks. If you have an extra week or two, spend more time with the resources listed at the end of Chapters 4–9.

| TIME | PREPARATION |
| --- | --- |
| Exam minus 14 days | Read Chapter 5, "Reading Comprehension," and work through the exercises. Use your reading comprehension skills as you review Chapter 9, "General Science Review." Work through the exercises in that chapter. |
| Exam minus 12 days | Read Chapters 7 and 8, "Biology Review" and "Chemistry Review," and work through the exercises. Use the resources listed at the end of the chapter, or your old textbooks, to review topics you're shaky on. |
| Exam minus 10 days | Read Chapter 6, "Math Review," and work through the exercises. |
| Exam minus 8 days | Read Chapter 4, "Verbal Ability," and work through the exercises. Go to bed early every night this week so you can be at your peak by test time. |
| Exam minus 6 days | Take the practice test in Chapter 10. Based on your scores, choose one or two areas to review until the day before the exam. Go back to the relevant instructional chapters and get the help of a teacher or friend. Go to bed early every night this week so you can be at your peak by test time. |
| Exam minus 4 days | Take the practice exam in Chapter 11 for extra practice. |
| Exam minus 1 day | Relax. Do something unrelated to your nursing school entrance exam. Eat a good meal and go to bed at your new early bedtime. |

## Step 4: Learn to Manage Your Time

**Activities: Practice these strategies as you take the sample tests in this book.**

Steps 4, 5, and 6 of the LearningExpress Test Preparation System put you in charge of your exam by showing you test-taking strategies that work. Practice these strategies as you take the sample tests in this book, and then you will be ready to use them on test day.

First, you will take control of your time on the exam. Most nursing school entrance exams have a time limit, which may give you more than enough time to complete all the questions. Then again, they may not. It is a terrible feeling to hear the examiner say, "Five minutes left," when you are only three-quarters of the way through the test. Here are some tips to keep that from happening to you:

- **Follow directions**. If the directions are given orally, listen to them. If they are written on the

exam booklet, read them carefully. Ask questions before the exam begins if there's anything you don't understand. If you are allowed to write in your exam booklet, write down the beginning time and the ending time of the exam.

- **Pace yourself**. Glance at your watch every few minutes, and compare the time to how far you have gotten in the test. When one-quarter of the time has elapsed, you should be a quarter of the way through the test, and so on. If you are falling behind, pick up the pace a bit.

- **Keep moving**. Don't dither around on one question. If you don't know the answer, skip the question and move on. Circle the number of the question in your test booklet in case you have time to come back to it later.

- **Keep track of your place on the answer sheet**. If you skip a question, make sure that you also skip the question on the answer sheet. Check yourself every five to ten questions to make sure that the number of the question still corresponds with the number on the answer sheet.

- **Don't rush.** Though you should keep moving, rushing won't help. Try to keep calm and work methodically and quickly.

# Step 5: Learn to Use the Process of Elimination

**Activity: Complete worksheet on Using the Process of Elimination (see page 22).**

After time management, your next most important tool for taking control of your exam is using the process of elimination wisely. It is standard test-taking wisdom that you should always read all the answer choices before choosing your answer. This helps you find the right answer by eliminating wrong answer choices. And, sure enough, that standard wisdom applies to your nursing school entrance exam, too.

Let's say you are facing a question that goes like this:

Which of the following lists of signs and symptoms indicates a possible heart attack?
   **a.** headache, nausea, confusion
   **b.** dull chest pain, sudden sweating, difficulty breathing
   **c.** wheezing, dizziness, chest pain
   **d.** difficulty breathing, high fever, chills

You should always use the process of elimination on a question like this, even if the right answer jumps out at you. Sometimes, the answer that jumps out isn't right after all. Let's assume, for the purpose of this exercise, that you are a little rusty on the signs and symptoms of a heart attack, so you need to use a little intuition to make up for what you don't remember. Proceed through the answer choices in order.

- **Start with choice a.** This one is pretty easy to eliminate; none of these signs and symptoms is likely to indicate a heart attack. Mark an **X** next to choice **a** so that you never have to look at it again.
- **On to choice b.** "Dull chest pain" looks good, though if you are not up on your cardiac signs and symptoms you might wonder if it should be "acute chest pain" instead. "Sudden sweating" and "difficulty breathing"? Check. And that's what you write next to choice **b**—a check mark, meaning "good answer; I might use this one."
- **Choice c is a possibility.** Maybe you don't really expect wheezing in a heart-attack victim, but you know "chest pain" is right, and let's say you are not sure whether "dizziness" is a sign of cardiac difficulty. Put a question mark next to choice **c**, meaning "well, maybe."
- **Choice d is also a possibility.** "Difficulty breathing" is a good sign of a heart attack. But wait a minute. "High fever"? Not really. "Chills"? Well, maybe. This doesn't really sound like a heart attack, and you already have a better answer picked out in choice **b**. If you are feeling sure of yourself, put an **X** next to this one. If you want to be careful, put a question mark. Now your question looks like this:

Which of the following lists of signs and symptoms indicates a possible heart attack?
   **X a.** headache, nausea, confusion
   **✓ b.** dull chest pain, sudden sweating, difficulty breathing
   **? c.** wheezing, dizziness, chest pain
   **? d.** difficulty breathing, high fever, chills

You have only one check mark for a good answer. If you are pressed for time, you should simply mark choice **b** on your answer sheet. If you have the time to be extra careful, you could compare your check-mark answer to your question-mark answers to make sure that it is better.

It is good to have a system for marking good, bad, and maybe answers. We recommend this one:

**X** = bad
**✓** = good
**?** = maybe

If you don't like these marks, devise your own system. Just make sure you do it long before test day—while you are working through the practice exams in this book—so you won't have to worry about it during the test.

### Key Words

Often, identifying key words in a question will help you in the process of elimination. Words such as *always, never, all, only, must,* and *will* often make statements incorrect. Here is an example of an incorrect statement:

*When a nurse is preparing to ambulate a client, making sure the client is wearing proper footwear will always prevent him or her from falling.*

The word *always* in this statement makes it incorrect. Nurses must also take other measures, in addition to providing proper footwear, when ambulating a resident, such as proper body mechanics and providing support to the client.

Words like *usually, may, sometimes,* and *most* may make a statement correct. Here is an example of a correct statement:

*Clients of healthcare facilities and hospitals may need help with tasks such as being fed and bathed.*

The word *may* makes this statement correct. There are clients in facilities who may be too ill or weak to perform daily tasks such as feeding and bathing themselves.

Even when you think you are absolutely clueless about a question, you can often use the process of elimination to get rid of at least one answer choice. If so, you are better prepared to make an educated guess, as you will see in Step 6. More often, you can eliminate answers until you have only two possible answers. Then you are in a strong position to guess.

Try using your powers of elimination on the questions in the worksheet *Using the Process of Elimination,* found on the previous pages. The questions are not about nursing; they are just designed to show you how the process of elimination works. The answer explanations for this worksheet show one possible way you might use this process to arrive at the right answer.

## Step 6: Know When to Guess

**Activity: Complete worksheet on Your Guessing Ability (see page 23).**

Armed with the process of elimination, you are ready to take control of one of the big questions in test taking: Should I guess? The first and main answer is *Yes.* Some exams have what's called a "guessing penalty," in which a fraction of your wrong answers is subtracted from your right answers, but nursing school entrance exams don't tend to work like that. The number of questions you answer correctly yields your raw score. So you have nothing to lose and everything to gain by guessing.

The more complicated answer to the question "Should I guess?" depends on you—your personality and your "guessing intuition." There are two things you need to know about yourself before you go into the exam:

Are you a risk-taker?
Are you a good guesser?

# USING THE PROCESS OF ELIMINATION

Use the process of elimination to answer the following questions.

1. Ilsa is as old as Meghan will be in five years. The difference between Ed's age and Meghan's age is twice the difference between Ilsa's age and Meghan's age. Ed is 29. How old is Ilsa?
   a. 4
   b. 10
   c. 19
   d. 24

2. "All drivers of commercial vehicles must carry a valid commercial driver's license whenever operating a commercial vehicle."

   According to this sentence, which of the following people need NOT carry a commercial driver's license?
   a. a truck driver idling his engine while waiting to be directed to a loading dock
   b. a bus operator backing her bus out of the way of another bus in the bus lot
   c. a taxi driver driving his personal car to the grocery store
   d. a limousine driver taking the limousine to her home after dropping off her last passenger of the evening

3. Smoking tobacco has been linked to
   a. increased risk of stroke and heart attack.
   b. all forms of respiratory disease.
   c. increasing mortality rates over the past ten years.
   d. juvenile delinquency.

4. Which of the following words is spelled correctly?
   a. incorrigible
   b. outragous
   c. domestickated
   d. understandible

## Answers

Here are the answers, as well as some suggestions as to how you might have used the process of elimination to find them.

**1. d.** You should have eliminated choice **a** off the bat. Ilsa can't be four years old if Meghan is going to be Ilsa's age in five years. The best way to eliminate other answer choices is to try plugging them in to the information given in the problem. For instance, for choice **b**, if Ilsa is 10, then Meghan must be 5. The difference in their ages is 5. The difference between Ed's age, 29, and Meghan's age, 5, is 24. Is 24 two times 5? No. Then choice **b** is wrong. You could eliminate choice **c** in the same way and be left with choice **d**.

**2. c.** Note the word *not* in the question, and go through the answers one by one. Is the truck driver in choice **a** "operating a commercial vehicle"? Yes, idling counts as "operating," so he needs to have a commercial driver's license. Likewise, the bus operator in choice **b** is operating a commercial vehicle; the question doesn't say the operator has to be on the street. The limo driver in choice **d** is operating a commercial vehicle, even if it doesn't have a passenger in it. However, the cabbie in answer **c** is not operating a commercial vehicle, but his own private car.

**3. a.** You could eliminate choice **b** simply because of the presence of the word *all*. Such absolutes hardly ever appear in correct answer choices. Choice **c** looks attractive until you think a little about what you know—aren't fewer people smoking these days, rather than more? So how could smoking be responsible for a higher mortality rate? (If you didn't know that mortality rate means the rate at which people die, you might keep this choice as a possibility, but you would still be able to eliminate two answers and have only two from which to choose.) And choice **d** is plain silly, so you could eliminate that one, too. You are left with the correct choice, **a**.

**4. a.** How you used the process of elimination here depends on which words you recognized as being spelled incorrectly. If you knew that the correct spellings were outrageous, domesticated, and understandable, then you were home free.

## YOUR GUESSING ABILITY

The following are ten really hard questions. You are not supposed to know the answers. Rather, this is an assessment of your ability to guess when you don't have a clue. Read each question carefully, just as if you did expect to answer it. If you have any knowledge of the subject, use that knowledge to help you eliminate wrong answer choices.

**1.** September 7 is Independence Day in
  **a.** India.
  **b.** Costa Rica.
  **c.** Brazil.
  **d.** Australia.

**2.** Which of the following is the formula for determining the momentum of an object?
  **a.** $p = MV$
  **b.** $F = ma$
  **c.** $P = IV$
  **d.** $E = mc^2$

**3.** Because of the expansion of the universe, the stars and other celestial bodies are all moving away from each other. This phenomenon is known as
  **a.** Newton's first law.
  **b.** the big bang.
  **c.** gravitational collapse.
  **d.** Hubble flow.

**4.** American author Gertrude Stein was born in
  **a.** 1713.
  **b.** 1830.
  **c.** 1874.
  **d.** 1901.

**5.** Which of the following is NOT one of the Five Classics attributed to Confucius?
  **a.** *I Ching*
  **b.** *Book of Holiness*
  **c.** *Spring and Autumn Annals*
  **d.** *Book of History*

**6.** The religious and philosophical doctrine that holds that the universe is constantly in a struggle between good and evil is known as
  **a.** Pelagianism.
  **b.** Manichaeism.
  **c.** neo-Hegelianism.
  **d.** Epicureanism.

**7.** The third Chief Justice of the U.S. Supreme Court was
   **a.** John Blair.
   **b.** Oliver Ellsworth.
   **c.** James Wilson.
   **d.** John Jay.

**8.** Which of the following is the most poisonous portion of a daffodil?
   **a.** the bulb
   **b.** the leaves
   **c.** the roots
   **d.** the flowers

**9.** The winner of the Masters golf tournament in 1953 was
   **a.** Sam Snead.
   **b.** Cary Middlecoff.
   **c.** Arnold Palmer.
   **d.** Ben Hogan.

**10.** The state with the highest per capita personal income in 1980 was
   **a.** Alaska.
   **b.** Connecticut.
   **c.** New York.
   **d.** Texas.

## Answers

Check your answers against the following correct answers.

**1. c.**
**2. a.**
**3. d.**
**4. c.**
**5. b.**
**6. b.**
**7. b.**
**8. a.**
**9. d.**
**10. a.**

## How Did You Do?

You may have simply gotten lucky and actually known the answer to one or two questions. In addition, your guessing was probably more successful if you were able to use the process of elimination on any of the questions. Maybe you didn't know who the third Chief Justice was (question 7), but you knew that John Jay was the first. In that case, you would have eliminated choice **d** and therefore improved your odds of guessing right from one in four to one in three.

According to probability, you should get two-and-a-half answers correct, so getting either two or three right would be average. If you got four or more right, you may be a really terrific guesser. If you got one or none right, you may be a really bad guesser.

Keep in mind, though, that this is only a small sample. You should continue to keep track of your guessing ability as you work through the sample questions in this book. Circle the numbers of questions you guess on as you make your guess; or, if you don't have time while you take the practice tests, go back afterward and try to remember which questions you guessed at. Remember, on a test with four answer choices, your chance of guessing correctly is one in four. So keep a separate "guessing" score for each exam. How many questions did you guess on? How many did you get right? If the number you got right is at least one-fourth of the number of questions you guessed on, you are at least an average guesser—maybe better—and you should always go ahead and guess on the real exam. If the number you got right is significantly lower than one-fourth of the number you guessed on, you would be safe in guessing anyway. However, you might feel more comfortable if you only guessed selectively when you can eliminate a wrong answer or when you have a good feeling about one of the answer choices.

Frankly, even if you are a play-it-safe person with lousy intuition, you are still safe guessing every time.

You will have to decide about your risk-taking quotient on your own. To find out if you are a good guesser, complete the worksheet, *Your Guessing Ability*, on page 23.

## Step 7: Reach Your Peak Performance Zone

**Activity: Complete the Physical Preparation Checklist.**
To get ready for a challenge like a big exam, you have to take control of your physical, as well as your mental, state. Exercise, proper diet, and rest in the weeks prior to the test will ensure that your body works with, rather than against, your mind during your preparation and on test day.

### Exercise

If you don't already have a regular exercise program going, the time during which you are preparing for an exam is an excellent time to start one. And if you are already keeping fit—or trying to get that way—don't let the pressure of preparing for an exam fool you into quitting now. Exercise helps reduce stress by pumping feel-good hormones, called endorphins, into your system. It also increases the oxygen supply throughout your body, including your brain, so you will be at peak performance on test day.

A half hour of vigorous activity—enough to raise a sweat—every day should be your aim. If you are really pressed for time, every other day is OK. Choose an activity you like and get out there and do it. Jogging with a friend or while listening to music always makes the time go faster.

But don't overdo it. You don't want to exhaust yourself. Moderation is the key.

### Diet

First, cut out the junk. Go easy on caffeine and nicotine, and eliminate alcohol from your system at least two weeks before the exam. What your body needs for peak performance is simply a balanced diet. Eat plenty of fruits and vegetables, along with protein and carbohydrates. Foods that are high in lecithin (an amino acid), such as fish and beans, are especially good "brain foods."

The night before the exam, you might "carbo-load" the way athletes do before a contest. Eat a big plate of spaghetti, rice and beans, or whatever your favorite carbohydrate is.

### Rest

You probably know how much sleep you need every night to be at your best, even if you don't always get it. Make sure you do get that much sleep, though, for at least a week before the exam. Moderation is important here, too. Extra sleep will just make you groggy.

If you are not a morning person and your exam will be given in the morning, you should reset your internal clock so that your body doesn't think you are taking an exam at 3 A.M. You have to start this process well before the exam. The way it works is to get up half an hour earlier each morning, and then go to bed half an hour earlier that night. Don't try it the other way around; you will just toss and turn if you go to bed early without having gotten up early. The next morning, get up another half an hour earlier, and so on. How long you will have to do this depends on how late you are used to getting up.

## Step 8: Get Your Act Together

**Activity: Complete Final Preparations worksheet on page 28.**
You are in control of your mind and body. You are in charge of test anxiety, your preparation, and your test-taking strategies. Now it is time to take charge of external factors, like the testing site and the materials you need to take the exam.

# PHYSICAL PREPARATION CHECKLIST

For the week before the test, write down 1) what physical exercise you engaged in and for how long and 2) what you ate for each meal. Remember, you're aiming for at least half an hour of exercise every other day (preferably every day) and a balanced diet that's light on junk food.

## Exam minus 7 days

Exercise: _____ for _____ minutes

Breakfast: _____

Lunch: _____

Dinner: _____

Snacks: _____

## Exam minus 6 days

Exercise: _____ for _____ minutes

Breakfast: _____

Lunch: _____

Dinner: _____

Snacks: _____

## Exam minus 5 days

Exercise: _____ for _____ minutes

Breakfast: _____

Lunch: _____

Dinner: _____

Snacks: _____

## Exam minus 4 days

Exercise: _____ for _____ minutes

Breakfast: _____

Lunch: _____

Dinner: _____

Snacks: _____

## Exam minus 3 days

Exercise: _____ for _____ minutes

Breakfast: _____

Lunch: _____

Dinner: _____

Snacks: _____

## Exam minus 2 days

Exercise: _____ for _____ minutes

Breakfast: _____

Lunch: _____

Dinner: _____

Snacks: _____

## Exam minus 1 day

Exercise: _____ for _____ minutes

Breakfast: _____

Lunch: _____

Dinner: _____

Snacks: _____

### Find Out Where the Test Is and Make a Trial Run

The testing agency or your nursing school advisor will notify you when and where your exam is being held. Do you know how to get to the testing site? Do you know how long it will take to get there? If not, make a trial run, preferably on the same day of the week at the same time of day. Make note on the worksheet *Final Preparations* on page 28 of the amount of time it will take you to get to the exam site. Plan on arriving at least ten to 15 minutes early so you can get the lay of the land, use the bathroom, and calm down. Then figure out how early you will have to get up that morning, and make sure you get up that early every day for a week before the exam.

### Gather Your Materials

The night before the exam, lay out the clothes you will wear and the materials you have to bring with you to the exam. Plan on dressing in layers; you won't have any control over the temperature of the examination room. Have a sweater or jacket you can take off if it is warm. Use the checklist on the worksheet *Final Preparations* on page 28 to help you pull together what you will need.

### Don't Skip Breakfast

Even if you don't usually eat breakfast, do so on exam morning. A cup of coffee doesn't count. Don't eat doughnuts or other sweet foods, either. A sugar high will leave you with a sugar low in the middle of the exam. A mix of protein and carbohydrates is best: Cereal with milk and just a little sugar, or eggs with toast, will do your body a world of good.

## Step 9: Do It!

**Activity: Ace the nursing school entrance exam!**
Fast forward to exam day. You are ready. You made a study plan and followed through. You practiced your test-taking strategies while working through this book. You are in control of your physical, mental, and emotional states. You know when and where to show up and what to bring with you. In other words, you are better prepared than most of the other people taking the nursing school entrance exam with you. You are psyched.

Just one more thing. . . . When you are done with the exam, you deserve a reward. Plan a celebration. Call up your friends and plan a party, or have a nice dinner for two—whatever your heart desires. Give yourself something to look forward to.

And then do it. Go into the exam, full of confidence, armed with test-taking strategies you have practiced until they are second nature. You are in control of yourself, your environment, and your performance on the exam. You are ready to succeed. So do it. Go in there and ace the exam. And look forward to your future career as a nurse!

## FINAL PREPARATIONS

### Getting to the Exam Site

Location of exam site: _____

Date: _____

Departure time: _____

Do I know how to get to the exam site?   Yes ___   No ___   (If no, make a trial run.)

Time it will take to get to exam site: _____

### Things to Lay Out the Night Before

Clothes I will wear        ___

Sweater/jacket             ___

Watch                      ___

Photo ID                   ___

Four #2 pencils            ___

### Other Things to Bring/Remember

_____        _____

_____        _____

_____        _____

_____        _____

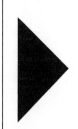

# 3 ▶ PRACTICE EXAM I

### *CHAPTER SUMMARY*

This is the first of three practice exams in this book based on actual nursing school entrance exams commonly used in the field today. Use this test to see how you would do if you had to take the test today.

**T**he practice test in this chapter is modeled on real entrance exams required by nursing education programs. Like many nursing school entrance exams, this practice test measures your skills, abilities, and knowledge of four core subjects: Verbal Ability, Math, Science, and Reading Comprehension. It uses a multiple-choice format, with four answer choices, **a** through **d**. The types of questions in the practice test reflect the kinds of test questions you will likely encounter on your entrance exam.

The practice test is divided into four sections, each covering the four main topics outlined above. On the actual test, each section will be timed separately, and the whole test will last about two to three hours. Here, you do not have to worry about timing—just try to relax and do your best. Remember: The goal of the practice test is to familiarize yourself with the test format and type of questions and to highlight the areas where you need to concentrate your study and preparation. Make sure that you have scheduled enough time to complete the test without major interruptions, taking only short breaks between sections.

On the following pages, you will find an answer sheet. Use this sheet to mark your answers, filling in the ovals that correspond with your answer choices. Each question has only one correct answer, so do not fill in more than one oval per item. The answer key is located on page 72. Although you should not refer to it while you take the practice test, be sure to review the answer explanations carefully after you have finished. A section about how to score your exam follows the answer key.

## Section 1: Verbal Ability

1. ⓐ ⓑ ⓒ ⓓ
2. ⓐ ⓑ ⓒ ⓓ
3. ⓐ ⓑ ⓒ ⓓ
4. ⓐ ⓑ ⓒ ⓓ
5. ⓐ ⓑ ⓒ ⓓ
6. ⓐ ⓑ ⓒ ⓓ
7. ⓐ ⓑ ⓒ ⓓ
8. ⓐ ⓑ ⓒ ⓓ
9. ⓐ ⓑ ⓒ ⓓ
10. ⓐ ⓑ ⓒ ⓓ
11. ⓐ ⓑ ⓒ ⓓ
12. ⓐ ⓑ ⓒ ⓓ
13. ⓐ ⓑ ⓒ ⓓ
14. ⓐ ⓑ ⓒ ⓓ
15. ⓐ ⓑ ⓒ ⓓ
16. ⓐ ⓑ ⓒ ⓓ
17. ⓐ ⓑ ⓒ ⓓ

18. ⓐ ⓑ ⓒ ⓓ
19. ⓐ ⓑ ⓒ ⓓ
20. ⓐ ⓑ ⓒ ⓓ
21. ⓐ ⓑ ⓒ ⓓ
22. ⓐ ⓑ ⓒ ⓓ
23. ⓐ ⓑ ⓒ ⓓ
24. ⓐ ⓑ ⓒ ⓓ
25. ⓐ ⓑ ⓒ ⓓ
26. ⓐ ⓑ ⓒ ⓓ
27. ⓐ ⓑ ⓒ ⓓ
28. ⓐ ⓑ ⓒ ⓓ
29. ⓐ ⓑ ⓒ ⓓ
30. ⓐ ⓑ ⓒ ⓓ
31. ⓐ ⓑ ⓒ ⓓ
32. ⓐ ⓑ ⓒ ⓓ
33. ⓐ ⓑ ⓒ ⓓ
34. ⓐ ⓑ ⓒ ⓓ

35. ⓐ ⓑ ⓒ ⓓ
36. ⓐ ⓑ ⓒ ⓓ
37. ⓐ ⓑ ⓒ ⓓ
38. ⓐ ⓑ ⓒ ⓓ
39. ⓐ ⓑ ⓒ ⓓ
40. ⓐ ⓑ ⓒ ⓓ
41. ⓐ ⓑ ⓒ ⓓ
42. ⓐ ⓑ ⓒ ⓓ
43. ⓐ ⓑ ⓒ ⓓ
44. ⓐ ⓑ ⓒ ⓓ
45. ⓐ ⓑ ⓒ ⓓ
46. ⓐ ⓑ ⓒ ⓓ
47. ⓐ ⓑ ⓒ ⓓ
48. ⓐ ⓑ ⓒ ⓓ
49. ⓐ ⓑ ⓒ ⓓ
50. ⓐ ⓑ ⓒ ⓓ

## Section 2: Reading Comprehension

1. ⓐ ⓑ ⓒ ⓓ
2. ⓐ ⓑ ⓒ ⓓ
3. ⓐ ⓑ ⓒ ⓓ
4. ⓐ ⓑ ⓒ ⓓ
5. ⓐ ⓑ ⓒ ⓓ
6. ⓐ ⓑ ⓒ ⓓ
7. ⓐ ⓑ ⓒ ⓓ
8. ⓐ ⓑ ⓒ ⓓ
9. ⓐ ⓑ ⓒ ⓓ
10. ⓐ ⓑ ⓒ ⓓ
11. ⓐ ⓑ ⓒ ⓓ
12. ⓐ ⓑ ⓒ ⓓ
13. ⓐ ⓑ ⓒ ⓓ
14. ⓐ ⓑ ⓒ ⓓ
15. ⓐ ⓑ ⓒ ⓓ

16. ⓐ ⓑ ⓒ ⓓ
17. ⓐ ⓑ ⓒ ⓓ
18. ⓐ ⓑ ⓒ ⓓ
19. ⓐ ⓑ ⓒ ⓓ
20. ⓐ ⓑ ⓒ ⓓ
21. ⓐ ⓑ ⓒ ⓓ
22. ⓐ ⓑ ⓒ ⓓ
23. ⓐ ⓑ ⓒ ⓓ
24. ⓐ ⓑ ⓒ ⓓ
25. ⓐ ⓑ ⓒ ⓓ
26. ⓐ ⓑ ⓒ ⓓ
27. ⓐ ⓑ ⓒ ⓓ
28. ⓐ ⓑ ⓒ ⓓ
29. ⓐ ⓑ ⓒ ⓓ
30. ⓐ ⓑ ⓒ ⓓ

31. ⓐ ⓑ ⓒ ⓓ
32. ⓐ ⓑ ⓒ ⓓ
33. ⓐ ⓑ ⓒ ⓓ
34. ⓐ ⓑ ⓒ ⓓ
35. ⓐ ⓑ ⓒ ⓓ
36. ⓐ ⓑ ⓒ ⓓ
37. ⓐ ⓑ ⓒ ⓓ
38. ⓐ ⓑ ⓒ ⓓ
39. ⓐ ⓑ ⓒ ⓓ
40. ⓐ ⓑ ⓒ ⓓ
41. ⓐ ⓑ ⓒ ⓓ
42. ⓐ ⓑ ⓒ ⓓ
43. ⓐ ⓑ ⓒ ⓓ
44. ⓐ ⓑ ⓒ ⓓ
45. ⓐ ⓑ ⓒ ⓓ

## Section 3: Quantitative Ability

| | | | |
|---|---|---|---|
| 1. | ⓐ | ⓑ | ⓒ | ⓓ |
| 2. | ⓐ | ⓑ | ⓒ | ⓓ |
| 3. | ⓐ | ⓑ | ⓒ | ⓓ |
| 4. | ⓐ | ⓑ | ⓒ | ⓓ |
| 5. | ⓐ | ⓑ | ⓒ | ⓓ |
| 6. | ⓐ | ⓑ | ⓒ | ⓓ |
| 7. | ⓐ | ⓑ | ⓒ | ⓓ |
| 8. | ⓐ | ⓑ | ⓒ | ⓓ |
| 9. | ⓐ | ⓑ | ⓒ | ⓓ |
| 10. | ⓐ | ⓑ | ⓒ | ⓓ |
| 11. | ⓐ | ⓑ | ⓒ | ⓓ |
| 12. | ⓐ | ⓑ | ⓒ | ⓓ |
| 13. | ⓐ | ⓑ | ⓒ | ⓓ |
| 14. | ⓐ | ⓑ | ⓒ | ⓓ |
| 15. | ⓐ | ⓑ | ⓒ | ⓓ |
| 16. | ⓐ | ⓑ | ⓒ | ⓓ |
| 17. | ⓐ | ⓑ | ⓒ | ⓓ |

| | | | |
|---|---|---|---|
| 18. | ⓐ | ⓑ | ⓒ | ⓓ |
| 19. | ⓐ | ⓑ | ⓒ | ⓓ |
| 20. | ⓐ | ⓑ | ⓒ | ⓓ |
| 21. | ⓐ | ⓑ | ⓒ | ⓓ |
| 22. | ⓐ | ⓑ | ⓒ | ⓓ |
| 23. | ⓐ | ⓑ | ⓒ | ⓓ |
| 24. | ⓐ | ⓑ | ⓒ | ⓓ |
| 25. | ⓐ | ⓑ | ⓒ | ⓓ |
| 26. | ⓐ | ⓑ | ⓒ | ⓓ |
| 27. | ⓐ | ⓑ | ⓒ | ⓓ |
| 28. | ⓐ | ⓑ | ⓒ | ⓓ |
| 29. | ⓐ | ⓑ | ⓒ | ⓓ |
| 30. | ⓐ | ⓑ | ⓒ | ⓓ |
| 31. | ⓐ | ⓑ | ⓒ | ⓓ |
| 32. | ⓐ | ⓑ | ⓒ | ⓓ |
| 33. | ⓐ | ⓑ | ⓒ | ⓓ |
| 34. | ⓐ | ⓑ | ⓒ | ⓓ |

| | | | |
|---|---|---|---|
| 35. | ⓐ | ⓑ | ⓒ | ⓓ |
| 36. | ⓐ | ⓑ | ⓒ | ⓓ |
| 37. | ⓐ | ⓑ | ⓒ | ⓓ |
| 38. | ⓐ | ⓑ | ⓒ | ⓓ |
| 39. | ⓐ | ⓑ | ⓒ | ⓓ |
| 40. | ⓐ | ⓑ | ⓒ | ⓓ |
| 41. | ⓐ | ⓑ | ⓒ | ⓓ |
| 42. | ⓐ | ⓑ | ⓒ | ⓓ |
| 43. | ⓐ | ⓑ | ⓒ | ⓓ |
| 44. | ⓐ | ⓑ | ⓒ | ⓓ |
| 45. | ⓐ | ⓑ | ⓒ | ⓓ |
| 46. | ⓐ | ⓑ | ⓒ | ⓓ |
| 47. | ⓐ | ⓑ | ⓒ | ⓓ |
| 48. | ⓐ | ⓑ | ⓒ | ⓓ |
| 49. | ⓐ | ⓑ | ⓒ | ⓓ |
| 50. | ⓐ | ⓑ | ⓒ | ⓓ |

## Section 4: General Science

| | | | |
|---|---|---|---|
| 1. | ⓐ | ⓑ | ⓒ | ⓓ |
| 2. | ⓐ | ⓑ | ⓒ | ⓓ |
| 3. | ⓐ | ⓑ | ⓒ | ⓓ |
| 4. | ⓐ | ⓑ | ⓒ | ⓓ |
| 5. | ⓐ | ⓑ | ⓒ | ⓓ |
| 6. | ⓐ | ⓑ | ⓒ | ⓓ |
| 7. | ⓐ | ⓑ | ⓒ | ⓓ |
| 8. | ⓐ | ⓑ | ⓒ | ⓓ |
| 9. | ⓐ | ⓑ | ⓒ | ⓓ |
| 10. | ⓐ | ⓑ | ⓒ | ⓓ |
| 11. | ⓐ | ⓑ | ⓒ | ⓓ |
| 12. | ⓐ | ⓑ | ⓒ | ⓓ |
| 13. | ⓐ | ⓑ | ⓒ | ⓓ |
| 14. | ⓐ | ⓑ | ⓒ | ⓓ |
| 15. | ⓐ | ⓑ | ⓒ | ⓓ |
| 16. | ⓐ | ⓑ | ⓒ | ⓓ |
| 17. | ⓐ | ⓑ | ⓒ | ⓓ |

| | | | |
|---|---|---|---|
| 18. | ⓐ | ⓑ | ⓒ | ⓓ |
| 19. | ⓐ | ⓑ | ⓒ | ⓓ |
| 20. | ⓐ | ⓑ | ⓒ | ⓓ |
| 21. | ⓐ | ⓑ | ⓒ | ⓓ |
| 22. | ⓐ | ⓑ | ⓒ | ⓓ |
| 23. | ⓐ | ⓑ | ⓒ | ⓓ |
| 24. | ⓐ | ⓑ | ⓒ | ⓓ |
| 25. | ⓐ | ⓑ | ⓒ | ⓓ |
| 26. | ⓐ | ⓑ | ⓒ | ⓓ |
| 27. | ⓐ | ⓑ | ⓒ | ⓓ |
| 28. | ⓐ | ⓑ | ⓒ | ⓓ |
| 29. | ⓐ | ⓑ | ⓒ | ⓓ |
| 30. | ⓐ | ⓑ | ⓒ | ⓓ |
| 31. | ⓐ | ⓑ | ⓒ | ⓓ |
| 32. | ⓐ | ⓑ | ⓒ | ⓓ |
| 33. | ⓐ | ⓑ | ⓒ | ⓓ |
| 34. | ⓐ | ⓑ | ⓒ | ⓓ |

| | | | |
|---|---|---|---|
| 35. | ⓐ | ⓑ | ⓒ | ⓓ |
| 36. | ⓐ | ⓑ | ⓒ | ⓓ |
| 37. | ⓐ | ⓑ | ⓒ | ⓓ |
| 38. | ⓐ | ⓑ | ⓒ | ⓓ |
| 39. | ⓐ | ⓑ | ⓒ | ⓓ |
| 40. | ⓐ | ⓑ | ⓒ | ⓓ |
| 41. | ⓐ | ⓑ | ⓒ | ⓓ |
| 42. | ⓐ | ⓑ | ⓒ | ⓓ |
| 43. | ⓐ | ⓑ | ⓒ | ⓓ |
| 44. | ⓐ | ⓑ | ⓒ | ⓓ |
| 45. | ⓐ | ⓑ | ⓒ | ⓓ |
| 46. | ⓐ | ⓑ | ⓒ | ⓓ |
| 47. | ⓐ | ⓑ | ⓒ | ⓓ |
| 48. | ⓐ | ⓑ | ⓒ | ⓓ |
| 49. | ⓐ | ⓑ | ⓒ | ⓓ |
| 50. | ⓐ | ⓑ | ⓒ | ⓓ |

## Section 5: Biology

1. ⓐ ⓑ ⓒ ⓓ
2. ⓐ ⓑ ⓒ ⓓ
3. ⓐ ⓑ ⓒ ⓓ
4. ⓐ ⓑ ⓒ ⓓ
5. ⓐ ⓑ ⓒ ⓓ
6. ⓐ ⓑ ⓒ ⓓ
7. ⓐ ⓑ ⓒ ⓓ
8. ⓐ ⓑ ⓒ ⓓ
9. ⓐ ⓑ ⓒ ⓓ
10. ⓐ ⓑ ⓒ ⓓ
11. ⓐ ⓑ ⓒ ⓓ
12. ⓐ ⓑ ⓒ ⓓ
13. ⓐ ⓑ ⓒ ⓓ
14. ⓐ ⓑ ⓒ ⓓ
15. ⓐ ⓑ ⓒ ⓓ
16. ⓐ ⓑ ⓒ ⓓ
17. ⓐ ⓑ ⓒ ⓓ
18. ⓐ ⓑ ⓒ ⓓ
19. ⓐ ⓑ ⓒ ⓓ
20. ⓐ ⓑ ⓒ ⓓ
21. ⓐ ⓑ ⓒ ⓓ
22. ⓐ ⓑ ⓒ ⓓ
23. ⓐ ⓑ ⓒ ⓓ
24. ⓐ ⓑ ⓒ ⓓ
25. ⓐ ⓑ ⓒ ⓓ
26. ⓐ ⓑ ⓒ ⓓ
27. ⓐ ⓑ ⓒ ⓓ
28. ⓐ ⓑ ⓒ ⓓ
29. ⓐ ⓑ ⓒ ⓓ
30. ⓐ ⓑ ⓒ ⓓ
31. ⓐ ⓑ ⓒ ⓓ
32. ⓐ ⓑ ⓒ ⓓ
33. ⓐ ⓑ ⓒ ⓓ
34. ⓐ ⓑ ⓒ ⓓ
35. ⓐ ⓑ ⓒ ⓓ
36. ⓐ ⓑ ⓒ ⓓ
37. ⓐ ⓑ ⓒ ⓓ
38. ⓐ ⓑ ⓒ ⓓ
39. ⓐ ⓑ ⓒ ⓓ
40. ⓐ ⓑ ⓒ ⓓ
41. ⓐ ⓑ ⓒ ⓓ
42. ⓐ ⓑ ⓒ ⓓ
43. ⓐ ⓑ ⓒ ⓓ
44. ⓐ ⓑ ⓒ ⓓ
45. ⓐ ⓑ ⓒ ⓓ
46. ⓐ ⓑ ⓒ ⓓ
47. ⓐ ⓑ ⓒ ⓓ
48. ⓐ ⓑ ⓒ ⓓ
49. ⓐ ⓑ ⓒ ⓓ
50. ⓐ ⓑ ⓒ ⓓ

## Section 6: Chemistry

1. ⓐ ⓑ ⓒ ⓓ
2. ⓐ ⓑ ⓒ ⓓ
3. ⓐ ⓑ ⓒ ⓓ
4. ⓐ ⓑ ⓒ ⓓ
5. ⓐ ⓑ ⓒ ⓓ
6. ⓐ ⓑ ⓒ ⓓ
7. ⓐ ⓑ ⓒ ⓓ
8. ⓐ ⓑ ⓒ ⓓ
9. ⓐ ⓑ ⓒ ⓓ
10. ⓐ ⓑ ⓒ ⓓ
11. ⓐ ⓑ ⓒ ⓓ
12. ⓐ ⓑ ⓒ ⓓ
13. ⓐ ⓑ ⓒ ⓓ
14. ⓐ ⓑ ⓒ ⓓ
15. ⓐ ⓑ ⓒ ⓓ
16. ⓐ ⓑ ⓒ ⓓ
17. ⓐ ⓑ ⓒ ⓓ
18. ⓐ ⓑ ⓒ ⓓ
19. ⓐ ⓑ ⓒ ⓓ
20. ⓐ ⓑ ⓒ ⓓ
21. ⓐ ⓑ ⓒ ⓓ
22. ⓐ ⓑ ⓒ ⓓ
23. ⓐ ⓑ ⓒ ⓓ
24. ⓐ ⓑ ⓒ ⓓ
25. ⓐ ⓑ ⓒ ⓓ
26. ⓐ ⓑ ⓒ ⓓ
27. ⓐ ⓑ ⓒ ⓓ
28. ⓐ ⓑ ⓒ ⓓ
29. ⓐ ⓑ ⓒ ⓓ
30. ⓐ ⓑ ⓒ ⓓ
31. ⓐ ⓑ ⓒ ⓓ
32. ⓐ ⓑ ⓒ ⓓ
33. ⓐ ⓑ ⓒ ⓓ
34. ⓐ ⓑ ⓒ ⓓ
35. ⓐ ⓑ ⓒ ⓓ
36. ⓐ ⓑ ⓒ ⓓ
37. ⓐ ⓑ ⓒ ⓓ
38. ⓐ ⓑ ⓒ ⓓ
39. ⓐ ⓑ ⓒ ⓓ
40. ⓐ ⓑ ⓒ ⓓ
41. ⓐ ⓑ ⓒ ⓓ
42. ⓐ ⓑ ⓒ ⓓ
43. ⓐ ⓑ ⓒ ⓓ
44. ⓐ ⓑ ⓒ ⓓ
45. ⓐ ⓑ ⓒ ⓓ
46. ⓐ ⓑ ⓒ ⓓ
47. ⓐ ⓑ ⓒ ⓓ
48. ⓐ ⓑ ⓒ ⓓ
49. ⓐ ⓑ ⓒ ⓓ
50. ⓐ ⓑ ⓒ ⓓ

## Section 1: Verbal Ability

Find the correctly spelled word in the following questions.

1. a. weigh
   b. wiegh
   c. weaigh
   d. wieigh

2. a. procede
   b. proceid
   c. proceed
   d. procied

3. a. portrit
   b. portrate
   c. portrait
   d. portiat

4. a. miscelaneous
   b. miscellaneous
   c. miscellaneus
   d. misellaneous

5. a. manageable
   b. managable
   c. manageble
   d. mannagable

6. a. catalog
   b. catolog
   c. catilog
   d. catologe

7. a. definately
   b. definitely
   c. defenately
   d. defanitely

8. a. errantt
   b. errant
   c. errent
   d. erant

9. a. obssession
   b. obsessian
   c. obsession
   d. obsessiun

10. a. jeoperdy
    b. jepardy
    c. jeapardy
    d. jeopardy

11. a. magnifisint
    b. magnifisent
    c. magnificent
    d. magnifficent

12. a. monotonous
    b. monotinous
    c. monotonus
    d. monotonos

13. a. eligable
    b. elligible
    c. eligibal
    d. eligible

14. a. inquiry
    b. inquirry
    c. enquirry
    d. enquery

15. a. terminated
    b. termenated
    c. terrminated
    d. termanated

**16. a.** persecution
   **b.** pursecution
   **c.** presecution
   **d.** persecusion

**17. a.** peculior
   **b.** peculiar
   **c.** peculliar
   **d.** piculear

**18. a.** psycology
   **b.** psycholigy
   **c.** psychollogy
   **d.** psychology

**19. a.** lisense
   **b.** lisence
   **c.** lycence
   **d.** license

**20. a.** credental
   **b.** credential
   **c.** credentshil
   **d.** credentile

**21. a.** necessatate
   **b.** necessitat
   **c.** necesitate
   **d.** necessitate

**22. a.** stabilize
   **b.** stablize
   **c.** stableize
   **d.** stabalize

**23. a.** irelevent
   **b.** irelevant
   **c.** irrelevant
   **d.** irrelevent

**24. a.** asspirations
   **b.** asparations
   **c.** aspirrations
   **d.** aspirations

**25. a.** excercise
   **b.** exercise
   **c.** exersize
   **d.** exercize

Find the misspelled word in the following questions.

**26. a.** friend
   **b.** feirce
   **c.** cried
   **d.** no mistakes

**27. a.** preperation
   **b.** government
   **c.** quiet
   **d.** no mistakes

**28. a.** propose
   **b.** rabble
   **c.** quadrupal
   **d.** no mistakes

**29. a.** cutlary
   **b.** donation
   **c.** insight
   **d.** no mistakes

**30. a.** obesity
   **b.** bees
   **c.** quaintly
   **d.** no mistakes

**31. a.** stein
   **b.** hieght
   **c.** perceive
   **d.** no mistakes

**32.** a. suite
b. tedium
c. emporer
d. no mistakes

**33.** a. incorporate
b. contridict
c. exhale
d. no mistakes

**34.** a. pertain
b. reversel
c. memorization
d. no mistakes

**35.** a. deceased
b. feroscious
c. evolve
d. no mistakes

**36.** a. inquire
b. monogram
c. restrain
d. no mistakes

**37.** a. phenomonal
b. emulate
c. misconception
d. no mistakes

**38.** a. mischief
b. temperture
c. lovable
d. no mistakes

**39.** a. dictionary
b. auditorium
c. biology
d. no mistakes

**40.** a. geometry
b. perimeter
c. circumferance
d. no mistakes

**41.** a. transparent
b. worrys
c. lightning
d. no mistakes

**42.** a. primarily
b. finallity
c. specifically
d. no mistakes

**43.** a. porridge
b. reprehensable
c. resonance
d. no mistakes

**44.** a. animosity
b. venture
c. caffiene
d. no mistakes

**45.** a. balcony
b. delenquent
c. emergency
d. no mistakes

**46.** a. gratitude
b. horrendous
c. forcast
d. no mistakes

**47.** a. rightious
b. strenuous
c. manageable
d. no mistakes

**48.** **a.** sincerly
    **b.** faithfully
    **c.** reliably
    **d.** no mistakes

**49.** **a.** label
    **b.** vacency
    **c.** medal
    **d.** no mistakes

**50.** **a.** digestion
    **b.** resperation
    **c.** circulation
    **d.** no mistakes

# Section 2:
# Reading Comprehension

Read each passage and answer the accompanying questions based solely on the information found in the passage. You have 45 minutes to complete this section.

No longer is asthma considered a condition with isolated, acute episodes of bronchospasm. Rather, asthma is now understood to be a chronic inflammatory disorder of the airways—that is, inflammation makes the airways chronically sensitive. When these hyper-responsive airways are irritated, air flow is limited, and attacks of coughing, wheezing, chest tightness, and difficulty in breathing occur.

Asthma involves complex interactions among inflammatory cells, mediators, and the cells and tissues in the airways. The interactions result in airflow limitation from acute bronchoconstriction, swelling of the airway wall, increased mucus secretion, and airway remodeling. The inflammation also causes an increase in airway responsiveness. During an asthma attack, the patient attempts to compensate by breathing at a higher lung volume in order to keep the air flowing through the constricted airways, and the greater the airway limitation, the higher the lung volume must be to keep airways open. The morphologic changes that occur in asthma include bronchial infiltration by inflammatory cells. Key effector cells in the inflammatory response are the mast cells, lymphocytes, and eosinophils. Mast cells and eosinophils are also significant participants in allergic responses, hence the similarities between allergic reactions and asthma attacks. Other changes include mucus plugging of the airways, interstitial edema, and microvascular leakage. Destruction

of bronchial epithelium and thickening of the subbasement membrane is also characteristic. In addition, there may be hypertrophy and hyperplasia of airway smooth muscle, increase in goblet cell number, and enlargement of submucous glands.

Although causes of the initial tendency toward inflammation in the airways of patients with asthma are not yet certain, to date the strongest identified risk factor is atopy. This inherited familial tendency to have allergic reactions includes increased sensitivity to allergens that are risk factors for developing asthma. Some of these allergens include domestic dust mites, animals with fur, cockroaches, pollens, and molds. Additionally, asthma may be triggered by viral respiratory infections, especially in children. By avoiding these allergens and triggers, a person with asthma lowers the risk of irritating sensitive airways. A few avoidance techniques include keeping the home clean and well-ventilated, using an air conditioner in the summer months when pollen and mold counts are high, and getting an annual influenza vaccination. Of course, asthma sufferers should avoid tobacco smoke altogether. Cigar, cigarette, and pipe smoke are triggers whether the patient smokes or breathes in the smoke from others. Smoke increases the risk of allergic sensitization in children and increases the severity of symptoms in children who already have asthma. Many of the risk factors for developing asthma may also provoke asthma attacks, and people with asthma may have one or more triggers, which vary from individual to individual. The risk can be further reduced by taking medications that decrease airway inflammation. Most exacerbations can be prevented by the combination of avoiding triggers and taking anti-inflammatory medications. An exception is physical activity, which is a common trigger of exacerbations in asthma patients. However, asthma patients should not necessarily avoid all physical exertion, because some types of activity have actually been proven to reduce symptoms. Rather, they should work in conjunction with a doctor to design a proper training regimen including the use of medication.

In order to diagnose asthma, a healthcare professional must appreciate the underlying disorder that leads to asthma symptoms and understand how to recognize the condition through information gathered from the patient's history, physical examination, measurements of lung function, and allergic status. Because asthma symptoms vary throughout the day, the respiratory system may appear normal during physical examination. Clinical signs are more likely to be present when a patient is experiencing symptoms; however, the absence of symptoms at the time of the examination does not exclude the diagnosis of asthma.

1. What is a symptom of a chronic inflammatory disorder of the airways?
   a. allergies
   b. influenza
   c. chest tightness
   d. lymphocyte swelling

2. Why does a person suffering from an asthma attack attempt to inhale more air?
   a. to prevent the loss of consciousness
   b. to keep air flowing through shrunken air passageways
   c. to prevent hyperplasia
   d. to compensate for weakened mast cells, lymphocytes, and eosinophils

3. The passage suggests that, in the past, asthma was regarded as
   a. a result of the overuse of tobacco products.
   b. a hysterical condition.
   c. mysterious, unrelated attacks affecting the lungs.
   d. a chronic condition.

4. Which of the following would be the best replacement for the word *exacerbations* in this passage?
   a. attacks
   b. allergies
   c. triggers
   d. allergens

5. The passage mentions all of the following allergens to which people with asthma may be particularly sensitive EXCEPT
   a. domestic dust mites.
   b. pollens.
   c. cockroaches.
   d. cigarette smoke.

6. Which of the following triggers, albeit surprising, is mentioned as possibly being able to reduce the symptoms of asthma in some patients?
   a. using a fan instead of an air conditioner
   b. second-hand cigarette smoke
   c. a family pet
   d. physical exercise

7. Why might a patient with asthma have an apparently normal respiratory system during an examination by a doctor?
   a. Asthma symptoms come and go throughout the day.
   b. Severe asthma occurs only after strenuous physical exertion.
   c. Doctors' offices are usually smoke-free and very clean.
   d. The pollen and mold count may be low that day.

**8.** Who might be the most logical audience for this passage?

  **a.** researchers studying the respiratory system

  **b.** healthcare professionals

  **c.** a mother whose child has been diagnosed with asthma

  **d.** an anti-smoking activist

**9.** What is the reason given for why second-hand smoke should be avoided by children?

  **a.** A smoke-filled room is most likely a breeding ground for viral respiratory infections.

  **b.** Smoke can stunt an asthmatic child's growth.

  **c.** Breathing smoke can lead to a fatal asthma attack.

  **d.** Smoke can heighten the intensity of asthma symptoms.

Today, food and color additives are more strictly studied, regulated, and monitored than at any other time in history. The Food and Drug Administration (FDA) has the primary legal responsibility for determining their safe use. To market a new food or color additive (or before using an additive already approved for one use in another manner not yet approved), a manufacturer or other sponsor must first petition the FDA for its approval. These petitions must provide evidence that the substance is safe for the ways in which it will be used. Since 1999, indirect additives have been approved via a pre-market notification process requiring the same data as was previously required by petition.

When evaluating the safety of a substance and whether it should be approved, the FDA considers: 1) the composition and properties of the substance, 2) the amount of the substance that would typically be consumed, 3) immediate and long-term health effects, and 4) various safety factors. The evaluation determines an appropriate level of use that includes a built-in safety margin—a factor that allows for uncertainty about the levels of consumption that are expected to be harmless. In other words, the levels of use that gain approval are much lower than what would be expected to have any adverse effect.

Because of inherent limitations of science, the FDA can never be *absolutely* certain of the absence of any risk from the use of any substance. Therefore, the FDA must determine—based on the best science available—if there is a *reasonable certainty of no harm* to consumers when an additive is used as proposed.

If an additive is approved, the FDA issues regulations that may include the types of foods in which the additive can be used, the maximum amounts to be used, and how it should be identified on food labels. In 1999, procedures changed so that the FDA now consults with the United States Department of Agriculture (USDA) during the review process for ingredients that are proposed for use in meat and poultry products. Federal officials then monitor the extent of Americans' consumption of the new additive and results of any new research on its safety to ensure its use continues to be within safe limits.

If new evidence suggests that a product already in use may be unsafe, or if consumption levels have changed enough to require another look, federal authorities may prohibit the use of that product or conduct further studies to determine if its use can still be considered safe.

Regulations known as Good Manufacturing Practices (GMP) limit the number of food ingredients used in foods to the amount necessary to achieve the desired effect.

**10.** Which of the following does the FDA take under consideration when evaluating a substance for possible approval?
   a. its cost
   b. its chemical makeup
   c. its palatability
   d. its possible appeal to the general public

**11.** According to the passage, which of the following is true?
   a. The FDA considers the properties of a substance when evaluating its safety.
   b. The FDA is in charge of developing new food and color additives.
   c. The FDA approves more new food and color additives than it rejects.
   d. The FDA is solely responsible for reviewing ingredients used in poultry products.

**12.** What does *reasonable certainty of no harm* mean?
   a. The FDA has only so much capability to test a substance fully before it is out on the commercial market.
   b. The FDA makes a notation of whether or not it feels a product is reasonable in the economic climate.
   c. An FDA seal of approval means that the government guarantees no danger will come from consumption.
   d. There is a 75% assurance that a product is safe for human consumption.

**13.** The FDA does NOT have the right to
   a. lower the amount of money charged for a food product using a recently approved additive.
   b. set limitations on the amount of a food dye that can be used in a certain product.
   c. determine the language used on a food's nutrition label.
   d. have a say in the way beef is commercially prepared.

**14.** At what point does the FDA issue regulations regarding an additive?
   a. as soon as the additive has been tested
   b. after the additive has been shown to be harmful
   c. before the additive has been submitted for testing
   d. after the additive has been approved

**15.** What is the main idea of the passage?
   a. Current dangerous food practices have caused increased FDA activity in recent years.
   b. The FDA is the organization responsible for making sure the substances you consume are safe.
   c. 1999 was a year of major change in the food and drug industry.
   d. The FDA is in charge of setting Good Manufacturing Practices for society.

Medical waste has been a growing concern because of recent incidents of public exposure to discarded blood vials, needles (sharps), empty prescription bottles, and syringes. Medical waste can typically include general refuse, human blood and blood products, cultures and stocks of infectious agents, laboratory animal carcasses, contaminated bedding material, and pathological wastes.

Wastes are collected by gravity chutes, carts, or pneumatic tubes. Chutes are limited to vertical transport, and there is some risk of exhausting contaminants into hallways if a door is left open during use. Another disadvantage of gravity chutes is that the waste container may get jammed while dropping or broken upon hitting the bottom. Carts are primarily for horizontal transport of bagged or containerized wastes. The main risk here is that bags may be broken or torn during transport, potentially exposing the worker to the wastes. Using automated carts can reduce the potential for exposure. Pneumatic tubes offer the best performance for waste transport in a large facility. Advantages include high-speed movement, movement in any direction, and minimal intermediate storage of untreated wastes. However, some objects cannot be conveyed pneumatically.

Off-site disposal of regulated medical wastes remains a viable option for smaller hospitals (those with fewer than 150 beds). Some preliminary on-site processing, such as compaction or hydropulping, may be necessary prior to sending the waste off-site. Compaction reduces the total volume of solid wastes, often reducing transportation and disposal costs, but it does not change the hazardous characteristics of the waste. However, compaction may not be economical if transportation and disposal costs are based on weight rather than volume.

Hydropulping involves grounding the waste in the presence of an oxidizing fluid, such as hypochlorite solution. The liquid is separated from the pulp and discharged directly into the sewer, unless local limits require additional pretreatment prior to discharge. The pulp can often be disposed of at a landfill. One advantage is that waste can be rendered innocuous and reduced in size within the same system. Disadvantages are the added operating burden, difficulty of controlling fugitive emission, and the difficulty of conducting microbiological tests to determine whether all organic matters and infectious organisms from the waste have been destroyed.

On-site disposal is a feasible alternative for hospitals generating two tons per day or more of total solid waste. Common treatment techniques include steam sterilization and incineration. Although other options are available, incineration is currently the preferred method for on-site treatment of hospital waste.

Steam sterilization is limited in the types of medical waste it can treat but is appropriate for laboratory cultures and/or substances contaminated with infectious organisms. The waste is subjected to steam in a sealed, pressurized chamber. The liquid that may form is drained off to the sewer or sent for processing. The unit is then reopened after a vapor release to the atmosphere, and the solid waste is taken out for further processing or disposal. One advantage of steam sterilization is that it has been used for many years in hospitals to sterilize instruments and containers and to treat small quantities of waste. However, since sterilization does not change the appearance of the waste, there could be a problem in gaining acceptance of the waste for landfilling.

A properly designed, maintained, and operated incinerator achieves a relatively high level of organism destruction. Incineration reduces the weight and volume of the waste as much as 95% and is especially appropriate for pathological wastes and sharps. The most common incineration system for medical waste is the controlled-air type. The principal advantage of this type of incinerator is low particulate emissions. Rotary kiln and grate-type units have been used, but use of grate-type units has been discontinued due to high air emissions. The rotary kiln also puts out high emissions, and the costs have been prohibitive for smaller units.

16. One disadvantage of the compaction method of waste disposal is that it
   a. cannot reduce transportation costs.
   b. reduces the volume of solid waste material.
   c. does not allow hospitals to confirm that organic matter has been eliminated.
   d. does not reduce the weight of solid waste material.

**17.** For small hospitals, medical wastes may be disposed
   **a.** in hydropulping facilities.
   **b.** off site.
   **c.** in compactors.
   **d.** on site.

**18.** Which of the following could be safely disposed of in a landfill but might not be accepted by landfill facilities?
   **a.** hydropulped material
   **b.** sterilized waste
   **c.** incinerated waste
   **d.** laboratory cultures

**19.** The two processes mentioned that involve the formation of liquid are
   **a.** compaction and hydropulping.
   **b.** incineration and compaction.
   **c.** hydropulping and sterilization.
   **d.** sterilization and incineration.

**20.** Two effective methods for treating waste caused by infectious matter are
   **a.** steam sterilization and incineration.
   **b.** hydropulping and steam sterilization.
   **c.** incineration and compaction.
   **d.** hydropulping and incineration.

**21.** Hospitals can minimize employee contact with dangerous waste by switching from
   **a.** a manual cart to a gravity chute.
   **b.** an automated cart to a hydropulping machine.
   **c.** a gravity chute to a manual cart.
   **d.** a manual cart to an automated cart.

**22.** The process that transforms waste from hazardous to harmless AND diminishes waste volume is
   **a.** sterilization.
   **b.** hydropulping.
   **c.** oxidizing.
   **d.** compacting.

**23.** As it is used in the fourth paragraph of the passage, the word *grounding* most nearly means
   **a.** confirming.
   **b.** descending.
   **c.** compressing.
   **d.** instructing.

**24.** Budgetary constraints have precluded some small hospitals from purchasing
   **a.** pneumatic tubes.
   **b.** rotary kilns.
   **c.** sterilization equipment.
   **d.** controlled-air kilns.

The immune system is equal in complexity to the combined intricacies of the brain and nervous system. The success of the immune system in defending the body relies on a dynamic regulatory-communications network consisting of millions and millions of cells. Organized into sets and subsets, these cells pass information back and forth like clouds of bees swarming around a hive. The result is a sensitive system of checks and balances, which produces an immune response that is prompt, appropriate, effective, and self-limiting.

At the heart of the immune system is the ability to distinguish between *self* and *nonself*. When immune defenders encounter cells or organisms carrying foreign or nonself molecules, the immune troops move quickly to eliminate the intruders. Virtually every body cell carries distinctive molecules that identify it as self. The body's immune defenses do not normally attack tissues that carry a self marker. Rather, immune cells and other body cells coexist peaceably in a state known as self-tolerance. When a normally functioning immune system attacks a nonself molecule, the system has the ability to "remember" the specifics of the foreign body. Upon subsequent encounters with the same species of molecules, the immune system reacts accordingly. With the possible exception of antibodies passed during lactation, this so-called immune system memory is not inherited. Despite the occurrence of a virus in your family, your immune system must "learn" from experience with the many millions of distinctive nonself molecules in the sea of microbes in which we live. Learning entails producing the appropriate molecules and cells to match up with and counteract each nonself invader.

Any substance capable of triggering an immune response is called an *antigen*. Antigens are not to be confused with *allergens*, which are most often harmless substances (such as ragweed pollen or cat hair) that provoke the immune system to set off the inappropriate and harmful response known as *allergy*. An antigen can be a virus, a bacterium, a fungus, a parasite, or even a portion or product of one of these organisms. Tissues or cells from another individual (except an identical twin, whose cells carry identical self markers) also act as antigens; because the immune system recognizes transplanted tissues as foreign, it rejects them. The body will even reject nourishing proteins unless they are first broken down by the digestive system into their primary, non-antigenic building blocks. An antigen announces its foreignness by means of intricate and characteristic shapes called *epitopes*, which protrude from its surface. Most antigens, even the simplest microbes, carry several different kinds of epitopes on their surface; some may even carry several hundred. Some epitopes will be more effective than

others at stimulating an immune response. Only in abnormal situations does the immune system wrongly identify self as nonself and execute a misdirected immune attack. The result can be a so-called autoimmune disease, such as rheumatoid arthritis or systemic lupus erythematosus. The painful side effects of these diseases are caused by a person's immune system actually attacking itself.

25. Which of the following is the analogy used in the passage to describe the communications network among the cells in the immune system?
    a. the immune system's memory
    b. immune troops eliminating intruders
    c. bees swarming around a hive
    d. a sea of microbes

26. One symptom of a person's immune system attacking itself is
    a. an excess of antigens.
    b. indigestion.
    c. rejection of foreign tissues.
    d. pain.

27. What is the specific term used in the passage for the substance capable of triggering an inappropriate or harmful immune response to a harmless substance such as ragweed pollen?
    a. antigen
    b. microbe
    c. allergen
    d. autoimmune disease

28. How do the cells in the immune system recognize an antigen as "foreign" or "nonself"?
    a. through an allergic response
    b. through blood type
    c. through fine hairs protruding from the antigen surface
    d. through characteristic shapes on the antigen surface

**29.** After you have had the chicken pox, your immune system will be able to do all of the following EXCEPT
   **a.** protect your offspring from infection by the chicken pox virus.
   **b.** distinguish between your body cells and those of the chicken pox virus.
   **c.** "remember" previous experiences with the chicken pox virus.
   **d.** match up and counteract nonself molecules in the form of the chicken pox virus.

**30.** Which of the following best expresses the main idea of this passage?
   **a.** The basic function of the immune system is to distinguish between self and nonself.
   **b.** An antigen is any substance that triggers an immune response.
   **c.** One of the immune system's primary functions is the allergic response.
   **d.** The human body presents an opportune habitat for microbes.

**31.** Based on the information in the passage, why would tissue transplanted from father to daughter have a greater risk of being detected as foreign than tissue transplanted between identical twins?
   **a.** The age of the twins' tissue would be the same and, therefore, less likely to be rejected.
   **b.** The twins' tissue would carry the same self markers and would therefore be less likely to be rejected.
   **c.** The difference in the sex of the father and daughter would cause the tissue to be rejected by the daughter's immune system.
   **d.** The twins' immune systems would "remember" the same encounters with childhood illnesses.

Notebooks, erasers, pencil sets, and backpacks are on most kids' back-to-school lists. But if your child has diabetes, you should add a few extra tasks to the list. At the top, put "good communication," with your child and with the school. Planning ahead, and getting help from others, will help pave the way for a successful year.

Diabetes is a serious and lifelong condition, and it's a growing problem among children and teens. About 186,000 Americans under age 20 have diabetes. Most have type 1 diabetes, which usually first appears during childhood. But in recent years a growing number of kids have been diagnosed with type 2 diabetes, a disease that in the past primarily struck adults over age 45. Excess weight and inactivity puts children and teens at risk for type 2 diabetes.

When you have diabetes, you have too much glucose in your blood. Over time, this excess glucose can damage both large and small blood vessels, leading to heart disease, stroke, nerve damage, blindness, and kidney disease. That's why people with diabetes must regularly check their blood glucose. They need to keep their levels from dropping by using strategies like snacking. When their glucose is too high, insulin can help to bring it down. Essentially, they have to manage their blood glucose level 24 hours a day, seven days a week.

This intensive management can be daunting to kids during school. They may wonder: What happens if I feel light-headed or need a snack in the middle of class? Will I be okay in gym class? When should I go to the nurse? These are all issues you should discuss ahead of time with school staff and with your child. Work with your child's healthcare team to develop a written diabetes management plan outlining your child's specific medical needs. Make sure key staff members, like your child's teacher, have a copy of the plan.

Heading back to school with diabetes can be a challenge. But by eating regular meals, making healthy food choices, staying active, and taking medications, kids with diabetes can do all the things their friends do and more. With planning and good communication, you can help your child have a healthy and happy school year.

**32.** What is a good title for the passage?
   **a.** The Obesity Epidemic: How Diabetes Is Affecting Youth in the Twenty-First Century
   **b.** Knowledge Is Power: Teaching Your Children about Their Diabetes
   **c.** Healthy and Happy: Good Living Tips for Children and Teens
   **d.** Snack Your Way to a Healthy Body

**33.** Which of the following put(s) children and teens at risk for type 2 diabetes?
   **a.** high estrogen levels
   **b.** excess weight and inactivity
   **c.** overactive thyroid
   **d.** being taller than average

**34.** According to the passage, which of the following is true?
   **a.** It is easier for a child to regulate his or her diabetes if he or she is homeschooled.
   **b.** Only people with diabetes have glucose in their system.
   **c.** Diabetes is a private disease that a child should learn to regulate on his or her own.
   **d.** Children with diabetes should pack snacks in their schoolbags.

**35.** Which of the following is not true about glucose?
   **a.** After a few years of healthy living, glucose levels even themselves out.
   **b.** Too much glucose can eventually destroy kidney function.
   **c.** Food is a way of raising glucose levels when they dip too low.
   **d.** Levels of blood glucose need to be monitored carefully.

**36.** According to the passage, children with diabetes
   **a.** should restrict calories and food intake in order to lose weight.
   **b.** must take care when playing team sports because they are susceptible to many diseases.
   **c.** need to become very familiar with their own blood glucose levels.
   **d.** contract the disease by eating too much sugar at an early age.

**37.** People with diabetes need insulin when
   **a.** their glucose levels are too low.
   **b.** their blood pressure is too low.
   **c.** their glucose levels are too high.
   **d.** their blood pressure is too high.

**38.** According to the passage, too much blood glucose can lead to all of the following health problems EXCEPT
   **a.** heart disease.
   **b.** kidney disease.
   **c.** stroke.
   **d.** paralysis.

**39.** What does the word *intensive* mean in the fourth paragraph?
   **a.** rigorous
   **b.** difficult
   **c.** painful
   **d.** confusing

**40.** According to the passage, the parents of children with diabetes should
  **a.** keep their child indoors at all times.
  **b.** make sure their child does not do any physical activity.
  **c.** develop a diabetes management plan.
  **d.** inject their child with insulin every hour.

There are two types of cell division: mitosis and meiosis. Most of the time when people refer to "cell division," they mean mitosis, the process of making new body cells. Meiosis is the type of cell division that creates gametes, or egg and sperm cells.

    Mitosis is a fundamental process for life. During mitosis, a cell duplicates all of its contents, including its chromosomes, and splits to form two identical daughter cells. Because this process is so critical, the steps of mitosis are carefully controlled by a number of genes. When mitosis is not regulated correctly, health problems, such as cancer, can result.

    The other type of cell division, meiosis, ensures that humans have the same number of chromosomes in each generation. It is a two-step process that reduces the chromosome number by half—from 46 to 23—to form sperm and egg cells. When the sperm and egg cells unite at conception, each contributes 23 chromosomes, so the resulting embryo will have the usual 46. Meiosis also allows genetic variation through processes of DNA shuffling during cell division.

**41.** What is the main idea of this passage?
  **a.** Meiosis is responsible for variations in physical characteristics.
  **b.** Mitosis can be the cause of fatal health problems.
  **c.** Cells divide through a pair of unique processes.
  **d.** Meiosis and mitosis are delicate biological processes that can lead to fatal disease.

**42.** According to the passage, which of the following is true?
  **a.** When a cell undergoes mitosis, the result is the same as its parent cell.
  **b.** The most important type of cell division is mitosis.
  **c.** Mitosis is responsible for forming the gametes that join to make an embryo.
  **d.** Meiosis creates two identical cells.

**43.** What is the meaning of the word *unite* in the passage?
  **a.** to get married
  **b.** to fight for a common cause
  **c.** to agree
  **d.** to join

**44.** What is a possible result of incorrectly regulated mitosis?
  **a.** cell duplication
  **b.** cancer
  **c.** meiosis
  **d.** twins

**45.** According to the information presented in the passage, which process is responsible for creating new skin cells when the skin has been cut?
  **a.** mitosis
  **b.** meiosis
  **c.** mitosis and meiosis
  **d.** neither mitosis nor meiosis

# Section 3: Quantitative Ability

Use scratch paper if needed to answer the following 50 questions. You have 45 minutes to complete this section.

1. What is the reciprocal of $3\frac{4}{5}$?
   a. $\frac{5}{19}$
   b. $\frac{19}{5}$
   c. $4\frac{1}{4}$
   d. $\frac{35}{4}$

2. What is the value of $y$ when $12y + 17 = 161$?
   a. 8.76
   b. 12
   c. 14.8
   d. 14

3. What is the circumference of a circle with a radius of 5?
   a. $5\pi$
   b. $10\pi$
   c. $25\pi$
   d. $50\pi$

4. A designer buys 180 square feet of wallpaper to cover a square wall with a length of 12 feet. How much wallpaper will be left over when he's done covering the wall?
   a. 6 sq. ft.
   b. 12 sq. ft.
   c. 36 sq. ft.
   d. 144 sq. ft.

5. A man is 6 feet 2 inches and his daughter is 4 feet 9 inches. How much taller is the man than his daughter?
   a. 1 ft., 3 in.
   b. 1 ft., 5 in.
   c. 2 ft., 3 in.
   d. 2 ft., 5 in.

6. A boy turned on his radio at 5:30 P.M. on Friday night while he was packing for a weekend trip. He forgot to switch it off, so it played the whole time he was gone. The boy finally turned it off on Sunday night at 8:15 P.M. In total, how long was the radio playing?
   a. 1 day, 3 hours
   b. 1 day, 2 hours, 45 minutes
   c. 2 days, 2 hours, 30 minutes
   d. 2 days, 2 hours, 45 minutes

7. A patient receives $2\frac{2}{5}$ grams of medication over 24 hours. If she is given 4 equal doses of medication over this time, how many grams of medication are in each dose?
   a. $\frac{1}{10}$
   b. $\frac{3}{20}$
   c. $\frac{3}{5}$
   d. $1\frac{2}{3}$

8. Sarah went to the mall and spent $25.20 on a shirt, $45.05 on a pair of pants, $3.25 on a smoothie, and $32.75 on a pair of shorts. In total, how much money did Sarah spend on clothes?
   a. $102.75
   b. $102.80
   c. $103.00
   d. $106.25

9. A clinic has enough flu vaccine this season to vaccinate 80% of its 30-person staff. How many staff members cannot be vaccinated this season?
   a. 2
   b. 6
   c. 11
   d. 24

**10.** Lara biked 12 miles per hour for the first two hours of a long ride through the country and 14 miles per hour for the last hour. What was her average speed for the trip in miles per hour?

a. $8\frac{2}{3}$

b. 12

c. $12\frac{2}{3}$

d. 13

**11.** Rosalind measured her temperature for five days and recorded these numbers: 99, 98, 97.9, 98.6, and 98.5. What was her average temperature during this time?

a. 97.9

b. 98.0

c. 98.4

d. 99.2

**12.** The perimeter of a rectangle is 148 feet. Its two longest sides add up to 86 feet. What is the length of each of its two shortest sides?

a. 31 ft.

b. 42 ft.

c. 62 ft.

d. 74 ft.

**13.** A hospital pays $15.50 for every new lab coat and $2.15 to wash each dirty one. If 50 new lab coats need to be purchased and 100 lab coats need to be washed, how much will the hospital spend in total?

a. $990.00

b. $1,215.00

c. $1,657.50

d. $1,730.65

**14.** If jogging for one mile uses 150 calories and brisk walking for one mile uses 100 calories, a jogger has to go how many times as far as a walker to use the same number of calories?

a. $\frac{1}{2}$

b. $\frac{2}{3}$

c. $\frac{3}{2}$

d. 2

**15.** A dosage of a certain medication is 12 cc per 100 pounds. What is the dosage for a patient who weighs 175 pounds?

a. 15 cc

b. 18 cc

c. 21 cc

d. 24 cc

**16.** A gram of fat contains 9 calories. An 1,800-calorie diet allows no more than 20% of calories from fat. How many grams of fat are allowed in that diet?

a. 40 g

b. 90 g

c. 200 g

d. 360 g

**17.** If $x = -1$, $y = 4$, and $z = -2$, what is the value of the expression $2x - yz$?

a. $-10$

b. $-4$

c. 6

d. 10

**18.** A 15 cc dosage must be increased by 20%. What is the new dosage?

a. 17 cc

b. 18 cc

c. 30 cc

d. 35 cc

**19.** What is the area of this triangle?

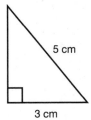

5 cm

3 cm

a. 6 sq. cm
b. 7.5 sq. cm
c. 12 sq. cm
d. 15 sq. cm

**20.** The following figure contains both a circle and a square. What is the area of the entire shaded figure?

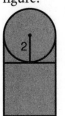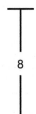

2

8

a. $16 + 4\pi$
b. $16 + 16\pi$
c. $24 + 2\pi$
d. $24 + 4\pi$

**21.** At a carnival, each ride costs $1.50. However, a dozen ride tickets can be bought for $15.50 at the park entrance. How much money can be saved by buying a dozen tickets at once rather than buying each ticket separately?

a. $2.50
b. $3.00
c. $10.30
d. $18.00

**22.** If Javier earns $3,500 a month and cannot spend more than 30% of his monthly income on rent, what is the highest monthly rent that he can afford?

a. $650
b. $900
c. $1,050
d. $1,260

**23.** If $t$ is 4 more than $s$, and $s$ is 2 less than $r$, what is $t$ when $r = 8$?

a. 2
b. 6
c. 10
d. 14

**24.** The percent increase from 8 to 10 is equal to the percent increase from 16 to what number?

a. 18
b. 20
c. 22
d. 24

**25.** If $(0.0013)x = 13$, then $x =$

a. 0.001
b. 0.01
c. 1,000
d. 10,000

**26.** $\frac{7}{40}$ is equal to

a. 0.0175
b. 0.175
c. 1.75
d. 17.5

**27.** A certain water pollutant is unsafe at a level above 20 ppm (parts per million). A city's water supply now contains 50 ppm of this pollutant. What percentage decrease will make the water safe?
a. 30%
b. 40%
c. 50%
d. 60%

**28.** In half of migraine sufferers, a certain drug reduces the number of migraines by 50%. Assuming all migraine sufferers experience the same number of migraines, what percentage of all migraines can be eliminated by this drug?
a. 25%
b. 50%
c. 75%
d. 100%

**29.** Nationwide, in one year, there were about 21,500 fire-related injuries associated with furniture. Of these, 11,350 were caused by smoking materials. About what percent of the fire-related injuries were smoking-related?
a. 47%
b. 49%
c. 51%
d. 53%

**30.** $0.08 \times 0.27$ is equal to
a. 0.00216
b. 0.0216
c. 2.16
d. 21.6

**31.** $\frac{2\frac{1}{4}}{\frac{2}{3}}$ is equal to
a. $\frac{8}{27}$
b. $1\frac{1}{2}$
c. $3\frac{3}{8}$
d. $3\frac{1}{2}$

**32.** $3\frac{9}{16} - 1\frac{7}{8}$ is equal to
a. $1\frac{11}{16}$
b. $2\frac{1}{8}$
c. $2\frac{1}{4}$
d. $2\frac{5}{16}$

**33.** If the average woman burns 8.2 calories per minute while riding a bicycle, how many calories will she burn if she rides for 35 minutes?
a. 286
b. 287
c. 387
d. 980

**34.** The basal metabolic rate (BMR) is the rate at which our body uses calories. The BMR for a man in his twenties is about 1,700 calories per day. If 204 of those calories should come from protein, about what percentage of this man's diet should be protein?
a. 1.2%
b. 8.3%
c. 12%
d. 16%

**35.** Four patients are being transferred from the hospital to a nursing home in an ambulance, one at a time. If the distance from the hospital to the nursing home is $10\frac{1}{5}$ miles, how many miles total does the ambulance travel after it drops off all the patients and returns to the hospital?
a. $40\frac{4}{5}$
b. $71\frac{2}{5}$
c. $80\frac{3}{5}$
d. $81\frac{3}{5}$

**36.** Down's syndrome occurs in about 1 in 1,500 children when the mothers are in their twenties. About what percentage of all children born to mothers in their twenties are likely to have Down's syndrome?
a. 0.0067%
b. 0.067%
c. 0.67%
d. 6.7%

**37.** If a population of yeast cells grows from ten to 320 in a period of five hours, what is the rate of growth?
a. It doubles its numbers every hour.
b. It triples its numbers every hour.
c. It doubles its numbers every two hours.
d. It triples its numbers every two hours.

**38.** Which value of $x$ will make this number sentence true? $x + 25 \leq 13$
a. −12
b. −11
c. 12
d. 38

**39.** A square with a side length of 6 has the same area as a rectangle with a length of 2 and a width of
a. 3.
b. 6.
c. 12.
d. 18.

**40.** If angle $r$ measures 52° and is supplementary to angle $s$, what is the measure of angle $s$?
a. 38°
b. 52°
c. 128°
d. 142°

**41.** Which of the following numbers is the smallest?
a. $\frac{8}{15}$
b. $\frac{6}{10}$
c. $\frac{33}{60}$
d. $\frac{11}{20}$

**42.** $2\frac{1}{4} + 4\frac{5}{8} + \frac{1}{2}$ is equal to
a. $6\frac{7}{8}$
b. $7\frac{1}{4}$
c. $7\frac{3}{8}$
d. $7\frac{3}{4}$

**43.** What percentage of 600 is 750?
a. 80%
b. 85%
c. 110%
d. 125%

**44.** Which of the following is the equivalent of $\frac{13}{25}$?
a. 0.38
b. 0.4
c. 0.48
d. 0.52

**45.** Dr. Slagle needs 4 m of plaster bandages to make a cast for a broken wrist. One roll of bandages is 250 cm long. How many rolls of bandages will she need?
a. 1
b. 2
c. 3
d. 4

**46.** Which of the following statements is true?
a. Parallel lines intersect at right angles.
b. Parallel lines never intersect.
c. Perpendicular lines never intersect.
d. Intersecting lines have two points in common.

**47.** 3.6 − 1.89 is equal to
  **a.** 1.47
  **b.** 1.53
  **c.** 1.71
  **d.** 2.42

**48.** If a particular woman's resting heartbeat is 72 beats per minute and she is at rest for $6\frac{1}{2}$ hours, about how many times will her heart beat during that period of time?
  **a.** 4,320
  **b.** 4,680
  **c.** 28,080
  **d.** 43,200

**49.** The number of red blood corpuscles in one cubic millimeter is about 5 million, and the number of white blood corpuscles in one cubic millimeter is about 8,000. What, then, is the ratio of white blood corpuscles to red blood corpuscles?
  **a.** 1:625
  **b.** 1:40
  **c.** 4:10
  **d.** 5:1,250

**50.** $\frac{5}{12} - \frac{3}{8}$ is equal to
  **a.** $\frac{1}{10}$
  **b.** $\frac{1}{24}$
  **c.** $\frac{5}{48}$
  **d.** $\frac{19}{24}$

# Section 4: General Science

This section will test your accumulated knowledge in general science.

1. Which of the following scientists is best known for describing the laws of planetary motion?
   a. Sir Charles Lyell
   b. Gregor Mendel
   c. Johann Kepler
   d. Robert Hooke

2. Suppose you conduct a scientific investigation to find out how daily intake of vitamin C affects a person's resistance to developing flu symptoms. You test 100 people, all of the same age and same general health. You give 25 people one vitamin tablet a day, another 25 people two vitamin tablets a day, another 25 people three vitamin tablets a day, and the final 25 people get four vitamin tablets a day. You carry this out for two months and observe the health of all 100 people over time. Which of the following is your experimental factor?
   a. number of people studied
   b. number of vitamin tablets a person gets each day
   c. the age of the people in the study
   d. the health of each person at the beginning of the study

3. Which of the following is the standard metric unit of volume?
   a. gram
   b. joule
   c. liter
   d. metric ton

4. How many micrograms are in one gram?
   a. 100
   b. 1,000
   c. 100,000
   d. 1,000,000

5. Which of the following statements correctly relates our present understanding of the universe?
   a. The universe is about five billion years old.
   b. The universe is getting smaller with time.
   c. The universe is expanding.
   d. The universe consists of only a few hundred galaxies.

6. Gregor Mendel studied plant variations using
   a. tomato plants.
   b. basil plants.
   c. geranium plants.
   d. pea plants.

7. What did Galileo do?
   a. first split light into its colors
   b. first used the $x$- and $y$-axis
   c. first realized the antiquity of Earth
   d. first observed the moons of Jupiter

8. If you want to test the effect of a new malaria vaccine, the group of people who receive shots that contain no vaccine is called the
   a. control group.
   b. experiment group.
   c. fake group.
   d. zero group.

9. How many milligrams are in one gram?
   a. 10
   b. 100
   c. 1,000
   d. 10,000

**10.** The biggest concepts in science are called
   **a.** predictions.
   **b.** theories.
   **c.** experiments.
   **d.** hypotheses.

**11.** Which of the following best describes the atmosphere of the planet Venus?
   **a.** very light and oxygen-rich
   **b.** filled with water vapor
   **c.** dominated by $CO_2$ (carbon dioxide)
   **d.** thin and cold

**12.** Which of the following is not a flavor of quark?
   **a.** up
   **b.** middle
   **c.** strange
   **d.** charm

**13.** What year was the first successful landing of a U.S. rover on Mars?
   **a.** 1969
   **b.** 1957
   **c.** 1997
   **d.** 2011

**14.** Two atoms both have 92 electrons as well as 92 protons in their nuclei, but one atom has 146 neutrons and the other has 144 neutrons. These two atoms are
   **a.** ions.
   **b.** compounds.
   **c.** molecules.
   **d.** isotopes.

**15.** If a substance gains electrons during a chemical reaction, the substance is said to be
   **a.** oxidized.
   **b.** acidified.
   **c.** reduced.
   **d.** fused.

**16.** The typical human hair is about 50 micrometers in diameter. That means it is 50 _____ of a meter.
   **a.** billionths
   **b.** thousandths
   **c.** parts
   **d.** millionths

**17.** Humans are putting about 6 billion tons of carbon into the atmosphere each year in the form of carbon dioxide. Another way of saying this number is how many tons of carbon?
   **a.** 6 megatons
   **b.** 6 kilotons
   **c.** 6 petatons
   **d.** 6 gigatons

**18.** Which of the following is the standard metric unit of energy?
   **a.** joule
   **b.** mole
   **c.** watt
   **d.** ampere

**19.** What exponent would you use to express how many meters are in a kilometer?
   **a.** $10^5$
   **b.** $10^3$
   **c.** $10^4$
   **d.** $10^2$

**20.** Compute the number of seconds in a year.
   **a.** about one million
   **b.** about thirty million
   **c.** about one hundred thousand
   **d.** about three million

**21.** If you feel waves of warmth coming from a campfire, which of the following means of heat transfer are you experiencing?
   **a.** conduction
   **b.** radiation
   **c.** electricity
   **d.** nuclear fusion

**22.** Which of the following is our best understanding of why the dinosaurs became extinct?
a. impact of a massive meteor on Earth
b. intense volcanic activity
c. disease
d. severe and prolonged storms

**23.** A rock that contains a fossil is most likely
a. igneous.
b. sedimentary.
c. volcanic.
d. metamorphic.

**24.** In which layer of the atmosphere does weather occur?
a. troposphere
b. stratosphere
c. mesosphere
d. thermosphere

**25.** Which of the following carry out photosynthesis?
a. nektons
b. heterotrophs
c. zooplanktons
d. autotrophs

**26.** In the electromagnetic spectrum, infrared wavelengths are slightly longer than those of visible red, and ultraviolet wavelengths are slightly shorter than those of visible blue. If an absorption spectrum from a calcium atom here on Earth has a characteristic pattern in the red wavelengths, looking at calcium in the absorption spectrum of a distant galaxy will show the same characteristic pattern shifted toward the
a. ultraviolet.
b. blue.
c. red (the same).
d. infrared.

**27.** In the stages of nuclear fusion inside stars, which element in the list, compared to the others, is formed last?
a. hydrogen
b. helium
c. carbon
d. oxygen

**28.** Which is the best answer for the events or processes that disperse elements born in the internal nuclear fires of stars, making those elements available for subsequent formations of new stars and planets?
a. supernovas
b. expanding universe
c. fusion reactions
d. red shift

**29.** Which element is not made in stars?
a. aluminum
b. boron
c. carbon
d. hydrogen

**30.** Which element in the universe (including inside our sun) is both primordial (meaning some of it was made shortly after the Big Bang, before any stars formed) and made inside stars during fusion reactions?
a. carbon
b. hydrogen
c. helium
d. iron

**31.** Which of the following increases in density as the universe ages?
a. energy
b. microwave radiation
c. hydrogen
d. carbon

**32.** The planet nearest to Earth is
a. Venus.
b. Jupiter.
c. Neptune.
d. Saturn.

**33.** Astronomers sometimes make units that fit the large scales of space and time. Consider the time interval from today back to the formation of Earth (in other words, Earth's condensation from the gas cloud that also formed the sun). For just this question, call this amount of time one Earth Formation Unit (1 EFU). About how many EFUs from today must you go back in time in order to reach the Big Bang?
a. 1 EFU
b. 3 EFUs
c. 8 EFUs
d. 15 EFUs

**34.** Our best dates for the origin of the solar system come from
a. rocks found on the moon.
b. the oldest rocks on Earth.
c. meteorites.
d. gases in the sun.

**35.** The planet nearest to the sun is
a. the asteroids.
b. Phobos.
c. Venus.
d. Mercury.

**36.** Humans are currently in space on the
a. Mir space station.
b. International Space Station.
c. space shuttle.
d. Apollo capsule.

**37.** Which of the following is considered a dwarf planet?
a. Mercury
b. Eris
c. Oort
d. Dysnomia

**38.** Which body in our solar system has very good evidence for the presence of liquid water at one time in the past?
a. the moon
b. Mars
c. Venus
d. Mercury

**39.** The Cassini space probe will explore the planet with rings. Before reaching that planet, Cassini has to pass the orbit of which planet?
a. Uranus
b. Saturn
c. Jupiter
d. Neptune

**40.** We know there is matter that cannot be seen by any means available to us, including the different wavelengths of the electromagnetic spectrum. Yet we know this so-called "dark matter" exists. How?
a. Black holes have consumed much of the matter that once existed.
b. At the origin of the universe, there was a large amount of antimatter that became hidden.
c. Einstein's equation shows us the equivalence of energy that could also be considered matter.
d. The spins of galaxies cannot be explained by the amount of known, ordinary matter.

**41.** Today, we know the composition of the universe fairly well in terms of types of matter (or types of energy that can be put into amounts of equivalent matter, using Einstein's equation $E = mc^2$). What percentage of the universe is dark energy?
   **a.** 98%
   **b.** 73%
   **c.** 23%
   **d.** 4%

**42.** One element crucial to life is carbon, which forms about 40% of our body's dry weight. If planets had formed around the very earliest stars in the universe, why would it have been unlikely for life to start on those earliest planets?
   **a.** Carbon is made slowly as the expanding energy is converted to matter.
   **b.** Carbon leaks into our universe through black holes.
   **c.** Carbon is made by fusion reactions in stars.
   **d.** Carbon is made by the fission of oxygen.

**43.** The geographical region of the ocean that meets the deep ocean floor is the
   **a.** continental alluvium.
   **b.** continental abyss.
   **c.** continental slope.
   **d.** continental shelf.

**44.** What word in ancient Greek means indivisible?
   **a.** atom
   **b.** molecule
   **c.** ion
   **d.** isotope

**45.** The radioactive isotope of carbon is
   **a.** carbon-11.
   **b.** carbon-12.
   **c.** carbon-13.
   **d.** carbon-14.

**46.** Protons and neutrons are made of what?
   **a.** electrons
   **b.** neutrinos
   **c.** quarks
   **d.** mesons

**47.** Parts of the atomic nucleus are sometimes collectively called *nucleons*. Nucleons are therefore
   **a.** protons and mesons.
   **b.** electrons and neutrons.
   **c.** mesons and electrons.
   **d.** neutrons and protons.

**48.** In measuring electricity, the unit of resistance is the
   **a.** volt.
   **b.** ohm.
   **c.** amp.
   **d.** watt.

**49.** Electromagnetism is the force that
   **a.** causes the interaction between electrically charged particles.
   **b.** binds protons and neutrons together to form the nucleus of an atom.
   **c.** is responsible for the radioactive decay of subatomic particles.
   **d.** causes dispersed matter to coalesce.

**50.** Which of the following scientists is known as the founder of modern genetics?
   **a.** Johann Kepler
   **b.** Sir Charles Lyell
   **c.** Gregor Mendel
   **d.** Robert Hooke

## Section 5: Biology

There are 50 questions in this section. You have 45 minutes to complete this section.

1. Which of the following represents a human nucleotide base pairing?
   a. T-U
   b. A-U
   c. G-T
   d. A-G

2. Adipose tissue is composed of
   a. amino acids.
   b. nucleotides.
   c. white blood cells.
   d. lipids.

3. Viruses appear to be living organisms with all of the following characteristics EXCEPT
   a. cellular reproduction.
   b. enzymes.
   c. adaptation.
   d. nucleic acids.

4. What is the correct order of classification from general to specific?
   a. Kingdom, Phylum, Class, Order, Genus, Family, Species
   b. Kingdom, Phylum, Class, Genus, Family, Order, Species
   c. Kingdom, Phylum, Order, Class, Family, Genus, Species
   d. Kingdom, Phylum, Class, Order, Family, Genus, Species

5. Which accessory organ detoxifies substances in the blood absorbed through the intestines?
   a. kidney
   b. liver
   c. pancreas
   d. spleen

6. The loop of Henle is part of which of the following organs?
   a. heart
   b. kidney
   c. pancreas
   d. liver

7. Which of the following organelles is found in plants, but not in animals or bacteria?
   a. mitochondria
   b. chloroplasts
   c. nucleus
   d. cell wall

8. What is $10^{-12}$ meters?
   a. a picometer
   b. a nanometer
   c. a micrometer
   d. a femtometer

9. Which of the following is an air- or fluid-filled space in the cytoplasm of a living cell?
   a. a vacuum
   b. a vacuole
   c. a centriole
   d. a centrosome

10. Which of the following structures is part of a plant cell but not of an animal cell?
    a. a mitochondrion
    b. a ribosome
    c. a chloroplast
    d. an endoplasmic reticulum

11. Which organelles generate the majority of ATP in eukaryotic cells?
    a. mitochondria
    b. chloroplasts
    c. ribosomes
    d. lysosomes

**12.** Cells of various organ systems
    **a.** have completely different DNA.
    **b.** have the same DNA.
    **c.** express different parts of their DNA.
    **d.** choices **b** and **c**

**13.** Which adaptation differentiates mammals from other animals?
    **a.** regulation of body temperature
    **b.** terrestrial mobility
    **c.** specialized communication
    **d.** mammary glands functional in mothers with offspring

**14.** The function of the lysosome is to
    **a.** contain the cell's genetic material.
    **b.** combine amino acids into proteins.
    **c.** break down waste material in the cell.
    **d.** generate ATP

**15.** Why might flowering plants' (angiosperms) recovery from a devastating environmental phenomenon be faster than conifers?
    **a.** Conifers require more sunlight.
    **b.** Angiosperms reproduce more quickly.
    **c.** Angiosperms depend on mammals to spread seeds.
    **d.** Conifers have tougher seeds.

**16.** What type of cell is shown in the following figure?

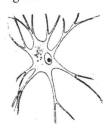

    **a.** a blood cell
    **b.** a fat cell
    **c.** a muscle cell
    **d.** a nerve cell

**17.** Hepatitis is an inflammation of the
    **a.** joints.
    **b.** lungs.
    **c.** liver.
    **d.** large intestine.

**18.** The process of cellular reproduction in bacteria is known as
    **a.** mitosis.
    **b.** meiosis.
    **c.** telophase.
    **d.** binary fission.

**19.** The principal function of blood platelets is to
    **a.** help clot blood.
    **b.** carry oxygen.
    **c.** produce antibodies.
    **d.** phagocytize bacteria.

**20.** The two or more related genes that control a trait are known as
    **a.** chromosomes.
    **b.** chromatids.
    **c.** phenotypes.
    **d.** alleles.

**21.** Once the amount of oxygen in the atmosphere was increased, which adaptation helped organisms evolve to more advanced forms?
    **a.** photosynthesis
    **b.** anaerobic respiration
    **c.** oxidation
    **d.** aerobic respiration

**22.** A fossil is found that is believed to be at least three billion years old. Which of the following modern organisms would it most likely resemble?
    **a.** primitive aquatic plants
    **b.** protists
    **c.** bacteria
    **d.** protozoa

23. A father presents an X-linked trait and a mother does not. What is the probability that the mother is a carrier of this trait if they produce a son who also presents the X-linked trait?
    a. 0%
    b. 25%
    c. 50%
    d. 100%

24. Which organ system is responsible for producing white blood cells in humans?
    a. skeletal
    b. immune
    c. circulatory
    d. integumentary

25. The term "biological catalyst" most closely describes
    a. RNA.
    b. DNA.
    c. a mitochondrion.
    d. an enzyme.

26. Which of the following is NOT a member of the class of fungi?
    a. common bread mold
    b. mushrooms
    c. kelp
    d. yeast

27. Which of the following is characteristic of viruses?
    I. Viruses lack most of the structural and functional features of a cell.
    II. Viruses can reproduce only when they are within living cells.
    III. Nearly all viruses cause diseases.
    a. I only
    b. II only
    c. I and II only
    d. I, II, and III

28. Initial classification of a bacterium is based on its
    a. size.
    b. shape.
    c. color.
    d. ability to cause disease.

29. Which of the following is NOT caused by a virus?
    a. polio
    b. rabies
    c. malaria
    d. cold sores (herpes simplex)

30. Which of the following is NOT true of most bacteria?
    a. They are single-celled.
    b. They belong to the Kingdom Bacteria.
    c. They are eukaryotes.
    d. They are systematically classified by their biochemical makeup.

31. The process of a complementary strand of RNA being made from a sequence of DNA is known as
    a. transcription.
    b. translation.
    c. mitosis.
    d. replication.

32. When part of a chromosome breaks off and attaches to another chromosome, some genetic information is transferred. What is this occurrence called?
    a. aneuploidy
    b. transcription
    c. translation
    d. translocation

**33.** The structure formed by the union of male and female gametes is the
a. zoospore.
b. zygote.
c. ova.
d. oocyte.

**34.** The metabolic pathway involving the degradation of glucose into pyruvate to produce ATP is known as
a. glycolysis.
b. gluconeogenesis.
c. the Calvin cycle.
d. the Krebs cycle.

**35.** During strenuous exercise, a build-up of what substance may cause muscle cramps?
a. lactic acid
b. lactose
c. adrenaline
d. serotonin

**36.** Which organ functions to absorb water and create feces from undigested food?
a. small intestine
b. liver
c. large intestine
d. stomach

**37.** During a latent period in muscle tissue, what is released from the sarcoplasmic reticulum?
a. calcium
b. sodium
c. lactic acid
d. acetylcholine

**38.** Beriberi is caused by a deficit of which vitamin?
a. vitamin $B_1$
b. vitamin C
c. vitamin E
d. vitamin D

**39.** The molecule responsible for the green color of leaves is
a. deoxyribonucleic acid.
b. adenosine triphosphate.
c. chlorophyll.
d. glucose.

**40.** Which of the following is NOT characteristic of anaphylaxis?
a. circulatory shock
b. bronchospasm
c. hives
d. hypertension

**41.** What is the generic term for any substance which blocks ONLY the sensory perception of pain?
a. analgesic
b. general anesthetic
c. local anesthetic
d. acetylcholine

**42.** Which of the following is NOT an amino acid?
a. tyrosine
b. tryptophan
c. thymine
d. threonine

**43.** Cells that remove dead and dying red blood cells from the liver are known as
a. leukocytes.
b. erythrocytes.
c. eosinophils.
d. Kupffer cells.

**44.** "Energy cannot be destroyed; it can only be transformed" is a statement of what physical law?
a. first law of thermodynamics
b. second law of thermodynamics
c. law of entropy
d. law of constant composition

**45.** In humans, an extra copy of chromosome 21 causes
   **a.** Turner's syndrome.
   **b.** Lesch-Nyhan syndrome.
   **c.** Down's syndrome.
   **d.** Klinefelter's syndrome.

**46.** The primary component of alcoholic beverages that acts as a central nervous system (CNS) depressant is
   **a.** isopropyl alcohol.
   **b.** methanol.
   **c.** methionine.
   **d.** ethanol.

**47.** Primary structure refers to a protein's
   **a.** amino acid sequence.
   **b.** $\alpha$-helices and $\beta$-sheets.
   **c.** shape.
   **d.** active site.

**48.** A benign tumor usually caused by a *papilloma-virus* is a
   **a.** wart.
   **b.** sarcoma.
   **c.** adenoma.
   **d.** cold sore.

**49.** What is the light-sensitive pigment found in the vertebrate retina?
   **a.** cytochrome
   **b.** hemoglobin
   **c.** rhodopsin
   **d.** melanin

**50.** What is another term for excessively high blood pressure?
   **a.** cardiomyopathy
   **b.** hypertension
   **c.** hypoglycemia
   **d.** hemophilia

# Section 6: Chemistry

There are 50 questions in this section. You have 45 minutes to complete this section. Use the periodic table on this page when necessary to help you answer the following questions.

| IA | | | | | | | | | | | | | | | | | VIIA | VIIIA |
|---|---|---|---|---|---|---|---|---|---|---|---|---|---|---|---|---|---|---|
| 1<br>**H**<br>1.00794 | | | | | | | | | | | | | | | | | 1<br>**H**<br>1.00794 | 2<br>**He**<br>4.002602 |
| 3<br>**Li**<br>6.941 | 4<br>**Be**<br>9.012182 | | | | | | | | | | | IIIA | IVA | VA | VIA | | | |
| 11<br>**Na**<br>22.989770 | 12<br>**Mg**<br>24.3050 | IIIB | IVB | VB | VIB | VIIB | | VIIIB | | | IB | IIB | 5<br>**B**<br>10.811 | 6<br>**C**<br>12.0107 | 7<br>**N**<br>14.00674 | 8<br>**O**<br>15.9994 | 9<br>**F**<br>18.9984032 | 10<br>**Ne**<br>20.1797 |
| 19<br>**K**<br>39.0983 | 20<br>**Ca**<br>40.078 | 21<br>**Sc**<br>44.955910 | 22<br>**Ti**<br>47.867 | 23<br>**V**<br>50.9415 | 24<br>**Cr**<br>51.9961 | 25<br>**Mn**<br>54.938049 | 26<br>**Fe**<br>55.845 | 27<br>**Co**<br>58.933200 | 28<br>**Ni**<br>58.6934 | 29<br>**Cu**<br>63.546 | 30<br>**Zn**<br>65.39 | 13<br>**Al**<br>26.981538 | 14<br>**Si**<br>28.0855 | 15<br>**P**<br>30.973761 | 16<br>**S**<br>32.066 | 17<br>**Cl**<br>35.4527 | 18<br>**Ar**<br>39.948 |
| 37<br>**Rb**<br>85.4678 | 38<br>**Sr**<br>87.62 | 39<br>**Y**<br>88.90585 | 40<br>**Zr**<br>91.224 | 41<br>**Nb**<br>92.90638 | 42<br>**Mo**<br>95.94 | 43<br>**Tc**<br>(98) | 44<br>**Ru**<br>101.07 | 45<br>**Rh**<br>102.90550 | 46<br>**Pd**<br>106.42 | 47<br>**Ag**<br>107.8682 | 48<br>**Cd**<br>112.411 | 31<br>**Ga**<br>69.723 | 32<br>**Ge**<br>72.61 | 33<br>**As**<br>74.92160 | 34<br>**Se**<br>78.96 | 35<br>**Br**<br>79.904 | 36<br>**Kr**<br>83.80 |
| 55<br>**Cs**<br>132.90545 | 56<br>**Ba**<br>137.327 | 57<br>**La***<br>138.9055 | 72<br>**Hf**<br>178.49 | 73<br>**Ta**<br>180.9479 | 74<br>**W**<br>183.84 | 75<br>**Re**<br>186.207 | 76<br>**Os**<br>190.23 | 77<br>**Ir**<br>192.217 | 78<br>**Pt**<br>195.078 | 79<br>**Au**<br>196.96655 | 80<br>**Hg**<br>200.59 | 49<br>**In**<br>114.818 | 50<br>**Sn**<br>118.710 | 51<br>**Sb**<br>121.760 | 52<br>**Te**<br>127.60 | 53<br>**I**<br>126.90447 | 54<br>**Xe**<br>131.29 |
| 87<br>**Fr**<br>(223) | 88<br>**Ra**<br>(226) | 89<br>**Ac****<br>(227) | 104<br>**Rf**<br>(261) | 105<br>**Db**<br>(262) | 106<br>**Sg**<br>(263) | 107<br>**Bh**<br>(262) | 108<br>**Hs**<br>(265) | 109<br>**Mt**<br>(266) | 110<br>**Ds**<br>(269) | 111<br>**Rg**<br>(281) | 112<br>**Cn**<br>(285) | 81<br>**Tl**<br>204.3833 | 82<br>**Pb**<br>207.2 | 83<br>**Bi**<br>208.98038 | 84<br>**Po**<br>(209) | 85<br>**At**<br>(210) | 86<br>**Rn**<br>(222) |
| | | | | | | | | | | | | | 113<br>**Uut**<br>(286) | 114<br>**Uuq**<br>(289) | 115<br>**Uup**<br>(289) | 116<br>**Uuh**<br>(289) | 117<br>**Uus**<br>(294) | 118<br>**Uuo**<br>(293) |

| * Lanthanide series | 58<br>**Ce**<br>140.116 | 59<br>**Pr**<br>140.90765 | 60<br>**Nd**<br>144.24 | 61<br>**Pm**<br>(145) | 62<br>**Sm**<br>150.36 | 63<br>**Eu**<br>151.964 | 64<br>**Gd**<br>157.25 | 65<br>**Tb**<br>158.92534 | 66<br>**Dy**<br>162.50 | 67<br>**Ho**<br>164.93032 | 68<br>**Er**<br>167.26 | 69<br>**Tm**<br>168.93421 | 70<br>**Yb**<br>173.04 | 71<br>**Lu**<br>174.967 |
|---|---|---|---|---|---|---|---|---|---|---|---|---|---|---|
| ** Actinide series | 90<br>**Th**<br>232.0381 | 91<br>**Pa**<br>231.03588 | 92<br>**U**<br>238.0289 | 93<br>**Np**<br>(237) | 94<br>**Pu**<br>(244) | 95<br>**Am**<br>(243) | 96<br>**Cm**<br>(247) | 97<br>**Bk**<br>(247) | 98<br>**Cf**<br>(251) | 99<br>**Es**<br>(252) | 100<br>**Fm**<br>(257) | 101<br>**Md**<br>(258) | 102<br>**No**<br>(259) | 103<br>**Lr**<br>(262) |

**1.** Which of the following substances has a pH closest to 7?

a. ammonia

b. blood

c. lemon juice

d. vinegar

**2.** What functional groups form a peptide bond?

a. amides

b. amines

c. esters

d. ethers

**3.** Which of the following groups is common to the majority of amino acids?

a. $CH_3$

b. $H_2O$

c. $NH_2$

d. $SO_4^{-2}$

**4.** When amino acids polymerize to make a protein, which of the following is produced as a byproduct?

a. $H_2O$

b. $H_2$

c. $O_2$

d. $CO_2$

**5.** The α-helices and β-sheets in a protein make up its
   **a.** primary structure.
   **b.** secondary structure.
   **c.** tertiary structure.
   **d.** quaternary structure.

**6.** $^{35}Cl$ has 17 protons. How many neutrons does it have?
   **a.** 17
   **b.** 18
   **c.** 35
   **d.** 52

**7.** The number of protons in an atom is always equal to its
   **a.** mass number.
   **b.** atomic number.
   **c.** number of isotopes
   **d.** number of neutrons

**8.** $NaOH + HCl \rightarrow NaCl + H_2O$
   The reaction shown here is best described as which of the following?
   **a.** base + acid → salt + water
   **b.** metal + acid → salt + hydrogen
   **c.** metal oxide + acid → salt + water
   **d.** metal carbonate + acid → salt + carbonate acid (unstable)

**9.** Chlorine, atomic number 17, becomes an ion when it bonds with sodium to form salt. How many electrons does that ion have?
   **a.** 0
   **b.** 1
   **c.** 17
   **d.** 18

**10.** Which of the following represents $t$-butane?
   **a.** $CH_3 - CH_2 - CH_2 - CH_3$
   **b.**
   $$CH_3 - \underset{\underset{CH_3}{|}}{\overset{\overset{CH_3}{|}}{C}} - CH_3$$
   **c.** $CH_3 - CH_2 - CH_3$
   **d.**
   $$CH_3 - \underset{\underset{CH_3}{|}}{\overset{\overset{H}{|}}{C}} - CH_3$$

**11.** $O^{2-}$ has how many electrons?
   **a.** 6
   **b.** 8
   **c.** 10
   **d.** 18

**12.** Which of the following is NOT a Lewis base?
   **a.** $C_6H_{10}O$
   **b.** H-O-$CH_3$
   **c.** Na
   **d.** $CH_3$-$CH_2$-$CH_2$-$CH(NH_2)$-$CH_3$

**13.** Which of the following is the correct, balanced equation for the combustion of propane?
   **a.** $C_3H_{8(g)} + 5O_{2(g)} + N_{2(g)} \rightarrow 3CO_{2(g)} + 2NO_{2(g)} + 4H_{2(g)}$
   **b.** $C_3H_{8(g)} + 5O_{2(g)} \rightarrow 3CO_{2(g)} + 4H_2O_{(g)}$
   **c.** $C_3H_{8(g)} + 6O_{2(g)} + 2H_{2(g)} \rightarrow 3CO_{2(g)} + 6H_2O_{(g)}$
   **d.** $C_3H_{8(g)} + O_{2(g)} + 4H_2O_{(g)} \rightarrow 3CO_{2(g)} + 6H_{2(g)}$

**14.** What is the electron configuration of a $Cl^-$ ion?
   **a.** $[Ne]3s^23p^5$
   **b.** $[Ne]3s^2p^63d^1$
   **c.** $[Ne]3s^23p^4$
   **d.** $[Ne]3s^23p^6$

**15.** Which of the following is the hybridization of the carbon atom in methane, $CH_4$?
a. $sp$
b. $sp^2$
c. $sp^3$
d. $sp^4$

**16.** Which of the following elements is the most electronegative?
a. Na
b. S
c. Cl
d. Br

**17.** When a liquid is at its boiling point, the vapor pressure of the liquid
a. is less than the external pressure on the liquid.
b. is equal to the external pressure on the liquid.
c. is greater than the external pressure on the liquid.
d. can be either less or greater than the external pressure on the liquid.

**18.** What is the oxidation state of iron in $Fe_2O_3$?
a. 0
b. +2
c. +3
d. +6

**19.** Which of the following is the empirical formula for ethylene glycol, $C_2H_6O_2$?
a. $CH_3O$
b. $C_2H_6O_2$
c. $C_4H_{12}O_4$
d. $CH_2$

**20.** What is the most likely oxidation state of Mg?
a. +2
b. +1
c. 0
d. −6

**21.** Which of the following is the chemical symbol for the species that has 16 protons, 17 neutrons, and 18 electrons?
a. $^{33}_{16}S$
b. $^{33}_{17}Cl$
c. $^{35}_{17}Cl$
d. $^{33}_{16}S^{2-}$

**22.** Which of the following equations correctly describes the reaction between $SO_{3(g)}$ and $KOH_{(aq)}$?
a. $4SO_{3(g)} + 4KOH_{(aq)} \rightarrow 2H_2SO_{4(aq)} + 4K_{(s)} + O_{2(g)}$
b. $SO_{3(g)} + 2KOH_{(aq)} \rightarrow K_2SO_{4(aq)} + H_2O_{(1)}$
c. $2SO_3 + 4KOH_{(aq)} \rightarrow 2K_2SO_{3(aq)} + 2H_2O_{(1)} + O_{2(g)}$
d. No reaction occurs.

**23.** Which of the following is a Lewis acid, but not a Brønsted acid?
a. HCl
b. $H_2SO_4$
c. $CH_4$
d. $AlCl_3$

**24.** Butane, $C_4H_{10}$, combusts to form $CO_2$ and $H_2O$. Which of the following is the balanced chemical equation that describes this reaction?
a. $C_4H_{10} + O_2 \rightarrow CO_2 + H_2O$
b. $C_4H_{10} + 7O_2 + H_2 \rightarrow 4CO_2 + 6H_2O$
c. $C_4H_{10} + 7O_2 \rightarrow 4CO_2 + 5H_2O$
d. $2C_4H_{10} + 13O_2 \rightarrow 8CO_2 + 10H_2O$

**25.** One liter of solution is made by dissolving 29.2 g of NaCl in water. What is the molarity of the solution?
a. 0.5 M
b. 2.0 M
c. 1.3 M
d. 0.82 M

**26.** Which of the following is an ether?
   **a.** $CH_3CH_2OCH_2CH_3$
   **b.** $CH_3CH_2COOH$
   **c.** $CH_3CH_2NH_2$
   **d.** $CH_3CH=CHCH_3$

**27.** Which of the following is the oxidation number of sulfur in the compound sodium thiosulfate, $Na_2S_2O_3$?
   **a.** +1
   **b.** −1
   **c.** +2
   **d.** −2

**28.** Two liters of air at a pressure of two atm are condensed to 0.5 liters. If the temperature is constant, what is the new pressure?
   **a.** 16 atm
   **b.** 8 atm
   **c.** 2 atm
   **d.** 0.5 atm

**29.** The composition of dry air consists of approximately 78% nitrogen, $N_2$, and 21% oxygen, $O_2$. If the air pressure of a 5-liter sample of dry air is 800 torr, what is the approximate partial pressure of oxygen?
   **a.** 620 torr
   **b.** 720 torr
   **c.** 210 torr
   **d.** 170 torr

**30.** What does the number 36 represent on the periodic table entry for krypton?
   **a.** atomic number
   **b.** relative atomic mass
   **c.** group number
   **d.** electron configuration

**31.** The electron configuration $1s^22s^22p^63s^23p^3$ describes which atom?
   **a.** N
   **b.** Ne
   **c.** Ar
   **d.** P

**32.** Which of the following is the best Lewis structure for methanol, $CH_3OH$?

   **a.**
```
        H
        | ..
  H – C – O – H
        | ..
        H
```

   **b.**
```
        H
        | ..
  C – O – H – H
        | ..
        H
```

   **c.**
```
   H
    \
     C = O – H :
    /   |
   H    H
```

   **d.**
```
        H
        | ..
  H – C – O – H
        |
        H
```

**33.** A single atom of an element in group VI is most likely to form an ionic bond with a single atom of an element in group
   **a.** I
   **b.** II
   **c.** III
   **d.** IV

**34.** What type of bond is responsible for water tension and the formation of water drops?
   **a.** ionic bond
   **b.** nuclear bond
   **c.** covalent bond
   **d.** hydrogen bond

**35.** Which of the following will do the least damage to the hemoglobin in blood?
   **a.** pH of 1.60
   **b.** pH of 2.50
   **c.** pH of 4.90
   **d.** pH of 7.40

**36.** Which of the following variables are inversely proportional for an ideal gas if all other conditions are constant?
   **a.** pressure and volume
   **b.** pressure and temperature
   **c.** pressure and the number of moles
   **d.** No two variables are inversely proportional.

Answer questions 37 and 38 based on the following phase diagram for an unknown compound.

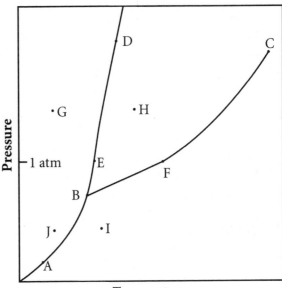

**37.** At which point is the compound a solid?
   **a.** F
   **b.** G
   **c.** H
   **d.** I

**38.** Sublimation occurs when moving from
   **a.** G to H.
   **b.** I to J.
   **c.** J to I.
   **d.** I to H.

**39.** Which of following is the balanced equation for the reaction between $NH_3$ and $O_2$?
   **a.** $4NH_3 + 5O_2 \rightarrow 4NO + 6H_2O$
   **b.** $2NH_3 + 3O_2 \rightarrow 2NO + 3H_2O$
   **c.** $2NH_3 + 2O_2 \rightarrow N_2O + 3H_2O$
   **d.** $NH_3 + O_2 \rightarrow N_2O + 3H_2O$

**40.** In the reaction $4Al + 3O_2 \rightarrow 2Al_2O_3$, how many grams of $O_2$ are needed to completely react with 1.5 moles of Al?

   **a.** 24 g
   **b.** 36 g
   **c.** 48 g
   **d.** 60 g

**41.** Appropriate protection from exposure to alpha particles is provided by

   **a.** thin clothing and breathing protection.
   **b.** thick layered clothing and breathing protection.
   **c.** concrete and/or lead walled containment.
   **d.** No material provides appropriate protection.

**42.** What is the hybridization of the carbon atoms in benzene, $C_6H_6$?

   **a.** s
   **b.** sp
   **c.** $sp^2$
   **d.** $sp^3$

**43.** Convert $8.26 \times 10^2$ nm to pm.

   **a.** $8.26 \times 10^3$ pm
   **b.** $8.26 \times 10^5$ pm
   **c.** $8.26 \times 10^{-3}$ pm
   **d.** $8.26 \times 10^{-5}$ pm

**44.** $HPO_4^{-2} + H^+ \rightarrow H_2PO^{-4}$
   The above system would be most effective for

   **a.** preventing a drop in blood pH below 7.40.
   **b.** preventing a rise in blood pH above 7.40.
   **c.** holding the blood pH significantly above 7.40.
   **d.** holding the blood pH significantly below 7.40.

**45.**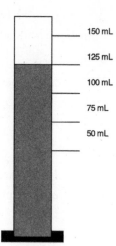

Which of these sets of measurements shows the greatest precision?

   **a.** 112 mL, 125 mL, 130 ml, 127 mL
   **b.** 122 mL, 121 mL, 121 mL, 121 mL
   **c.** 125 mL, 123 mL, 126 mL, 125 mL
   **d.** 132 mL, 126 mL, 124 mL, 122 mL

**46.** Which of the following is most reactive with water?

   **a.** Cs
   **b.** Ba
   **c.** Fr
   **d.** Ra

**47.** Electronegativity increases on the periodic table travelling

   **a.** down and to the left.
   **b.** down and to the right.
   **c.** up and to the left.
   **d.** up and to the right.

**48.** Which of the following ions is essential in the clotting of blood?

   **a.** $Ca^{2+}$
   **b.** $F^-$
   **c.** $Na^+$
   **d.** $OH^-$

**49.** What is the empirical formula for glucose, $C_6H_{12}O_6$?

    **a.** $CH_2O$

    **b.** CHO

    **c.** $C_3H_4O_3$

    **d.** $[CH_2O]_6$

**50.** A fatty acid with no double bonds is known as a

    **a.** polyunsaturated fatty acid.

    **b.** monounsaturated fatty acid.

    **c.** saturated fatty acid.

    **d.** trans fatty acid.

# Answers

## Section 1: Verbal Ability

1. **a.** weigh
2. **c.** proceed
3. **c.** portrait
4. **b.** miscellaneous
5. **a.** manageable
6. **a.** catalog
7. **b.** definitely
8. **b.** errant
9. **c.** obsession
10. **d.** jeopardy
11. **c.** magnificent
12. **a.** monotonous
13. **d.** eligible
14. **a.** inquiry
15. **a.** terminated
16. **a.** persecution
17. **b.** peculiar
18. **d.** psychology
19. **d.** license
20. **b.** credential
21. **d.** necessitate
22. **a.** stabilize
23. **c.** irrelevant
24. **d.** aspirations
25. **b.** exercise
26. **b.** The correct spelling is fierce.
27. **a.** The correct spelling is preparation.
28. **c.** The correct spelling is quadruple.
29. **a.** The correct spelling is cutlery
30. **d.** no mistakes
31. **b.** The correct spelling is height.
32. **c.** The correct spelling is emperor.
33. **b.** The correct spelling is contradict.
34. **b.** The correct spelling is reversal.
35. **b.** The correct spelling is ferocious.
36. **d.** no mistakes
37. **a.** The correct spelling is phenomenal.
38. **b.** The correct spelling is temperature.
39. **d.** no mistakes
40. **c.** The correct spelling is circumference.
41. **b.** The correct spelling is worries.
42. **b.** The correct spelling is finality.
43. **b.** The correct spelling is reprehensible.
44. **c.** The correct spelling is caffeine.
45. **b.** The correct spelling is delinquent.
46. **c.** The correct spelling is forecast.
47. **a.** The correct spelling is righteous.
48. **a.** The correct spelling is sincerely.
49. **b.** The correct spelling is vacancy.
50. **b.** The correct spelling is respiration.

## Section 2: Reading Comprehension

1. **c.** A common symptom of a chronic inflammatory disorder of the airways, such as asthma, is chest tightness. The first paragraph lists chest tightness among the symptoms that also include coughing, wheezing, and difficulty in breathing.
2. **b.** The second paragraph explains that during an attack, the asthmatic will compensate for constricted airways by breathing a greater volume of air.
3. **c.** The first sentence of the passage begins, *No longer . . .*, indicating that in the past, asthma was considered an anomalous inflammation of the bronchi. Now asthma is considered a chronic condition of the lungs.
4. **a.** An *exacerbation* is usually defined as an aggravation of symptoms or increase in the severity of a disease. However, in this passage, *exacerbations* is interchangeable with *asthma attacks*.
5. **d.** Although people with asthma should avoid cigarette smoke, it is not specifically listed among the allergens to which people with asthma may be particularly sensitive in paragraph 3 of the passage.
6. **d.** The third paragraph discusses triggers in detail. Only physical activity is listed as also being a possible symptom reducer.
7. **a.** Since asthma symptoms vary throughout the day, relying on the presence of an attack or even just on the presence of a respiratory ailment to diagnose asthma is flawed logic.

**8. b.** All of the individuals listed would glean a certain amount of knowledge from the passage; however, a healthcare professional would find the broad overview of the effects of asthma, combined with the trigger-avoidance and diagnosis information, most relevant.

**9. d.** According to the third paragraph, second-hand smoke can increase the risk of allergic sensitization in children.

**10. b.** According to paragraph 2, when reviewing a new substance, the FDA considers its safety in terms of factors like *the composition and properties of the substance.*

**11. a.** See the first sentence of paragraph 2, which states that *When evaluating the safety of a substance and whether it should be approved, the FDA considers: 1) the composition and properties of the substance . . .*

**12. a.** According to paragraph 3, the limitations of science mean that the FDA can never be 100% sure of the absence of any risk from the use of any substance.

**13. a.** Nowhere in the passage is the FDA's involvement in the amount of money charged for products using their approved additives discussed.

**14. d.** See the first sentence of paragraph 4, which states that *If an additive is approved, the FDA issues regulations that may include the types of foods in which the additive can be used, the maximum amounts to be used, and how it should be identified on food labels.*

**15. b.** The passage as a whole introduces the FDA and talks about its function in society.

**16. d.** See the last sentence of the third paragraph. Compaction may well reduce transportation costs (choice **a**) according to the third paragraph. That it reduces the volume of waste (choice **b**) is an advantage, not a disadvantage. Compaction is not designed to eliminate organic matter, so confirming that it has been eliminated (choice **c**) is not an issue.

**17. b.** See the first sentence of paragraph 3. Hydropulping (choice **a**) and compacting (choice **c**) are processing methods, not disposal methods. On-site disposal (choice **d**) is not usually an option for small hospitals with limited resources.

**18. b.** See the last sentence of the sixth paragraph, which points out that steam sterilization does not change the appearance of the waste, thus perhaps raising questions at a landfill.

**19. c.** The fourth paragraph states that liquid is separated from pulp in the hydropulping process. The sixth paragraph says that liquid may form during the sterilization process.

**20. a.** This response relies on an understanding of pathological wastes, which are wastes generated by infectious materials. The seventh paragraph points out that incineration is especially appropriate for pathological wastes. Previously, the sixth paragraph states that steam sterilization is appropriate for substances contaminated with infectious organisms.

**21. d.** The second paragraph says that the main risk of manual carts is potential exposure from torn bags, but also that automated carts can reduce that potential.

**22. b.** See the next-to-last sentence of the fourth paragraph. Sterilization does not change the volume of waste. While compacting does change the volume of the waste, it is not appropriate for eliminating hazardous materials.

**23. c.** See the first sentence of the fourth paragraph: *Hydropulping involves grounding the waste in the presence of an oxidizing fluid, such as hypochlorite solution*, meaning that hydropulping involves compressing the waste.

**24. b.** See the last sentence of the passage, which states, regarding the rotary kiln, that *the costs have been prohibitive for smaller units.*

**25. c.** In the first paragraph, the communication network of the millions of cells in the immune system is compared to bees swarming around a hive.

**26. d.** See the final sentence of the passage: *The painful side effects of these diseases are caused by a person's immune system actually attacking itself.*

**27. c.** See the last paragraph. Allergens are responsible for triggering an inappropriate immune response to otherwise harmless substances such as ragweed pollen or cat hair.

**28. d.** The last paragraph of the passage mentions that an antigen *announces its foreignness* with intricate shapes called *epitopes* that protrude from its surface.

**29. a.** Every individual's immune system must learn to recognize and deal with nonself molecules through experience. However, the last section of the second paragraph mentions that the immune system is capable of choices **b**, **c**, and **d**.

**30. a.** According to the second paragraph, the ability to distinguish between self and nonself is the heart of the immune system. This topic is further elucidated throughout the body of the passage.

**31. b.** The last paragraph mentions that tissues or cells from another individual may act as antigens *except* in the case of identical twins, whose cells carry identical self markers.

**32. b.** The passage is a message to parents about how important it is to inform their children about their condition and how best to handle it.

**33. b.** According to paragraph 2, excess weight and inactivity put children and teens at risk for type 2 diabetes.

**34. d.** According to paragraph 3, people with diabetes need to keep their glucose levels from dropping by snacking.

**35. a.** The passage does not say anything about glucose levels regulating themselves. It makes a point to say that managing blood glucose levels must be done 24 hours a day, seven days a week.

**36. c.** Paragraph 3 makes a point to specify that *people with diabetes must regularly check their blood glucose.*

**37. c.** People with diabetes have too much glucose in their blood. As stated in paragraph 3, insulin is used to help bring blood glucose levels down.

**38. d.** Paragraph 3 states that excess glucose can lead to heart disease, stroke, nerve damage, blindness, and kidney disease because of damage to large and small blood vessels. Paralysis is not listed as an ailment.

**39. a.** Managing diabetes is an *intensive*, or rigorous, process.

**40. c.** According to paragraph 4, parents should develop a diabetes management plan with their child's healthcare team that outlines the child's specific medical needs. Nowhere in the passage does it say that children with diabetes need to stay indoors, avoid physical activity, or inject insulin every hour.

**41. c.** As a whole, the passage introduces and explains meiosis and mitosis, the two types of cell division.

**42. a.** According to paragraph 2, *During mitosis, a cell duplicates all of its contents, including its chromosomes, and splits to form two identical daughter cells.*

**43. d.** When the sperm and the egg *unite* during conception, they physically come together, or join.

**44. b.** See the second paragraph, which explains that *When mitosis is not regulated correctly, health problems, such as cancer, can result.*

**45. a.** According to paragraph 1, mitosis is the process responsible for making new body cells; meiosis is the process responsible for creating egg and sperm cells.

## Section 3: Quantitative Ability

**1. a.** First, change $3\frac{4}{5}$ into an improper fraction: $3\frac{4}{5} = \frac{19}{5}$. The reciprocal of $\frac{19}{5}$ is $\frac{5}{19}$.

**2. b.** To solve for $y$, you must isolate it on one side of the equation. Subtract 17 from both sides to get $12y = 144$. Divide both sides by 12 to find that $y = 12$.

**3. b.** The formula for circumference is $2\pi r$. Since the radius is 5, the circumference is $2\pi(5)$, or $10\pi$.

**4. c.** First, find the total area of the wall. Since the wall is square, all sides are the same. The area of a square is length $\times$ width, so the area of the wall is $12 \times 12 = 144$ square feet. If the designer buys 180 square feet and only uses 144, he has $180 - 144 = 36$ square feet left.

**5. b.** Be careful to keep track of the units in which you are working. An easy way to compute is to change all units to inches: 6 feet, 2 inches = $6(12) + 2 = 74$ inches. 4 feet, 9 inches = $4(12) + 9 = 57$ inches. 74 inches − 57 inches = 17 inches, or 1 foot 5 inches.

**6. d.** First, find the number of complete days—all day Saturday is one full day. Next, subtract 5:30 from the 12:00 (midnight) that follows to get 6 hours 30 minutes for Friday. Next, add 8:15 to the 12 hours from midnight to noon on Sunday to get 20 hours 15 minutes for the whole day. Add them all together: 1 day + 6 hours 30 minutes + 20 hours 15 minutes = 1 day + 26 hours 45 minutes = 2 days, 2 hours, 45 minutes.

**7. c.** Read the question carefully; it asks how much medication is given in every dose, not at every hour. First change the total grams of medication into an improper fraction: $2\frac{2}{5} = \frac{12}{5}$. Then divide by 4 by multiplying by its reciprocal and reduce to get the final answer: $\frac{12}{5} \div 4 = \frac{12}{5} \times \frac{1}{4} = \frac{12}{20} = \frac{3}{5}$

**8. c.** Read the question carefully; it asks how much Sarah spent on *clothes* only: $25.20 + $45.05 + $32.75 = $103.00.

**9. b.** Be careful to answer what the question asks, which is how many staff members *cannot* be vaccinated. $30 \times 0.80 = 24$ people can be vaccinated, so $30 - 24 = 6$ cannot be vaccinated.

**10. c.** Add together her miles per hour for each hour traveled and then divide by 3 (total hours traveled) to get the average speed: 12 for hour one + 12 for hour two + 14 for hour three = $\frac{38}{3} = 12\frac{2}{3}$.

**11. c.** You may have been able to estimate that 99.2 is too high to be the average, since all the numbers given are less than 99.2, and that 97.9 and 98.0 are too low, since most of the numbers are greater than 98. You can also calculate the answer by adding all the numbers together and dividing by 5: $\frac{99 + 98 + 97.9 + 98.6 + 98.5}{5} = \frac{492}{5} = 98.4$.

**12. a.** The first step in solving the problem is to subtract 86 from 148. The remainder, 62, is then divided by 2 to get 31.

**13. a.** The hospital will spend $50(\$15.50) + 100(\$2.15) = \$775 + \$215 = \$990.00$ on lab coats.

**14. b.** $150x = (100)(1)$, where $x$ is the part of a mile a jogger has to go to burn the calories a walker burns in 1 mile. If you divide both sides of this equation by 150, you get $x = \frac{100}{150}$. Cancel 50 from the numerator and denominator to get $\frac{2}{3}$. This means that a jogger has to jog only $\frac{2}{3}$ of a mile to burn the same number of calories a walker burns in a mile of brisk walking.

**15. c.** The ratio is $\frac{12\,cc}{100\,lbs.} = \frac{x\,cc}{175\,lbs.}$, where $x$ is the number of cc's per 175 lbs. Multiply both sides by 175 in order to get $175 \times \frac{12}{100} = x$, so $x = 21$.

**16. a.** 20% of $1,800 = (0.2)(1,800) = 360$ calories from fat. Since there are 9 calories in each gram of fat, you should divide 360 by 9 to find that 40 grams of fat are allowed.

**17. c.** Plug in the given values, being careful with the signs: $2x - yz = 2(-1) - (4)(-2) = -2 - (-8) = -2 + 8 = 6$.

**18. b.** 20% of 15 cc $= (0.20)(15) = 3$. Adding 3 to 15 gives 18 cc.

**19. a.** The area of a triangle equals $\frac{1}{2}(base \times height)$ but only the base is given. Since this is a right triangle, we can find the height $h$ using the Pythagorean theorem. $h^2 + 3^2 = 5^2$; $h^2 + 9 = 25$; $h^2 = 16$; $h = 4$. Thus, the area is $\frac{1}{2}(3)(4) = \frac{1}{2}(12) = 6$.

**20. c.** The easiest way to calculate the area is to realize that in order to include the shaded areas between the circle and the square, the entire shaded figure must be made up of half a circle of diameter 4, or radius 2, on top of a rectangle that is 4 units wide and 6 units tall. The area of a rectangle is *length* × *width*. The area of a circle is $\pi r^2$. So the area of the shaded area $= (4)(6) + \frac{1}{2}\pi(2)^2 = 24 + 2\pi$.

**21. a.** First, find out what 12 rides would cost if you bought each ride individually: $12 \times \$1.50 = \$18.00$. $\$18.00 - \$15.50 = \$2.50$.

**22. c.** The highest monthly rent that Javier can afford is 30% of his monthly income, or $0.30(\$3,500) = \$1,050$.

**23. c.** Write out the words into equations. $t = s + 4$; $s = r - 2$. When $r = 8$, then $s = 6$. When $s = 6$, then $t = 6 + 4 = 10$.

**24. b.** First, find the percent increase from 8 to 10. $10 - 8 = 2$. $\frac{2}{8} = \frac{1}{4} = 25\%$. How do you increase 16 by 25%? Find 25% of 16: $16 \times 0.25 = 4$. Add this 25% to 16: $16 + 4 = 20$.

**25. d.** Solve the equation by isolating $x$: $13 \div 0.0013 = 10,000$.

**26. b.** Simply estimating the value of $\frac{7}{40}$ will probably let you know that 0.0175 is much too small, and 1.75 and 17.5 are much too large. If that did not work for you, however, you could divide 7 by 40 in order to get 0.175.

**27. d.** 30 ppm of the pollutant would have to be removed to bring 50 ppm down to 20 ppm; 30 ppm represents 60% of 50 ppm.

**28. a.** The drug is 50% effective for half (or 50%) of migraine sufferers, so it eliminates $(0.50)(0.50) = 0.25 = 25\%$ of all migraines.

**29. d.** Division is used to arrive at a decimal, which can then be rounded to the nearest hundredth and converted to a percentage: $11,350 \div 21,500 = 0.5279$; 0.5279 rounded to the nearest hundredth is 0.53, or 53%.

**30. b.** Since there are two digits after the decimal point in each number you are multiplying, there will be four digits after the decimal point in the correct answer: 0.0216.

**31. c.** First, change $2\frac{1}{4}$ to an improper fraction: $\frac{9}{4}$. Next, in order to divide by $\frac{2}{3}$, invert that fraction to $\frac{3}{2}$ and multiply: $\frac{9}{4} \times \frac{3}{2} = \frac{27}{8} = 3\frac{3}{8}$.

**32. a.** First, find the least common denominator, 16; $\frac{7}{8} = \frac{14}{16}$, so you can rewrite the problem as $(3 + \frac{9}{16}) - (1 + \frac{14}{16})$. To get a large enough numerator from which to subtract 14, you borrow 1 from the 3 to rewrite the problem as $2\frac{25}{16} - 1\frac{14}{16} = 1\frac{11}{16}$.

**33. b.** This is a simple multiplication problem, which is solved by multiplying $35 \times 8.2$ in order to get 287.

**34. c.** The problem is solved by dividing 204 by 1,700. The answer, 0.12, is then converted to a percentage, 12%.

**35. d.** The patients are being transferred from the hospital to the nursing home, and the question asks for total miles traveled by the time the ambulance returns to the hospital. Since the ambulance is starting and ending at the hospital, it will be making 4 round trips total with 4 patients, or traveling $8 \times 10\frac{1}{5} = 80\frac{8}{5} = 81\frac{3}{5}$ miles.

**36. b.** The simplest way to solve this problem is to divide 1 by 1,500, which is 0.0006667, and then count off two decimal places to arrive at the percentage 0.06667%. Since the question asks *about what percentage,* the nearest value is 0.067%.

**37. a.** You can use trial and error to arrive at a solution to this problem. Using choice **a**, after the first hour, the number would be 20, after the second hour 40, after the third hour 80, after the fourth hour 160, and after the fifth hour 320. The other answer choices do not have the same outcome.

**38. a.** Since the solution to the problem $x + 25 \le 13$ is $x \le -12$, choices **b**, **c**, and **d** are all too large to be correct.

**39. d.** The area formula for both a square and a rectangle is $A = length \times width$. Since all sides of a square are equal, a square of side length 6 has an area of $6^2 = 36$. To have the same area, a rectangle of length 2 must have a width $w$ such that $2w = 36$, or $w = 18$.

**40. c.** The measures of supplementary angles add up to 180°, so $r + s = 180°$. Therefore, $52° + s = 180°$, and $s = 128°$.

**41. a.** Fractions must be converted to the lowest common denominator, which is 60; $\frac{6}{10} = \frac{36}{60}$; $\frac{11}{20} = \frac{33}{60}$; $\frac{8}{15} = \frac{32}{60}$, which is the smallest fraction.

**42. c.** Add the whole numbers: $2 + 4 = 6$. Use the least common denominator of 8 to add the fractions: $\frac{2}{8} + \frac{5}{8} + \frac{4}{8} = \frac{11}{8} = 1\frac{3}{8}$. Add 1 to the whole number sum: $1 + 6 = 7$, and then add the fraction to get $7\frac{3}{8}$.

**43. d.** 750 is $n$% of 600, which, expressed as an equation, is $750 = (\frac{n}{100})(600)$. Cancel 100 in the right side of the equation: $750 = 6n$. Divide both sides by 6 to arrive at $n = 125$. Therefore, 750 is 125% of 600.

**44. d.** Multiply the numerator and denominator of $\frac{13}{25}$ by 4 to get $\frac{52}{100}$ or 0.52.

**45. b.** Make sure to convert the given numbers to the same units. Convert the length of bandages needed into centimeters: $4 \text{ m} \times 100 \text{ cm/m} = 400 \text{ cm}$. One 250 cm roll of bandages will not be enough, but two rolls will provide 500 cm of bandages, which will fulfill the doctor's needs with 100 cm left over.

**46. b.** Because parallel lines never intersect, choice **a** is incorrect. Perpendicular lines do intersect, so choice **c** is incorrect. Choice **d** is incorrect because intersecting lines have only one point in common.

**47. c.** This is a simple subtraction problem, as long as the decimals are lined up correctly: $3.60 - 1.89 = 1.71$.

**48.** **c.** This is a two-step multiplication problem. To find out how many heartbeats there would be in one hour, you must multiply 72 beats per minute by 60 minutes per hour, and then multiply this result, 4,320, by 6.5 hours in order to get 28,080.

**49.** **a.** The unreduced ratio is 8,000:5,000,000 or 8:5,000; $5,000 \div 8 = 625$, for a ratio of 1:625.

**50.** **b.** Before subtracting, you must convert both fractions to 24ths: $\frac{5}{12} - \frac{3}{8} = \frac{10}{24} - \frac{9}{24} = \frac{1}{24}$.

## Section 4: General Science

**1.** **c.** Johann Kepler gave us the laws of planetary motion. Lyell studied changes in the Earth over time; Mendel studied the heredity of plants; and Hooke studied biological cells.

**2.** **b.** The experimental factor is the one you change or manipulate. All the others are held constant.

**3.** **c.** The standard metric unit of volume is the liter.

**4.** **d.** There are 1,000,000 micrograms in one gram. The prefix *micro-* means million.

**5.** **c.** The universe is expanding outward.

**6.** **d.** Mendel used pea plants to conduct his research in trait inheritance. He grew and studied nearly 30,000 pea plants.

**7.** **d.** Galileo made himself a small—but for that time, powerful—telescope, turned it skyward, and made many discoveries, including the moons of Jupiter, craters of our moon, and sunspots.

**8.** **a.** The control in an experiment is the baseline that is not subjected to the variable under study. Choices **c** and **d** are made up.

**9.** **c.** One gram is equal to 1,000 milligrams. The prefix *milli-* means thousandth.

**10.** **b.** Theories, such as Einstein's theory of relativity or Darwin's theory of evolution, are the biggest concepts in science. Theories can contain more detailed hypotheses, and good theories make predictions.

**11.** **c.** The atmosphere of Venus is dominated by $CO_2$. It has no water vapor and is very thick.

**12.** **b.** There are six flavors of quark: up, down, bottom, top, charm, and strange.

**13.** **c.** Mars Pathfinder successfully landed on Mars in 1997.

**14.** **d.** If atoms have the same number of protons but different numbers of neutrons, they are isotopes.

**15.** **c.** If a substance gains electrons, it is reduced. If it loses electrons, it is said to be oxidized (because its oxidation state is decreased).

**16.** **d.** The prefix *micro-* refers to millionths.

**17.** **d.** The prefix *giga-* refers to billions.

**18.** **a.** The standard metric unit of energy is the joule.

**19.** **b.** There are 1,000, or $10^3$, meters in a kilometer.

**20.** **b.** Multiplying 60 seconds per minute by 60 minutes per hour times 24 hours per day by 365 days in a year (actually 365.25) yields the answer of between 31 and 32 million seconds per year.

**21.** **b.** Radiation is the means of heat transfer by which heat moves outward from a hot body.

**22.** **a.** We believe the dinosaurs became extinct because of a massive meteor that impacted the Earth. Evidence for this includes a layer of iridium in the rock layer from the same time period, with iridium being found primarily in meteorites. Also, a giant impact crater has been found from that time.

**23.** **b.** If a rock contains fossils, it is most likely sedimentary. Igneous, metamorphic, and volcanic rocks have been exposed to too much heat and/or pressure for any traces of life to be left behind.

**24.** **a.** Weather occurs in the troposphere.

**25.** **d.** Autotrophs are plants, algae, and bacteria that produce their own food through photosynthesis. The other choices are all animals, which do not carry out photosynthesis.

**26. d.** Patterns from distant galaxies are shifted "red," which means toward longer wavelengths. In this case, going from a pattern in the red toward a pattern in longer wavelengths means the infrared.

**27. d.** Oxygen is formed last because it is the most massive and complex of the four elements listed. Fusion reactions build from the simplest to the most complex, and the stages of fusion take hydrogen and then the other elements built in sequence as starting points for more complex elements.

**28. a.** Supernova explosions, which are catastrophic events at the end of the lives of giant stars, scatter elements previously made by fusion reactions in the star over their lifetimes, as well as elements born in the intense temperatures and pressures of the supernova explosion itself.

**29. d.** Hydrogen is primordial and was made shortly after the Big Bang when the universe cooled enough for atoms to condense. The other elements are all made by nuclear fusion reactions in stars. These reactions consume hydrogen.

**30. c.** Helium is both primordial and made during fusion reactions when two hydrogen nuclei are fused together inside stars. This fusion reaction is the main source of energy for stars.

**31. d.** Carbon increases in density because as time passes, more and more carbon is made in the fusion reactions inside stars. Choices **a** and **b** actually decrease in density as the universe expands, and choice **c** also decreases in density as hydrogen is consumed in fusion reactions.

**32. a.** Venus is the closest planet to Earth. It is 38 million kilometers from Earth at its closest approach. Mars, the second-nearest planet to Earth, is 54 million kilometers at its closest approach.

**33. b.** If the time when the Big Bang occurred was 13.7 billion years ago, the formation of Earth occurred about 4.5 billion years ago. Therefore, taking 1 EFU as 4.5 billion years (by definition from the question), there were $\frac{13.7}{4.5}$, or about 3, EFUs back to the Big Bang.

**34. c.** Meteorites formed along with Earth at the beginning of the solar system. But on Earth, no rocks go back that far. The dates from meteorites give us the best estimate of the origin of our solar system.

**35. d.** Mercury is the nearest planet to the sun. The asteroids are between Mars and Jupiter. Phobos is a moon of Mars.

**36. b.** Of the possibilities, the only one in space right now is the International Space Station. The space shuttles have been taken out of active service, so Russian rockets are taking new astronauts to the space station at this time.

**37. b.** Eris is the most massive known dwarf planet in the Solar System.

**38. b.** In 2004, rovers on the surface of Mars discovered types of minerals that, as far as we know, could have been formed only with the activity of water. Also, channels on Mars had previously been seen that looked much like the branching slow patterns of Earth's rivers.

**39. c.** Jupiter comes before the planet with rings, Saturn. Choices **a** and **d** are planets farther away than Saturn. And obviously, Saturn itself (choice **b**) makes no sense.

**40. d.** The spins of galaxies cannot be explained by the amount of known, ordinary matter. Something out there (the "dark matter") is creating more gravity than we can account for with the known, ordinary matter.

**41. b.** 73% of the universe is dark energy.

**42. c.** Carbon is made by fusion reactions in stars. Therefore, before stars and supernovas can disperse that carbon, there would have been no carbon in the earliest planets (in fact, planets as solid bodies could not have formed either). Life is so dependent on carbon that without carbon is seems likely there could not have been life.

**43. c.** The continental slope is still part of the continent, but it does head downward to the ocean floor itself.

**44. a.** The word *atom* comes from the Greek word that means indivisible. Though atoms are now known to have parts (they are divisible), they still are the fundamental units of any element.

**45. d.** Carbon-14 is the radioactive form of carbon (the most common form is carbon-12). Carbon-14 is formed in the atmosphere when cosmic rays hit nitrogen and convert small amounts of it by changing a proton to a neutron—a nuclear change. Using its half-life decay rate, we can measure the amount of carbon-14 in ancient wood to determine the dates of wood architecture of ancient peoples, as well as their campfires and even bones.

**46. c.** Quarks are the constituents of protons and neutrons.

**47. d.** Neutrons and protons are the parts of the nucleus of an atom.

**48. b.** The unit of resistance is the ohm.

**49. a.** Electromagnetism describes the interaction between charged particles. Answers **b**, **c**, and **d** correspond to the strong, weak, and gravitational forces, respectively.

**50. c.** Mendel is known as the founder of modern genetics because of his work showing how the inheritance of certain traits in pea plants follows a pattern. This is now called Mendelian Inheritance.

## Section 5: Biology

**1. b.** A-U is a nucleotide base pairing. This represents the pairing in RNA with tyrosine (T) replaced by uracil (U).

**2. d.** Adipose tissue is the connective tissue otherwise known as fat. Adipose is made up of lipids, also referred to as fatty acids or triglycerides.

**3. a.** Viruses are unable to reproduce because they lack cells. Viruses rely on host cells to express their genetic material. Viruses contain enzymes and nucleic acid and have evolved through natural selection.

**4. d.** Kingdoms are general categories and species are very specific groups.

**5. b.** One of the primary functions of the liver is to process toxins absorbed in the digestive system.

**6. b.** The loop of Henle is a component of the nephron of the kidney, the excretory organ in vertebrates.

**7. b.** Chloroplasts are found only in plants. Both plants and animals have mitochondria and nuclei, and bacteria and plants possess cell walls.

**8. a.** The following are the SI units: $10^{-1} = deci$; $10^{-2} = centi$; $10^{-3} = milli$; $10^{-6} = micro$; $10^{-9} = nano$; $10^{-12} = pico$; $10^{-15} = femto$; $10^{-18} = atto$.

**9. b.** A compartment filled with air or watery fluid in the cytoplasm is referred to as a vacuole. Centrioles and centrosomes are associated with the process of cell division.

**10. c.** Chloroplasts contain chlorophyll and are found only in plant cells.

**11. a.** Mitochondria are known as the power plants of the cell and are responsible for most ATP generation.

**12. d.** All cells undergo mitosis to reproduce into identical cells with the same DNA. Cells specialize into different tissue by expressing different parts of their DNA. Only gametes may have different DNA from their parent cells due to meiosis.

**13. d.** Mammals are differentiated from other animals by their mammary glands, which females use to nurse their young. Birds can also regulate their body temperatue, so that is not the correct answer.

**14. c.** The lysosome is the garbage truck of the cell, handling waste and breaking it down.

**15. b.** Flowering plants (angiosperms) might reproduce faster because their reproductive process involves flowers, which attract insects to help spread pollen and other animals to spread seeds. Also, the seeds of angiosperms have a tough skin, which may help them tolerate harsh conditions.

**16. d.** The figure shows a nerve cell. Note the long extensions (axons and dendrites) unique to neurons. Blood, fat, and muscle cells have very different shapes.

**17. c.** Hepatitis is a disease marked by a inflammation of the liver, as indicated by the Greek roots *hepato* meaning liver and *itis* meaning inflammation.

**18. d.** Bacteria reproduce by binary fission. All other choices relate to eukaryotic cell division.

**19. a.** The primary function of a blood platelet is to aid in the blood clotting process. Platelets scrape against the rough edges of broken tissue and release a substance to promote clotting. Red blood cells carry oxygen. Antibodies are produced by B lymphocytes. Phagocytic cells include neutrophils and macrophages (monocytes).

**20. d.** An expressed trait is determined by two alleles. A phenotype is the physical or visual expression of the genotype.

**21. d.** Organisms that adapted to use oxygen through aerobic respiration made energy more efficiently than those that used anaerobic respiration, giving them an evolutionary advantage.

**22. c.** Early cells were prokaryotic and resemble the bacteria found today. The other options are simple life forms that evolved from single-celled prokaryotes.

**23. d.** The father gives only his Y chromosome to the son, so the mother must have given the son the X-linked trait. Because the mother does not show the X-linked trait, she is considered a carrier of the trait.

**24. a.** Marrow produces red and white blood cells and platelets and is located in the bones of the skeletal system.

**25. d.** Enzymes are catalysts that allow chemical reactions to proceed more rapidly.

**26. c.** Kelp is a brown algae; the others are fungi.

**27. c.** Viruses are noncellular, and they must enter a living cell to replicate. However, not all viruses are disease-causing; many viruses do no apparent harm.

**28. b.** Bacteria can be placed in three groups (cocci, bacilli, spirilla) based on their shape.

**29. c.** Malaria is caused by *Plasmodium*, which is a protist. The others are viruses.

**30. c.** All bacteria are prokaryotes, meaning that they lack a nucleus. Eukaryotes contain a nucleus and other organelles. Some eukaryotes are single-celled (protists).

**31. a.** Transcription describes the copying of DNA to messenger RNA, which travels out of the nucleus before being translated into proteins.

**32. d.** Translocation is a type of mutation in which a section of one chromosome breaks off and joins with another. In aneuploidy, an individual has an abnormal number of chromosomes. Transcription is the process in which genetic information is transferred from DNA to mRNA. Translation is a process used in the synthesis of new proteins on ribosomes.

**33. b.** A zygote is the product of a sperm nucleus fused with an ovum nucleus. A zoospore is found in certain fungi. Ova is the plural of ovum, a female egg, while an oocyte is a cell in the ovary that produces an ovum after undergoing meiosis.

**34. a.** Glycolysis is a combination of "glucose" and "lysis" (meaning breakdown).

**35. a.** When there is a shortage of oxygen in muscle tissue, pyruvic acid produces lactic acid to be converted to glucose by the liver. Lactose is milk sugar. Adrenaline is a hormone produced in the adrenal medulla that stimulates the sympathetic nervous system, while serotonin, also a hormone, is produced in many parts of the body.

**36. c.** The large intestine's main functions are water absorption and feces production. The large intestine consists of the rectum, colon, and caecum. Almost all the digestion and absorption of nutrients occurs in the small intestine. The liver has numerous functions, including the metabolism of carbohydrates, lipids, and proteins, as well as the removal of drugs and hormones and the production of bile. The stomach is the holding reservoir in which saliva, food, and gastric juices mix prior to continuing the digestive process in the small intestine.

**37. a.** Calcium ions are released in the interim between the time when a stimulus is received and a response occurs in muscle tissue.

**38. a.** Beriberi, most common in countries where white rice is the main food source, is caused by a lack of vitamin $B_1$. Deficiencies in vitamin C can cause scurvy, and deficiencies in vitamin D can cause rickets. Hemolytic anemia is a possible consequence of vitamin E deficiency.

**39. c.** Chlorophyll is the pigment that absorbs light energy and is critical to photosynthesis. It is green in color.

**40. d.** Anaphylaxis is an immune system response such as that which occurs in a person who gets stung by a bee and is allergic to the venom. Hypertension is another term for high blood pressure and is not a common characteristic of anaphylaxis.

**41. a.** The correct answer is analgesic. Anesthetics block perception of *all* sensory stimuli either generally (all over) or locally (in a specific area). Acetycholine is a neurotransmitter.

**42. c.** Thymine is a DNA nucleobase that pairs with adenine.

**43. d.** Kupffer cells remove red blood cells, otherwise known as erythrocytes, and other degenerating matter from the liver. Leukocytes and eosinophils are white blood cells.

**44. a.** The first law of thermodynamics describes the conservation of energy.

**45. c.** Down's syndrome is also known as trisomy 21 syndrome.

**46. d.** Ethanol, or ethyl alcohol, depresses the CNS, thereby affecting the neural activity of the consumer. Isopropyl alcohol is for external use only and is found in cosmetics. Methanol is wood alcohol used as a solvent. Methionine is an organic compound used in dietary supplements.

**47. a.** The primary structure describes a protein's amino acid sequence. Choices **b** and **c** describe a protein's secondary and tertiary structures, respectively.

**48. a.** Warts are usually insignificant growths caused by a virus. Sarcomas are malignant tumors arising from connective tissue, while adenomas are glandlike benign tumors. A cold sore is a lesion caused by the herpes simplex virus.

**49. c.** Rhodopsin, or visual purple, is the light-sensitive pigment in vertebrate eyes. Cytochrome is a respiratory enzyme, hemoglobin is the oxygen-bearing protein in red blood cells that gives them their red color, and melanin is the dark pigment found in skin, hair, and the retina.

**50. b.** People suffering from high blood pressure, or hypertension, have an increased risk of stroke and heart attack. Cardiomyopathy is a form of muscle damage that leads to heart failure.

## Section 6: Chemistry

**1. b.** It is very important for blood to be close to neutral pH, as variance outside a small pH range can cause death. Ammonia is a well-known base, while lemon juice and vinegar contain citric and acetic acids, respectively, giving them low pH.

**2. a.** The condensation of two amino acids occurs when amine and carboxylic acid groups combine to form an amide bond.

**3. c.** $NH_2$ is an amino group, which gives an amino acid the first part of its name. It is found in 19 of the 20 amino acids. The other prevalent group is carboxylic acid, or COOH, which is not one of the answer choices.

**4. a.** When two amino acids come together, the carboxylic acid group of one reacts with the amine group of the other. An $OH^-$ from the carboxylic acid combines with an $H^+$ from the amine group to form $H_2O$. The remaining C=O of the carboxylic acid then bonds with the remaining N-H of the amine to form a peptide bond.

**5. b.** The secondary structure describes the geometry of segments of the protein, such as α-helices and β-sheets. The amino acid sequence describes the primary structure, while the 3-dimensional fold of the protein describes the tertiary structure. Quaternary structure is the arrangement of multiple protein subunits into a larger protein complex.

**6. b.** The mass number (35) is equal to the number of protons + neutrons. $35 - 17 = 18$ neutrons.

**7. b.** The atomic number is the number of protons in any given element.

**8. a.** Sodium hydroxide, a strong base, forms sodium chloride (table salt) and water when combined with hydrochloric acid, a strong acid.

**9. d.** According to the octet rule, the atom tends to be most stable when it has eight valence electrons. Chlorine, a group VII element on the periodic table, will have to gain one electron to have eight valence electrons. This gives it a total of 18 electrons.

**10. d.** A butane is an alkane with four carbon atoms. The *t* in *t*-butane stands for a tertiary carbon. The central carbon of choice **d** is tertiary because it has three other carbon atoms bonded to it. Choice **a** is also a butane molecule, but it is *n*-butane. Choices **b** and **c** are not butanes.

**11. c.** Neutral oxygen possesses 8 electrons (same as the number of protons). The $-2$ charge on the ion means that there are 2 additional electrons for 10 total.

**12. c.** A Lewis base is defined as a species that has a nonbonding pair or pairs of electrons that it can donate to form new bonds. Sodium is the only choice that does not have at least one lone pair of electrons.

**13. b.** Combustion is a reaction in which an alkane burns in excess oxygen to give off carbon dioxide and water. Hydrogen gas, present in all three incorrect equations, is not a participant in combustion reactions.

**14. d.** The configuration of a chlorine atom in the ground state is [Ne]$3s^2 3p^5$. A Cl$^-$ ion has an additional electron, giving it the same electron configuration as an argon atom in the ground state, which can also be written as [Ne]$3s^2 3p^6$.

**15. c.** The carbon atom in methane has four sigma bonds around it, meaning that it uses its $s$ atomic orbital and all three $p$ atomic orbitals to form four $sp^3$ molecular orbitals. The number of atomic orbitals combining always equals the number of molecular orbitals formed.

**16. c.** Electronegativity is a measure of the ability of an atom to attract shared electrons to itself. It increases going across rows of the periodic table to the right and decreases going down columns of the table. Na, S, and Cl are all in the same row of the table, with Cl being rightmost. Cl is also above Br, so it is the most electronegative atom.

**17. b.** This is the definition of the boiling point. At temperatures higher than the boiling point, the vapor pressure of the liquid is greater than external pressure, and molecules begin to escape in the gaseous phase.

**18. c.** $Fe_2O_3$ contains 3 O atoms, each with a $-2$ charge. To balance this $-6$ overall charge, each iron atom must have an oxidation state of $+3$.

**19. a.** The empirical formula of a compound is the formula written in the simplest form possible. $C_2H_6O_2$ has one molecule of both C and O for every three molecules of H, so the empirical formula is $CH_3O$.

**20. a.** Neutral magnesium possesses 2 valence electrons. To reach its nearest full valence shell, it loses those electrons, giving it an oxidation state of $+2$.

**21. d.** The complete chemical symbol includes two numbers. The lower number is the atomic number, or the number of protons in the nucleus. The upper number is the mass number, or the sum of the protons and neutrons in the nucleus. Therefore, the answer is $^{33}_{16}S^{2-}$ because there are 18 electrons present.

**22. b.** Nonmetal oxides ($SO_3$) and bases (KOH) react to form salts and water. The solution in choice **a** forms an acid, and that in choice **c** forms a salt, but such a reaction would not give off oxygen.

**23. d.** Lewis acids are electron-pair acceptors, while Brønsted acids are proton donors. HCl and $H_2SO_4$ are proton donors. $CH_4$ is not an acid of any type. $AlCl_3$ has the ability to accept 2 electrons (to give it 8 in its valence shell), making it a Lewis acid.

**24. d.** This problem is simply an equation-balancing problem. The number of molecules of each element must be the same on each side of the equation. Choice **d** has 8 carbons, 20 hydrogens, and 26 oxygens on each side of the equation.

**25. a.** The molar mass of the compound NaCl is approximately 58.4 g/mol; 29.2 grams is one-half the molar mass of NaCl, so the solution is 0.5 M because there is one liter of the solution. Molarity is moles/liter.

**26. a.** Ethers have the formula $R_1$–O–$R_2$. Choices **b**, **c**, and **d** are a carboxylic acid, an amine, and an alkene, respectively.

**27. c.** The sum of the oxidation numbers must be equal to the net charge on the compound, so the sum must be equal to zero. The charge on the cation is the same as its oxidation number, so the oxidation number of Na is +1 and the oxidation number for $S_2O_3$ is −2. Oxygen almost always has an oxidation number of −2, so the oxidation number of sulfur must be +2.

**28. b.** The formula $P_1V_1 = P_2V_2$ must be used. Solving 2 atm(2 L) = $P_2$(0.5 L) for $P_2$ gives 8 atm.

**29. d.** The sum of the partial pressures is the total pressure, or, in this case, the air pressure. Since the sample is 21% oxygen, and there is a total pressure of 800 torr, the partial pressure is 800 × 0.21, or 170 torr.

**30. a.** 36 is the atomic number of krypton. The atomic mass of krypton is 83.80, and the electron configuration is represented by the period numbers listed on the left of the periodic table. The group number refers to the element's placement on a vertical column on the periodic table.

**31. d.** P possesses 15 total electrons and this electronic structure, according to Hund's rule.

**32. a.** Only choice **a** has all the octets filled and no formal charges. Other choices leave impossible or unstable structures (i.e., choice **b**), unfilled octets (i.e., choice **d**), or formal charges.

**33. b.** Group VI elements will fill their outer shells by gaining two electrons, giving them a charge of −2. They will most likely form ionic bonds with atoms from group II, which will lose two electrons to have a full outer shell and a charge of +2.

**34. d.** The hydrogen bond causes an attraction between the positive and negative poles of water molecules, making the surface of water sticky.

**35. d.** The pH of blood is naturally 7.40 and must always remain near that pH to prevent shock and/or death.

**36. a.** This question refers to the ideal gas law, or the equation PV = nRT. Solving for P gives P = nRT/V. Therefore, pressure is inversely proportional to volume.

**37. b.** Compounds are solids in the upper left portion of the diagram.

**38. c.** To sublime is to go directly from the solid to the gas state. The gas state is the farthest down on the phase diagram.

**39. a.** $NH_3$ and $O_2$ form NO. Choice **a** is the only equation that forms this molecule and is balanced.

**40. b.** 36 grams of $O_2$ are needed; the molar mass of $O_2$ is 32 g/mol.
$$1.5 \text{ mole Al} \times \frac{3 \text{ moles } O_2}{4 \text{ moles Al}} \times \frac{32 \text{ g } O_2}{\text{mole } O_2} = 36 \text{ g } O_2$$

**41. a.** Only a thin layer of clothing and breathing protection are necessary to protect the body from exposure to alpha particles.

**42. c.** Each carbon atom in benzene has 3 σ bonds (2 to other carbons and 1 to hydrogen), meaning that it must use 1 s atomic orbital and 2 of its p orbitals to form 3 $sp^2$ molecular orbitals.

**43. b.** $8.26 \times 10^2 \times 10^3$ pm = $8.26 \times 10^5$ pm

**44. a.** This system shows one of the blood's acid buffers preventing a rise in acidity, which also means that it is preventing a drop in pH. This system is preventing the pH from dropping below 7.40, which is the pH of blood.

**45. b.** Precision is the degree of closeness to which the measurements are repeated, regardless of how close those measurements are to the true value. The group of measurements closest to each other, although not necessarily 125, are 122 mL, 121 mL, 121 mL, and 121 mL.

**46. c.** Reactivity with water increases going down and to the left on the periodic table.

**47. d.** Electronegativity increases on the periodic table travelling up and to the right, making F the most electronegative element.

**48. a.** Calcium ions convert prothrombin to thrombin, which causes fibrinogen to convert to fibrin. Fibrin causes coagulation of the blood.

**49. a.** The empirical formula describes the simplest relative ratios of the atoms in a molecule.

**50. c.** The definition of a saturated fatty acid is a fatty acid with no double bonds.

# Scoring

Your score on each section is reported both as a raw score, the number of questions you got right in that section, and as a percentile, a number that indicates what percent of other test takers scored lower than you did on this section. No total score is reported, only scores for individual sections. Furthermore, there is no such thing as a "passing" raw or percentile score. Individual schools set their own standards.

For purposes of comparison, you'll work with raw scores in this book. So the first thing you should do is count up the number of questions you got right in each section and record them in the following blanks.

**Section 1:** _____ of 50 questions right
**Section 2:** _____ of 45 questions right
**Section 3:** _____ of 50 questions right
**Section 4:** _____ of 50 questions right
**Section 5:** _____ of 50 questions right
**Section 6:** _____ of 50 questions right

Your purpose in taking this first practice exam—in addition to getting practice in answering the kinds of questions found on nursing school entrance exams—is to identify your strengths and weaknesses.

In order to do so, convert your raw scores above into percentages. (Note that this *percentage* is not the same as the *percentile* that will appear on your score report. The percentage is simply the number you would have gotten right if there had been 100 questions in the section; it will enable you to compare your raw scores among the various sections. The percentile compares your score with that of other candidates.)

To get percentages for the sections with 50 questions, simply multiply your raw score by two. (Since each section has 50 questions, your percentage is twice your raw score.)

For section 2, divide your raw score by 45, and then move the decimal point two places to the right to arrive at a percentage.

Now that you know what percentage of the questions on each section you got right, you're ready to outline your study plan. The sections on which you got the lowest percentages are the ones that you should plan on studying hardest. Sections on which you got higher percentages may not need as much of your time. However, unless you scored over 95% on a given section, you can't afford to skip studying that section altogether. After all, you want the highest score you can manage in the time left before the exam.

Use your percentage scores in conjunction with the Nursing School Entrance Exam Planner in Chapter 1 of this book to help you devise a study plan. Then turn to the chapters that follow this one, which cover each of the areas tested on the nursing school entrance exam. These chapters contain valuable information on each section of the exam, along with study and test-taking tips and lots of practice questions to help you score your best.

# 4 ▶ VERBAL ABILITY

### *CHAPTER SUMMARY*

In order to be a successful health professional, you have to express ideas clearly and accurately. Because written expression is an important part of your ability to communicate, your nursing school entrance exam will contain a spelling section. In the Verbal Ability section, you will not be required to spell out words, but rather, you will be asked to *identify* the correct spelling of a word from four choices.

**T**his chapter is designed to help you refresh your spelling skills by teaching you rules you can use to spell your best. You'll learn strategies to help you spell words with tricky letter combinations, unusual plurals, prefixes, and hyphenated and compound words.

## What Spelling Questions Are Like

The spelling part of the Verbal Ability section of your exam will test your capacity to spell correctly and recognize properly and improperly spelled words. For example, you may be given four differently spelled versions of the same word and asked to find the choice that is spelled correctly.

**1.** Select the correctly spelled word.
   **a.** peice
   **b.** piece
   **c.** peece
   **d.** peise

The correct answer is choice **b**, *piece*. Knowing the rule for when to use *ie* or *ei* could have helped you answer this question. Read on to learn the rule.

Your exam might also present you with a set of different words and ask you to pick out the one word that is spelled incorrectly. For example:

**2.** Choose the misspelled word.
  **a.** destructive
  **b.** decisive
  **c.** distinguished
  **d.** There is no misspelled word.

If your spelling skills are sharp, you know that the correct answer is choice **d**; all three choices are spelled correctly.

Another version of this question type may ask you to find the *correctly* spelled word from a group of misspelled words. When you are taking your exam, always be sure to read each question carefully so that you know exactly what the question is asking.

## How to Prepare for Spelling Questions

Reading as much as you can, looking at words carefully, visualizing the words, listening for the sounds of words, and learning the most common prefixes, suffixes, and roots are all simple and effective ways to improve your spelling skills naturally. But if you want to ensure that you ace the spelling portion of your entrance exam, nothing beats learning the rules.

## Spelling Rules

Most of the spelling questions found on your nursing school entrance exam will test your knowledge of spelling rules, so getting a good grasp on these rules is essential. The most common rules the test will cover are:

## ie *and* ei

If you've never heard the old rhyme, "I before e except after c, or when sounding like a as in *neighbor* or *weigh*," be sure to learn it now—it works. Another way to think about *ie* vs. *ei* is to remember that you use *ie* to make a long e sound and *ei* to make a long a sound. Words with the long e sound include: *wield*, *fierce*, and *cashier*. Words with the long a sound include: *eight*, *vein*, and *deign*.

**3.** Choose the correctly spelled word.
  **a.** yeild
  **b.** mischeivous
  **c.** achieve
  **d.** percieve

If you remember the rhyme and the long a/long e rule above, it's easy to see the correct answer is choice **c**, *achieve*.

But beware! There are some words that are exceptions to this rule. Memorize the following words so you'll recognize them if they come up on the exam:

| | | |
|---|---|---|
| *friend* | *piety* | *fiery* |
| *quiet* | *notoriety* | *society* |
| *science* | *ancient* | *deficient* |
| *conscience* | *either* | *seize* |
| *weird* | *sheik* | *seizure* |
| *leisure* | *height* | *sleight* |
| *stein* | *seismology* | *heifer* |
| *their* | *foreign* | *forfeit* |
| *neither* | *protein* | *Fahrenheit* |
| *Codeine* | | |

## ia *and* ai

Use *ai* when the vowel combination makes the sound "uh," like the word *villain*. Use *ia* when each vowel is pronounced separately, like the word *median*.

**4.** Which of the following words is misspelled?
  **a.** guardain
  **b.** Britain
  **c.** controversial
  **d.** There is no misspelled word.

Choice **a** is spelled incorrectly. In the word *guardian*, the *i* and *a* are pronounced separately—*guard-I-an*. Therefore, *ia* should be used.

## Other Two-Vowel Combinations

Another grade-school rhyme will help you here: "When two vowels go walking, the first one does the talking." This holds true *most* of the time. Let's break down the rhyme to fully understand it. "When two vowels go walking" refers to a two-vowel combination in a word. For example, abst*ai*n, ch*ea*p, and f*oe*. "The first one does the talking" means that in the two-vowel combinations, only the first vowel is pronounced, and the second one is silent. In the case of our examples, you hear the long *a* in *abstain*, but not the *i*. In *cheap*, you hear the long *e* but not the *a*. Similarly, in *foe*, you hear the long *o* but not the *e*.

Here are some more examples of words that follow the two-vowels rule:

| | |
|---|---|
| *plead* | *float* |
| *woe* | *repeat* |
| *boat* | *gear* |
| *treat* | *suit* |
| *steal* | *read* |
| *chaise* | *bead* |
| *moat* | *heat* |

**5.** Choose the correctly spelled word.
   **a.** nuisance
   **b.** niusance
   **c.** nuicanse
   **d.** niucanse

The correct answer is choice **a**, *nuisance*. Say this word out loud. It sounds like *new-sance*, right? You hear the long *u*, but not the *i*, The first vowel does the talking here, so the correct combination must be *ui*.

## When to Drop the Final e

Drop the final *e* before adding any ending that begins with a vowel, such as *-ed*, *-ing*, and *-able*. Some examples are *biked* and *baking*. Keep the final *e* when adding endings that begin with consonants, such as *-ly* or *-ful*. Some examples are *carefully* and *gamely*.

There are a few exceptions to this rule. You keep the final *e* when adding an ending that begins with a vowel if:

- You need to protect pronunciation (show that a preceding vowel should be long, for example, as in *hoe + ing = hoeing*, not *hoing*).

You will drop the final *e* when adding an ending that begins with a consonant if:

- The *e* follows a *u* or *w*.

**6.** Choose the misspelled word.
   **a.** placed
   **b.** woeful
   **c.** truely
   **d.** There is no misspelled word.

The misspelled word is found in choice **c**, *truely*. The correct spelling is *truly*. This word is an example of an exception to the rule. Usually, when adding an ending that begins with a consonant (in this case, *-ly*), you keep the final *e*, unless it follows a *u* or *w*. In the word *true*, the letter *e* does indeed follow the letter *u*, so when adding *true + ly*, drop the final *e*: *truly*.

## When to Keep a Final y or Change It to i

When a final *y* follows a consonant, change the *y* to *i* when adding any ending except *-ing*. When the final *y* follows a vowel, it does not change. This rule applies to **all** endings, even plurals.

Change the *y* to an *i*:

| | |
|---|---|
| *early—earlier* | *fly—flier, flies* |
| *party—partied,* | *weary—wearied, wearies* |
| *partier, parties* | *pretty—prettier,* |
| *sorry—sorrier* | *prettiness* |
| *worry—worried,* | *try—tried, tries* |
| *worrier, worries* | |

Remember to keep the *y* when adding *-ing*:

| | |
|---|---|
| *fly—flying* | *party—partying* |
| *weary—wearying* | *worry—worrying* |
| *try—trying* | |

When the final *y* is preceded by a vowel, you do not change it to an *i*. For example:

| | |
|---|---|
| *enjoy—enjoyed,* | *employ—employed,* |
| *enjoying, enjoys* | *employing, employs* |
| *pray—prayed,* | *delay—delayed,* |
| *praying, prays* | *delaying, delays* |

**7.** Find the misspelled word.
   **a.** holiness
   **b.** queasyness
   **c.** spying
   **d.** There is no misspelled word.

The rule states that when a final *y* follows a consonant, you must change the *y* to *i* when adding any ending except *-ing*. The final *y* in *queasy* is preceded by a consonant (letter *s*), so when the ending *-ness* is added, the *y* should change to *i*: *queasiness*. Therefore, choice **b** is misspelled.

## Adding Endings to Words with a Final c

Add a *k* after a final *c* before any ending that begins with *e, i,* or *y*. All other endings do not require a *k*.

For example:

traffic + *-er* = trafficker
traffic + *-able* = trafficable

Other examples of when to add a *k* are:

*panic—panicking, panicked, panicky*
*mimic—mimicking, mimicked, mimicker*
*picnic—picnicking, picnicked, picnicker*

**8.** Choose the correctly spelled word.
   **a.** trafficer
   **b.** panicy
   **c.** historical
   **d.** havoced

Only choice **c**, *historical*, is spelled correctly. Remember, a *k* is required after a final *c* when an ending that begins with *e, i,* or *y* is added. So the other choices should be *trafficker*, *panicky*, and *havocked*.

One of the difficulties of spelling in English is creating plurals. Unfortunately, you can't always simply add the letter *-s* to the end of the word to signal more than one.

## When to Use -s or -es to Form Plurals

There are two simple rules that govern most plurals.

1. Most nouns add *-s* to make plurals.
2. If a noun ends in a sibilant sound (*s, ss, z, ch, x, sh*), add *-es*.

The following are some examples of plurals:

| | | |
|---|---|---|
| *cars* | *faxes* | *dresses* |
| *computers* | *indexes* | *churches* |
| *books* | *lunches* | *guesses* |
| *skills* | *dishes* | *buzzes* |

## Exceptions

Remember from the last lesson that when a word ends in a *y* preceded by a consonant, the *y* changes to *i* when you add *-es*.

| SINGULAR | PLURAL |
|---|---|
| fly | flies |
| rally | rallies |

## Plurals for Words That End in *o*

If a final *o* follows another vowel, you need to add only an *-s*.

Here are some examples:

| | |
|---|---|
| *patios* | *radios* |
| *studios* | *videos* |

When the final *o* follows a consonant rather than a vowel, there is no rule to guide you in choosing *-s* or *-es*. You just have to learn the individual words.

The following words form a plural with *-s* alone:

| | |
|---|---|
| *albinos* | *pianos* |
| *altos* | *silos* |
| *banjos* | *sopranos* |
| *logs* | *broncos* |

The following words take *-es*:

| | |
|---|---|
| *heroes* | *tomatoes* |
| *potatoes* | *vetoes* |

When in doubt about whether to add *-s* or *-es* to a word, look it up in the dictionary.

## Plurals That Don't Use -s or -es

There are many words that don't use *-s* or *-es* to form plurals. These are usually words that still observe the rules of the languages from which they were adopted. For instance, in Latin words, *-um* becomes *-a*, *-us* becomes *-i*, and in Greek words, *-sis* becomes *-ses*. Most of these plurals are part of your reading, speaking, and listening vocabularies. A good way to remember these plurals is by saying the words aloud, because you may remember them more easily if you listen to the sound of the spelling.

| SINGULAR | PLURAL |
|---|---|
| child | children |
| deer | deer |
| goose | geese |
| man | men |
| mouse | mice |
| ox | oxen |
| woman | women |
| alumnus | alumni |
| curriculum | curricula |
| datum | data |
| fungus | fungi |
| medium | media |
| stratum | strata |
| analysis | analyses |
| axis | axes |
| basis | bases |
| oasis | oases |
| parenthesis | parentheses |
| thesis | theses |

**9.** Choose the correctly spelled word.
  **a.** pianoes
  **b.** tomatos
  **c.** deers
  **d.** spies

Only choice **d**, *spies*, is spelled correctly. The correct spelling of choices **a** and **b** is *pianos* and *tomatoes*. These words belong to the group of plurals that has to be learned individually. Choice **c** is an exception. It belongs to the group of plurals that do not use *-s/-es* endings. The plural form of *deer* is *deer*.

## Homonyms

Homonyms are words that sound the same but are spelled differently. Many of these words have just one change in the vowel or vowel combination. There's no rule about these words, so you'll simply have to memorize them.

Here are some examples of word pairs that can be troublesome. Often, the two words in a homophone pair are a different part of speech. Take a look at the following examples:

| | |
|---|---|
| *affect/effect* | *led/lead* |
| *altar/alter* | *minor/miner* |
| *bare/bear* | *passed/past* |
| *bloc/block* | *peal/peel* |
| *cite/site* | *piece/peace* |
| *cord/chord* | *sheer/shear* |
| *coarse/course* | *stationery/stationary* |
| *descent/dissent* | *weak/week* |
| *dual/duel* | *which/witch* |
| *heal/heel* | *write/right* |

Since the meanings of these homonyms are usually very different, context within a sentence is probably the best way to differentiate between these words.

### Examples in Context

He led a **dual** (*adjective*) life as a spy.
He fought a **duel** (*noun*) with his great enemy.

He had to **alter** (*verb*) his clothes after he lost weight.
The bride smiled as she walked toward the **altar** (*noun*).

## Prefixes

Generally, when you add a prefix to a root word, neither the root nor the prefix changes spelling:

*un-* + prepared = unprepared
*mal-* + nutrition = malnutrition
*sub-* + traction = subtraction
*mis-* + informed = misinformed

This rule applies even when the root word begins with the last letter of the prefix. Generally, you use both consonants, but let your eye be your guide. If it looks funny, it's probably not spelled correctly. The following are some examples of double consonants that are correct:

| | |
|---|---|
| *dissatisfied* | *irreverent* |
| *disservice* | *misspelled* |
| *illegible* | *misstep* |
| *irrational* | *unnatural* |

**10.** Choose the correctly spelled word.
  **a.** ilogical
  **b.** illogicall
  **c.** illogicle
  **d.** illogical

Only choice **d**, *illogical*, is spelled correctly. Remember that in the majority of cases, when you add a prefix to a root word (*il-* + logical), neither the root nor the prefix changes spelling, even when the root word begins with the last letter of the prefix.

## Practice Questions

Here are some practice spelling questions. The answers follow.

Choose the correctly spelled word in questions 11–15.

11. **a.** magically
    **b.** magickelly
    **c.** majicelly
    **d.** magicaly

12. **a.** beleif
    **b.** bilief
    **c.** belief
    **d.** beleaf

13. **a.** nieghbor
    **b.** neihbor
    **c.** niehbor
    **d.** neighbor

14. **a.** eficient
    **b.** eficeint
    **c.** efficient
    **d.** efficeint

15. **a.** collaborate
    **b.** colaborate
    **c.** collaborat
    **d.** colabarate

Find the misspelled word in questions 16–20.

16. **a.** women
    **b.** people
    **c.** babys
    **d.** There is no misspelled word.

17. **a.** radios
    **b.** leaves
    **c.** alumni
    **d.** There is no misspelled word.

18. **a.** anouncement
    **b.** advisement
    **c.** description
    **d.** There is no misspelled word.

19. **a.** omission
    **b.** aisle
    **c.** litrature
    **d.** There is no misspelled word.

20. **a.** oases
    **b.** tomatoes
    **c.** heroes
    **d.** gooses

### Answers to Practice Questions

11. **a.** magically
12. **c.** belief
13. **d.** neighbor
14. **c.** efficient
15. **a.** collaborate
16. **c.** The correct spelling is babies.
17. **d.** There is no misspelled word.
18. **a.** The correct spelling is announcement.
19. **c.** The correct spelling is literature.
20. **d.** The correct spelling is geese.

# Tips for Answering Verbal Ability Questions

- **Practice** using the sample questions in this chapter.
- **Read widely** to improve your general vocabulary and spelling.
- **Say the words** silently to yourself. If it sounds wrong, it probably is wrong.
- **Dissect the words** to find their roots, prefixes, and suffixes.
- **Learn the rules** of spelling and memorize words that are exceptions.

## Additional Resources

If you'd like to improve your verbal ability, your best resource is your public or college library. Any challenging reading will improve your vocabulary and spelling. The following are some LearningExpress books specifically about building those skills.

- *Vocabulary and Spelling Success in 20 Minutes a Day, 5th Edition*
- *501 Synonym and Antonym Questions*

# 5▶

# READING COMPREHENSION

## CHAPTER SUMMARY

Because reading is such a vital skill, many nursing school entrance exams include a reading comprehension section that tests your ability to understand what you read. The tips and exercises in this chapter will help you improve your comprehension of written passages so that you can increase your score in this area.

A s a nursing professional, you will do a lot of reading—memos, policies, and manuals, as well as medical and technical reports, charts, and procedures. Understanding written material is a key part of the job. Reading comprehension is also an essential skill for students of nursing programs—most likely, you will need to read and understand scientific and medical textbooks as part of the training for your career. As a result, nursing school entrance exams attempt to measure how well applicants understand what they read.

The reading comprehension section of your test will look much like reading comprehension segments you have encountered before on other standardized tests. You read a passage one to five paragraphs long, usually scientific in nature, and then answer one or more questions based on what you have read. You do not need to have any prior or specific knowledge to answer the questions—you need *only* the information presented in the passage. You will be asked to interpret passages, identify the author's purpose, look at how ideas are organized and presented, and draw conclusions based on the information in the passage.

# Types of Reading Comprehension Questions

As a test taker, you have two advantages when answering multiple-choice questions about reading passages:

1. Before you start reading, you don't have to know anything about the topic of the passage.
2. You're being tested *only* on the information the passage provides.

The disadvantage is that you have to know where and how to find that information quickly in an unfamiliar text. This makes it easy to fall for one of the wrong answer choices, especially since they are designed to mislead you.

The best way to do well on this passage/question format is to be very familiar with the kinds of questions that are typically asked on the test. Questions most frequently ask you to:

- Identify a specific **fact or detail** in the passage.
- Note the **main idea** of the passage.
- Make an **inference** based on the passage.
- Define a **vocabulary** word from the passage.

**Facts and details** are the specific pieces of information that support the passage's **main idea**. The main idea is the thought, opinion, or attitude that governs the whole passage. Generally speaking, facts and details are indisputable—things that don't need to be proven, like statistics (18 million people) or descriptions (a green overcoat). Let's say, for example, you read a sentence that says, "After the department's reorganization, workers were 50% more productive." A sentence like this, which gives you the **fact** that 50% of workers were more productive, might support a **main idea** that says, "Every department should be reorganized." Notice that this main idea is not something indisputable; it is an opinion. The writer thinks all departments should be reorganized, and because this

is his opinion (and not everyone shares it), he needs to support his opinion with facts and details.

An **inference** is a conclusion that can be drawn based on facts or evidence. For example, you can infer based on the fact that workers became 50% more productive after the reorganization, which is a dramatic change, that prior to the reorganization, the department had not been efficiently organized. The fact sentence, "After the department's reorganization, workers were 50% more productive," also implies that the reorganization of the department was the reason workers became more productive. There may, of course, have been other reasons, but we can infer only one from this sentence.

As you might expect, **vocabulary** questions ask you to determine the meanings of particular words. If you have read carefully, you can determine the meaning of a word from its context—that is, how the word is used in the sentence or paragraph.

Because most of the texts you will read as a nursing student and professional are scientific in nature, you are most likely to find fact or detail and vocabulary questions on your entrance exam. However, because all four types of questions are important to reading comprehension (because not all scientific texts are objective, and analysis and interpretation are important parts of the scientific process), you will find main idea and inference questions on the tests as well.

The following is a sample test passage, followed by four questions. Read the passage carefully, and then answer the questions based on your reading of the text by circling your choice. Note under your answer which type of question has been asked (fact or detail, main idea, inference, or vocabulary). Correct answers appear immediately after the questions.

## Practice Passage 1: Using the Four Question Types

The immune system, which protects the body from infections, diseases, and other injuries, is composed of the lymphatic system and the skin. Lymph nodes, which measure about 1 to

25 centimeters across, and small vessels called lymphatics compose the lymphatic system. The nodes are located in the groin, armpits, throat, and trunk, and are connected by the lymphatics. The nodes work with the body's immune system to fight off infectious agents, like bacteria and fungus. When infected, the lymph nodes are often swollen and sensitive. The skin, the largest organ of the human body, is also considered part of the immune system. Hundreds of small nerves in the skin send messages to the brain to communicate pressure, pain, and other sensations. The skin encloses the organs to prevent injuries and forms a protective barrier that repels dirt and water and stops the entry of most harmful chemicals. Sweat glands in the skin help regulate the body's temperature, and other glands release oils that can kill or impede the growth of certain bacteria. Hair follicles in the skin also provide protection, especially of the skull and groin.

1. Lymph nodes are connected by
   a. blood vessels.
   b. smaller nodes.
   c. nerves.
   d. small vessels.
   Question type: _____

2. According to the passage, pain in the lymph nodes most likely indicates that the
   a. skin is dirty or saturated with water.
   b. nodes are battling an infection.
   c. brain is not responding properly to infection.
   d. lymphatics are not properly connected to the nodes.
   Question type: _____

3. Which of the following best expresses the main idea of the passage?
   a. The immune system is very sensitive and registers minute sensations.
   b. The skin and its glands are responsible for preventing most infections.
   c. The lymphatic system and the skin work together to protect the body from infection.
   d. Communication between the lymphatic system and the brain is essential in preventing and fighting infection.
   Question type: _____

4. As it is used in this passage, the word *compose* most nearly means
   a. create, construct.
   b. arrange, put in order.
   c. control, pull together.
   d. form, constitute.
   Question type: _____

## Answers and Explanations for Practice Passage 1

Don't just look at the right answers and move on. The explanations are the most important part, so read them carefully. Use these explanations to help you understand how to tackle each kind of question the next time you come across it.

1. **d.** Question type: fact or detail. The third sentence of the passage says that the nodes *are connected by the lymphatics*, which are defined in the second sentence as *small vessels*. You may know that nerves and blood vessels make a web of connections in our bodies, but the passage specifically states that lymphatics—*small* vessels, not *blood* vessels (choice **a**)—connect the nodes.

**2. b.** Question type: inference. The passage says that when lymph nodes are infected, they are *often swollen and sensitive*. Thus, if nodes are painful, they are probably swollen and sensitive, and they are swollen and sensitive because they are fighting an infection. This is also the best answer because none of the other answers are clearly connected to pain in the lymph nodes. Dirty or saturated skin (choice **a**) may indeed result in infection, but that is not what the question is asking. Choices **c** and **d** describe malfunctions of the immune system, a subject that is not discussed in the passage.

**3. c.** Question type: main idea. The idea that the lymphatic system and the skin work together to protect the body from infection is the only answer that can serve as a "net" for the whole passage. The other three answers are limited to specific aspects of the immune system and, therefore, are too restrictive to be the *main* idea. For example, choice **b** refers only to the skin, so it does not encompass all of the ideas in the passage.

**4. d.** Question type: vocabulary. Although all of the answers can mean *compose* in certain circumstances, choice **d** is the only meaning that really works in the context of the passage, which says that the lymph nodes and the lymphatics "*compose* the lymphatic system." The passage makes it clear that the lymph nodes and the lymphatics are the two parts of the lymphatic system. Thus, they *form* or *constitute* the lymphatic system. They don't create it, arrange it, or control it; they are it.

# Detail and Main Idea Questions

Detail or fact questions and main idea questions both ask you for information that is right there in the passage. All you have to do is find it.

## Detail or Fact Questions

In detail or fact questions, you have to identify a specific item of information from the text. This is usually the simplest kind of question. You just have to be able to separate important information from less important information. However, the choices may often be very similar, so you must be careful not to get confused.

Be sure you read the passage and questions carefully. In fact, it is usually a good idea to read the questions first, *before* you even read the passage, so you will know what details to look out for.

## Main Idea Questions

The main idea of a passage, like that of a paragraph or a book, is what it is *mostly* about. The main idea is like an umbrella that covers all of the ideas and details in the passage, so it is usually something general, not specific. For example, in Practice Passage 1, question 3 asked about the main idea, and the correct answer was the choice that said the skin and the lymphatic system work together to prevent infection. This is the best answer because it is the only one that includes both the skin and the lymphatic system, both of which are discussed in the passage.

Sometimes, the main idea is stated clearly, often in the first or last sentence of the passage. The main idea is expressed in the first sentence of Practice Passage 1, for example. The sentence that expresses the main idea is often referred to as the **topic sentence**.

At other times, the main idea is not stated in a topic sentence but is *implied* in the overall passage, and you will need to determine the main idea by inference. Because there may be a lot of information given in the passage, the trick is to understand what all that information adds up to—the gist of what the author wants you to know. Often, some of the wrong answers on main idea questions are specific facts or details from the passage. A good way to test yourself is to ask, "Can this answer serve as a *net* to hold the whole passage together?" If not, chances are you have chosen a fact or detail, not a main idea.

Practice answering main idea and detail questions by working on the questions that follow this passage. Check your answers against the key that appears immediately after the questions.

### Practice Passage 2: Detail and Main Idea Questions

Because the body responds differently to different allergens, allergic reactions have been divided into four categories. Type I allergies, the most common, are characterized by the production of immunoglobulin E (IgE), a type of antibody that the immune system releases when it thinks a substance is a threat to the body. IgE releases chemicals called mediators, like histamine, which cause blood vessels to dilate and release fluid into the surrounding tissues, usually resulting in a runny nose and sneezing. Type I allergies include allergic asthma and hay fever, as well as reactions to insect stings and dust. Type II allergies, which are far more rare, are usually reactions to medications and can cause liver and kidney damage or anemia. The body sends immunoglobulin M (IgM) and immunoglobulin G (IgG) to the site to fight the infection. Type III allergies are usually caused by reactions to drugs like penicillin. The body releases IgM and IgG, but these allergens cause IgM and IgG to bind away from cell surfaces. This creates clumps of allergens and antibodies that get caught in the tissues and cause swelling, which can affect the kidneys, joints, and skin. Type IV allergies cause the release of mediators that create swelling as well as itchy rashes. These are usually skin reactions to irritants like poison ivy, soaps, cosmetics, and other contact allergens.

1. Which type(s) of allergic reactions result in swelling?
   a. Types I and III
   b. Types III and IV
   c. Type III only
   d. Types II and IV

2. IgE, IgG, and IgM can be classified as
   a. allergens.
   b. mediators.
   c. antibodies.
   d. medications.

3. Which of the following would be the best title for this passage?
   a. Preventing Allergic Reactions
   b. Determining the Causes of Allergies
   c. Allergens and the Human Body
   d. Four Types of Allergic Reactions

4. Which of the following best expresses the main idea of the passage?
   a. Allergies cause different responses in the body.
   b. People should avoid things that may cause allergic reactions.
   c. Type I allergies affect the most people.
   d. Mediators play an important role in allergic reactions.

### Answers and Explanations for Practice Passage 2

1. **b.** The passage says that both Type III and Type IV allergic reactions cause swelling. In Type III allergies, IgM and IgG *bind away from cell surfaces. This creates clumps of allergens and antibodies that . . . cause swelling.* Type IV allergies also *cause the release of mediators that create swelling as well as itchy rashes.*

**2. c.** The passage says that immunoglobulin E (IgE) is *a type of antibody that the immune system releases*. The Ig in IgE, IgG, and IgM stands for immunoglobulin; all three are different types of immunoglobulin and, therefore, different types of antibodies. The immunoglobulins then release the mediators, like histamine, so choice **b** is incorrect. Further, immunoglobulins are produced in response to allergens, so choice **a** cannot be correct. And the passage clearly indicates that immunoglobulins are produced by the body, so choice **d** is also incorrect.

**3. d.** Titles generally reflect the main idea of a passage and must therefore be general enough to cover everything in that passage. The passage does not discuss how to prevent allergic reactions, so choice **a** is not a good answer. The passage does discuss what causes allergic reactions, but that is only part of what the passage covers, and it does not discuss how to determine the specific causes of a reaction, so choice **b** is incorrect. Choice **c** is not right because the passage does not focus on allergens; in fact, specific allergens aren't even mentioned for Type II allergies. Finally, it is clear that choice **d** is the best answer because the first sentence in the passage is a topic sentence: *Because the body responds differently to different allergens, allergic reactions have been divided into four categories.* This indicates that the passage is primarily about the four types of allergic reactions and not about allergens.

**4. a.** This choice best expresses the main idea of the passage because it restates the topic sentence, which tells us that the body *responds differently* to different allergens. Choice **b** is not a good answer because the passage does not discuss ways to avoid allergic reactions, and although choices **c** and **d** are mentioned in the passage, they are too specific to encompass the whole passage. Remember, the

main idea should be general enough to include all of the ideas in the passage.

# Inference and Vocabulary Questions

Questions that ask you about the meaning of vocabulary words in the passage and those that ask what the passage *suggests* or *implies* (inference questions) are different from detail or main idea questions. In vocabulary and inference questions, you usually have to pull ideas that are not expressly stated in the passage, sometimes from more than one place in the passage.

## Inference Questions

Inference questions can be the most difficult to answer because they require you to draw meaning from the text when that meaning is implied rather than directly stated. Inferences are conclusions that we draw based on the clues the writer has given us. When you draw inferences, you have to be something of a detective, looking for clues such as word choice, tone, and specific details that suggest a certain conclusion, attitude, or point of view. You have to read between the lines in order to make a judgment about what an author is implying in the passage.

A good way to test whether you have drawn an acceptable inference is to ask, "What evidence do I have for this inference?" If you can't find any, you probably have the wrong answer. You need to be sure that your inference is logical and that it is based on something that is suggested or implied in the passage itself—*not* by what you or others might think. Like a good detective, you need to base your conclusions on evidence—facts, details, and other information—*not* on random hunches or guesses.

## Vocabulary Questions

There are generally two types of vocabulary questions. The first tests how carefully you have read a passage that may contain a number of new or technical terms and definitions. If you see that a passage has a number of unfamiliar terms, mark each term as it is defined.

This will make it easier for you to go back and find the right answer.

The second type of vocabulary question is designed to measure how well you can figure out the meaning of a word from its context. *Context* refers to how the word is used in the sentence—how it works with the words and ideas that surround it. If the context is clear enough, you should be able to substitute a nonsense word for the one being sought and still make the right choice because you could determine its meaning strictly from the sense of the sentence. For example, you should be able to determine the meaning of the following italicized nonsense word based on its context:

The speaker noted that it gave him great *terivinix* to announce the winner of the Outstanding Leadership Award.

In this sentence, *terivinix* most likely means
  a. pain.
  b. sympathy.
  c. pleasure.
  d. anxiety.

Clearly, the context of an award makes choice **c**, *pleasure*, the best answer. Awards don't usually bring pain, sympathy, or anxiety.

When confronted with an unfamiliar word, try substituting a nonsense word and see if the context gives you the clue. If you are familiar with prefixes, suffixes, and word roots, you can also use this knowledge to help you determine the meaning of an unfamiliar word.

More often, however, you will be asked about how familiar words or phrases are used in context. These questions can be very tricky because words often have more than one acceptable meaning. Your job is to figure out which meaning makes the most sense in the context of the sentence. For example, the word *manipulate* can mean either (**a**) *to handle or manage skillfully* or (**b**) *to arrange or influence cleverly or craftily*. The meaning of this word depends entirely upon the con-

text in which it is used, as you can see from the following sentences.

  **a.** The patient *manipulated* the wheelchair around the obstacles.
  **b.** The media's *manipulation* of the facts has a powerful effect on politics.

Sentence **a** uses the first definition of the word, while sentence **b** uses the second.

When you are confronted with this type of question, your best bet is to take each possible answer and substitute it for the word in question in the sentence. Whichever answer makes the most sense in the context of the sentence should be the correct answer.

The questions that follow this passage are strictly vocabulary and inference questions. Circle the answers to the questions, and then check your answers against the key that appears immediately after the questions.

## Practice Passage 3: Inference and Vocabulary Questions

The rise of science in the seventeenth century ushered in the modern world. Four men are primarily responsible for the discoveries that form the foundation of scientific and philosophical thought today: Copernicus, Kepler, Galileo, and Newton. Copernicus overthrew the geocentric notion of the universe which held that the earth—and therefore humanity—was at the center of the universe and showed that the planets revolve around the sun. Kepler, the first major astronomer to adopt Copernicus's heliocentric theory, discovered three laws of planetary motion that helped validate Copernicus's theory. Galileo revealed the role of acceleration in dynamics and established the law of falling bodies. Finally, Newton's studies of motion—made possible only by the work of the three scientists before him—led to his laws of motion and the universal law of gravitation: "Every body attracts every other body with a force directly proportional to the product of their masses and inversely proportional to the square of the distance between them." Much of modern science is based upon these theories.

1. As it is used in the passage, the word "adopt" most nearly means to
   a. take and use as one's own.
   b. approve or accept.
   c. make suitable for a new situation.
   d. take guardianship for.

2. From the passage, which of the following can be inferred about Copernicus's heliocentric theory?
   a. It supported the religious doctrine of the time.
   b. It was accepted only because of Kepler.
   c. It went against established ideas.
   d. It revealed the laws of planetary motion.

3. Information contained in the passage supports which of the following statements about the four scientists?
   a. Their scientific discoveries contributed to the philosophical and social changes of the seventeenth century.
   b. Of the four, Newton's theories have been most instrumental in modern science.
   c. Their primary goal was to refute the theory that Earth was the center of the universe.
   d. They recognized that their achievements were based on the achievements of those before them.

4. As it is used in the passage, the word *established* most nearly means
   a. instituted or ordained by law or agreement.
   b. set up permanently or brought into existence.
   c. settled in a place or position.
   d. introduced and secured acceptance of.

## Answers and Explanations for Practice Passage 3

1. **b.** Look at how *adopt* is used in the sentence: *Kepler, the first major astronomer to* adopt *Copernicus's heliocentric theory, discovered three laws of planetary motion that helped validate Copernicus's theory.* Because Kepler helped validate this theory, choice **a** can't be correct, and neither can choice **d**; the passage clearly indicates that it's Copernicus's theory, not Kepler's. Furthermore, there's no indication from the context that Kepler changed the theory to make it suitable for another situation, so choice **c** cannot be correct either.

2. **c.** We can infer that Copernicus's theory went against established ideas because the passage says that Copernicus *overthrew* the notion that humanity was at the center of the universe, suggesting that the geocentric theory was the accepted theory of the time and that Copernicus's idea was revolutionary. There is no suggestion in the passage that Copernicus's theory supported the religious doctrine of the time, so choice **a** cannot be correct. Furthermore, the passage says that Kepler's discovery *helped* validate Copernicus's theory, but this does not imply that it was accepted only because of Kepler (choice **b**). Finally, the laws of planetary motion were discovered by Kepler, not Copernicus, so choice **d** cannot be correct.

3. **a.** The passage discusses scientific discoveries that challenged and changed the way human beings saw themselves in the universe and how the motion of bodies on Earth and in the universe was understood. We can thus infer that these discoveries greatly altered ideas in both philosophy and, of course, science. Again, the word *overthrew* suggests upheaval, so choice **a** is the best answer. Choice **b** cannot be correct because the passage does not favor one scientist over the others; in fact, the passage tells us that Newton could not have

done his work without those who came before him. Furthermore, although these men did refute the theory that Earth was the center of the universe, there's no indication in this passage that that was what the men were out to prove, as in choice **c**. Finally, while the *writer* of the passage recognizes that the achievements of these men were based only on the achievements of the others before them, there is no indication here of what the men themselves thought, so choice **d** cannot be correct.

**4. d.** If you insert the possible answers into the sentence, it should be clear that choice **d** makes the most sense in context. Galileo *"established the law of falling bodies"*—a law of gravity and motion that naturally exists in the universe—so he could not have personally instituted these laws by law or agreement (choice **a**), set them up or brought them into existence (choice **b**), or settled them in a place or position (choice **c**). Instead, he introduced them to the public and secured acceptance of them by revealing the role of acceleration in dynamics (choice **d**).

## If English Is Not Your First Language

A major problem for non-native English speakers is difficulty in recognizing vocabulary and idioms (expressions like "chewing the fat") that assist comprehension. In order to read with good understanding, it's important to have an immediate grasp of as many words as possible in the text. Test takers need to be able to recognize vocabulary and idioms immediately so that the ideas those words and phrases express are clear.

## The Day-to-Day

Read newspapers, magazines, and other periodicals that deal with current events and matters of local, state, and national importance. Pay special attention to articles related to the career you want to pursue.

Be alert to new or unfamiliar vocabulary or terms that occur frequently in the popular press. Use a highlighter pen to mark new or unfamiliar words as you read. Keep a list of those words and their definitions. Review them for 15 minutes each day. Though at first you may find yourself looking up a lot of words, don't be frustrated—you will look up fewer and fewer words as your vocabulary expands.

## During the Test

When you are taking the test, make a picture in your mind of the situation being described in the passage. Ask yourself, "What did the writer want me to think about this subject?"

Locate and underline the topic sentence that carries the main idea of the passage. Remember that the topic sentence—if there is one—may not always be the first sentence. If there doesn't seem to be one, try to determine what idea summarizes the whole passage.

# Review: Putting It All Together

A good way to solidify what you have learned about reading comprehension questions is for *you* to write the questions. Here is a passage, followed by space for you to write your own questions. Write one question of each of the four types: fact or detail, main idea, inference, and vocabulary.

In the years since it was first proposed, the free radical theory of aging has gained wide acceptance. But hypotheses that attempt to explain exactly how free radicals are involved in the aging process are muddled by the lack of a clear definition of aging. Is aging a programmed stage of cellular differentiation, or is it the result of physiological processes impaired by free radical or other damage to cells? Despite the want of a clear definition, few people question that free radical damage to cell nucleic acids and lipids is an important factor in aging. A recent study shows that oxygen-free radicals cause approximately 10,000 DNA base modifications per cell per day. Perhaps the accumulation of unrepaired damage of this type accounts for the deterioration of physiological function. A new theory, however, indicates that free radicals also damage cell proteins, and that the accumulation of oxidized protein is an important factor in aging.

1. Detail question: _____
   _____
   a.
   b.
   c.
   d.

2. Main idea question: _____
   _____
   a.
   b.
   c.
   d.

3. Inference question: _____
   _____
   a.
   b.
   c.
   d.

4. Vocabulary question: _____
   _____
   a.
   b.
   c.
   d.

## Possible Questions

Here is one question of each type based on the previous passage. Your questions may be very different, but these will give you an idea of the kinds of questions that could be asked.

1. **Detail:** DNA modification can occur
   a. 10,000 times in the life of a cell.
   b. 1,000 times every second.
   c. thousands of times a day.
   d. once a day.

2. **Main idea:** Which sentence best sums up this passage?
   a. There are many theories, but no one knows how free radicals really affect aging.
   b. Free radicals are deadly.
   c. Scientists need a clearer definition of aging.
   d. Free radicals will lead scientists to the fountain of youth.

3. **Inference:** The passage suggests which of the following about the aging process?
   a. A clear definition of aging must be found in order to determine the cause of aging.
   b. DNA controls the aging process.
   c. Free radical damage to proteins increases with age.
   d. Aging is somehow related to free radical damage to cells.

4. **Vocabulary:** The phrase *want of* as used in the fourth sentence most nearly means
   a. desire for.
   b. lack of.
   c. requirement of.
   d. request for.

## Answers
1. c.
2. a.
3. d.
4. b.

## Additional Resources

Here are some other ways you can build the vocabulary and knowledge that will help you do well on reading comprehension questions.

- Practice asking the four sample question types about passages you read for information or pleasure.
- Using a computer search engine such as Google or Yahoo!, search out articles and forums related to the career you would like to pursue. Exchange views with others through online forums and message boards. All of these exchanges will help expand your knowledge of job-related material that may appear in a passage on the test.
- Begin now to build a broad knowledge of your potential profession. Get in the habit of reading articles in newspapers and magazines on job-related issues. Keep a clipping file of those articles. This will help keep you informed of trends in the profession and familiarize you with pertinent vocabulary.
- Consider reading or subscribing to professional journals. They are usually available for a reasonable annual fee. They may also be available in your library.
- If you need more help building your reading skills and taking reading comprehension tests, consider *Reading Comprehension Success in 20 Minutes a Day, 4th Edition*, published by LearningExpress.

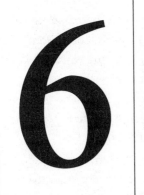

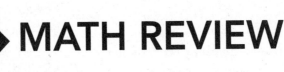

# MATH REVIEW

### *CHAPTER SUMMARY*

This chapter gives you important tips for dealing with math questions on your nursing school entrance exam and reviews some of the most commonly tested concepts. If you have forgotten most of your high school math or have math anxiety, this chapter is for you.

The math section of any nursing school entrance exam covers concepts that you probably studied in high school, with an emphasis on arithmetic, algebra, and geometry. Nurses need to be comfortable with numbers and be able to compute sums quickly. Both your ability to learn the scientific concepts that form the foundation of your work and your on-the-job performance will depend on your ability to reason logically using numbers.

For an entrance exam to the educational program of your choice, you need to know how to work not only with whole numbers, but also with fractions and decimals. You will have to be able to figure percentages, solve algebraic equations, and work with geometric figures. The tests assume that you know some basic terminology—words such as *sum* and *perimeter*—and some basic formulas, such as the area of a square or circle. Some admissions tests have a separate analytical reasoning section that measures your ability to recognize relationships between shapes or objects through visualization. This chapter will also prepare you for these types of questions.

Before you review those concepts, however, take a look at some strategies you can use to help you answer multiple-choice math questions.

# Math Strategies

- **Don't work in your head! Use your test book or scratch paper to take notes, draw pictures, and calculate.** Although you might think that you can solve math questions more quickly in your head, that's a good way to make mistakes. Write out each step.

- **Read a math question in *chunks* rather than straight through from beginning to end.** As you read each chunk, stop to think about what it means and make notes or draw a picture to represent that chunk.

- **When you get to the actual question in the middle of a word problem, circle it.** This will keep you more focused as you solve the problem.

- **Glance at the answer choices for clues.** If they're fractions, you should probably do your work in fractions; if they're decimals, you should probably work in decimals; etc.

- **Before you begin doing any math, make a plan of attack to help you solve the problem.**

- **If a question stumps you, try one of the backdoor approaches explained in the next section.** These are particularly useful for solving word problems.

- **When you get your answer, reread the circled question to make sure you've answered it.** This helps avoid the careless mistake of answering the wrong question.

- **Check your work after you get an answer.** Test takers get a false sense of security when they get an answer that matches one of the multiple-choice answers. Here are some good ways to check your work *if you have time*:
  - Ask yourself if your answer is reasonable and if it makes sense.
  - Plug your answer back into the problem to make sure the problem holds together.
  - Do the question a second time, but use a different method.

- **Approximate when appropriate.** For example:
  - $5.98 + $8.97 is a little less than $15. (Add: $6 + $9)
  - 0.9876 × 5.0342 is close to 5. (Multiply: 1 × 5)

- **Skip hard questions and come back to them later.** Mark them in your test book so you can find them quickly. Make sure you also skip the question on your answer sheet!

## Backdoor Approaches for Answering Questions

Remember those word problems you dreaded in high school? Many of them are actually easier to solve using backdoor approaches. The two techniques that follow are terrific ways to solve multiple-choice word problems. The first technique, *nice numbers*, is useful when there are unknowns (like $x$) in the text of the word problem, making the problem abstract. The second technique, *working backward*, presents a quick way to substitute numeric answer choices into the problem to see which one works.

### Nice Numbers

1. When a question contains unknowns, like $x$, plug "nice numbers" in for the unknowns. A nice number is one that is easy to calculate with and makes sense in the problem.

2. Read the question with the nice numbers in place. Then solve it.

3. If the answer choices are all numbers, the choice that matches your answer is the right one.

4. If the answer choices contain unknowns, substitute the **same** nice numbers into **all** of the answer choices. The choice that matches your answer is the right one. If more than one answer matches, do the problem again with different nice numbers. You'll only have to check the answer choices that have already matched.

**Example**

Judi went shopping with $p$ dollars in her pocket. If the price of shirts was $s$ shirts for $d$ dollars, what is the maximum number of shirts Judi could buy with the money in her pocket?

a. $psd$

b. $\frac{ps}{d}$

c. $\frac{pd}{s}$

d. $\frac{ds}{p}$

To solve this problem, let's try these nice numbers: $p = \$100$, $s = 2$ shirts; $d = \$25$. Now reread it with the numbers in place:

Judi went shopping with **$100** in her pocket. If the price of shirts was **2** shirts for **$25**, what is the maximum number of shirts Judi could buy with the money in her pocket?

Since 2 shirts cost $25, that means that 4 shirts cost $50, and 8 shirts cost $100. So our answer is 8. Let's substitute the nice numbers into all four answers:

a. $100 \times 2 \times 25 = 5{,}000$

b. $\frac{100 \times 2}{25} = 8$

c. $\frac{100 \times 25}{2} = 1{,}250$

d. $\frac{25 \times 2}{100} = \frac{1}{2}$

The answer is choice **b** because it is the only one that matches our answer of **8**.

## Working Backward

You can frequently solve a word problem by plugging the given answer choices into the text of the problem to see which one fits all the facts stated in the problem. The process is faster than you think because you'll

probably only have to substitute one or two answers to find the right one.

This approach works only when:

- All of the answer choices are numbers.
- You're asked to find a simple number—*not* a sum, product, difference, or ratio.

Here's what to do:

1. Look at all the answer choices and begin with the one in the middle of the range. For example, if the answers are 14, 8, 2, 20, and 25, begin by plugging 14 into the problem.
2. If your choice doesn't work, eliminate it. Determine if you need a bigger or smaller answer.
3. Plug in one of the remaining choices.
4. If none of the answers works, you may have made a careless error. Begin again or look for your mistake.

**Example**

Juan ate $\frac{1}{3}$ of the jelly beans. Maria then ate $\frac{3}{4}$ of the remaining jelly beans, which left 10 jelly beans. How many jelly beans were there to begin with?

a. 60

b. 80

c. 90

d. 120

e. 140

Starting with the middle answer, let's assume there were 90 jelly beans to begin with:

Since Juan ate $\frac{1}{3}$ of them, that means he ate 30 ($\frac{1}{3} \times 90 = 30$), leaving 60 of them ($90 - 30 = 60$). Maria then ate $\frac{3}{4}$ of the 60 jelly beans, or 45 of them ($\frac{3}{4} \times 60$ = 45). That leaves 15 jelly beans (60 − 45 = 15).

The problem states that there were **10** jelly beans left, and we wound up with **15** of them. That indicates that we started with too big a number. Thus, 90, 120, and 140 are all wrong! With only two choices left, let's use common sense to decide which one to try. The next lower answer is only a little smaller than 90 and may not be small enough. So, let's try 60:

Since Juan ate $\frac{1}{3}$ of them, that means he ate 20 ($\frac{1}{3}$ × 60 = 20), leaving 40 of them (60 − 20 = 40). Maria then ate $\frac{3}{4}$ of the 40 jelly beans, or 30 of them ($\frac{3}{4} \times 40$ = 30). That leaves 10 jelly beans (40 − 30 = 10).

Because this result of 10 remaining jelly beans agrees with the original problem, the right answer is choice **a**.

## GLOSSARY OF TERMS

| | |
|---|---|
| **Denominator** | the bottom number in a fraction. *Example:* 2 is the denominator in $\frac{1}{2}$. |
| **Difference** | the answer you get when you subtract. The difference of two numbers means to subtract one number from the other. |
| **Divisible by** | a number is divisible by a second number if that second number divides evenly into the original number. *Example:* 10 is divisible by 5 (10 ÷ 5 = 2, with no remainder). However, 10 is not divisible by 3. (See *multiple of*) |
| **Even Integer** | integers that are divisible by 2, like . . . −4, −2, 0, 2, 4, . . . (See *integer*) |
| **Integer** | numbers along the number line, like . . . −3, −2, −1, 0, 1, 2, 3, . . . Integers include the whole numbers and their opposites. (See *whole number*) |
| **Multiple of** | a number is a multiple of a second number if that second number can be multiplied by an integer to get the original number. *Example:* 10 is a multiple of 5 (10 = 5 × 2); however, 10 is not a multiple of 3. (See *divisible by*) |
| **Negative Number** | a number that is less than zero, like . . . −1, −18.6, $-\frac{3}{4}$, . . . |
| **Numerator** | the top part of a fraction. *Example:* 1 is the numerator of $\frac{1}{2}$. |
| **Odd Integer** | integers that aren't divisible by 2, like . . . −5, −3, −1, 1, 3, . . . |
| **Positive Number** | a number that is greater than zero, like . . . 2, 42, $\frac{1}{2}$, 4.63, . . . |
| **Prime Number** | an integer that is divisible only by 1 and itself, like . . . 2, 3, 5, 7, 11, . . . |
| **Product** | the answer you get when you multiply. The product of two numbers means the numbers are multiplied together. |
| **Quotient** | the answer you get when you divide. *Example:* 10 divided by 5 is 2; the quotient is 2. |
| **Real Number** | all the numbers you can think of, like . . . 17, −5, $\frac{1}{2}$, −23.6, 3.4329, 0, . . . Real numbers include integers, fractions, and decimals. (See *integer*) |
| **Remainder** | the number left over after division. *Example:* 11 divided by 2 is 5, with a remainder of 1. |
| **Sum** | the answer you get when you add. The sum of two numbers means the numbers are added together. |
| **Whole Number** | numbers you can count on your fingers, like . . . 1, 2, 3, . . . All whole numbers are positive. |

# Word Problems

Many of the math problems on tests are word problems. A word problem can include any kind of math, including simple arithmetic, fractions, decimals, percentages, and even algebra and geometry.

The hardest part of any word problem is translating English into math. When you read a problem, you can frequently translate it *word for word* from English statements into mathematical statements. At other times, however, a key word in the word problem only hints at the mathematical operation to be performed. Here are the translation rules:

**EQUALS keywords: is, are, has**

| English | Math |
|---|---|
| Bob **is** 18 years old. | $b = 18$ |
| There **are** 7 hats. | $h = 7$ |
| Judi **has** 5 cats. | $c = 5$ |

**ADDITION keywords: sum, more than, greater than, older than, total, altogether**

| English | Math |
|---|---|
| The **sum** of two numbers is 10. | $x + y = 10$ |
| Karen has $5 **more than** Sam. | $k = 5 + s$ |
| The base is 3 inches **greater than** the height. | $b = 3 + h$ |
| Judi is 2 years **older than** Tony. | $j = 2 + t$ |
| The **total** of three numbers is 25. | $a + b + c = 25$ |
| How much do Joan and Tom have **altogether**? | $j + t = ?$ |

**SUBTRACTION keywords: difference, fewer than, less than, younger than, remain, left over**

| English | Math |
|---|---|
| The **difference** between two numbers is 17. | $x - y = 17$ |
| Mike has 5 **fewer** cats **than** twice the number Jan has. | $m = 2j - 5$ |
| Jay is 2 years **younger than** Brett. | $j = b - 2$ |
| After Carol ate 3 apples, $r$ apples **remained**. | $r = a - 3$ |

**MULTIPLICATION keywords: of, product, times, each, at**

| English | Math |
|---|---|
| 20% **of** the samples | $0.20 \times s$ |
| Half **of** the bacteria | $\frac{1}{2} \times b$ |
| The **product** of two numbers is 12. | $a \times b = 12$ |

**DIVISION keyword: per**

| English | Math |
|---|---|
| 15 drops **per** teaspoon | $\frac{15 \text{ drops}}{\text{teaspoon}}$ |
| 22 miles **per** gallon | $\frac{22 \text{ miles}}{\text{gallon}}$ |

## DISTANCE FORMULA: DISTANCE = RATE × TIME

You know you will need to use the distance formula when you see movement words like: plane, train, boat, car, walk, run, climb, or swim.

- How far did the **plane** travel in 4 hours if it averaged 300 miles per hour?

  $D = 300 \times 4$

  $D = 1,200$ miles

- Ben **walked** 20 miles in 4 hours. What was his average speed?

  $20 = r \times 4$

  5 miles per hour $= r$

### Solving a Word Problem Using the Translation Table

Remember the problem at the beginning of this chapter about the jelly beans?

Juan ate $\frac{1}{3}$ of the jelly beans. Maria then ate $\frac{3}{4}$ of the remaining jelly beans, which left 10 jelly beans. How many jelly beans were there to begin with?

**a.** 60
**b.** 80
**c.** 90
**d.** 120

We solved it by *working backward*. Now let's solve it using our translation rules.

Assume Juan started with $J$ jelly beans. If Juan ate $\frac{1}{3}$ **of** them, that means there were $\frac{2}{3}$ of them left, or $\frac{2}{3} \times J$ jelly beans. Maria ate a fraction of the **remaining** jelly beans, which means we must **subtract** to find out how many are left. Maria ate $\frac{3}{4}$, leaving $\frac{1}{4}$ **of** the $\frac{2}{3} \times J$ jelly beans, or $\frac{1}{4} \times \frac{2}{3} \times J$ jelly beans. Multiplying out $\frac{1}{4} \times \frac{2}{3} \times J$ gives $\frac{1}{6}J$ as the number of jelly beans left. The problem states that there were 10 jelly beans left, meaning that we set $\frac{1}{6} \times J$ **equal** to 10:

$$\frac{1}{6} \times J = 10$$

Solving this equation for $J$ gives $J = 60$. Thus, the right answer is choice **a** (the same answer we got when we *worked backward*). As you can see, both methods—working backward and translating from English to math—work. You should use whichever method is more comfortable for you.

### Practice Word Problems

You will find word problems using fractions, decimals, and percentages as these specific sections come up later in this chapter. For now, practice using the translation table on problems that just require you to work with basic arithmetic. Answers are at the end of the chapter.

_____ **1.** Joan went shopping with $100 and returned home with only $18.42. How much money did she spend?

  **a.** $81.58
  **b.** $72.68
  **c.** $72.58
  **d.** $71.68
  **e.** $71.58

_____ **2.** Each of five physical therapists at the therapy center works six hours per day. Each therapist can work with three patients per hour. In total, how many patients can be seen each day at the center?

  **a.** 18
  **b.** 30
  **c.** 60
  **d.** 75
  **e.** 90

_____ **3.** The office secretary can type 80 words per minute on his word processor. How many minutes will it take him to type a report containing 760 words?

a. 8

b. $8\frac{1}{2}$

c. 9

d. $9\frac{1}{2}$

e. 10

_____ **4.** Mr. Wallace is writing a budget request to upgrade his personal computer system. He wants to purchase a cable modem, which will cost $100, two new software programs at $350 each, a color printer for $249, and an additional color cartridge for $25. What is the total amount Mr. Wallace should write on his budget request?

a. $724

b. $974

c. $1,049

d. $1,064

e. $1,074

# Fraction Review

Problems involving fractions may be straightforward calculation questions, or they may be word problems. Typically, they ask you to add, subtract, multiply, divide, or compare fractions.

## *Working with Fractions*

A fraction is a part of something.

### Example

Let's say that a pizza was cut into 8 equal slices and you ate 3 of them. The fraction $\frac{3}{8}$ tells you what part of the pizza you ate. The following pizza shows 3 of the 8 pieces (the ones you ate) shaded.

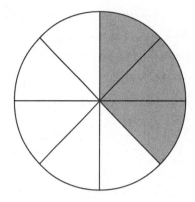

## Three Kinds of Fractions

**Proper fraction:** The top number (numerator) is less than the bottom number (denominator):

$$\frac{1}{2}, \frac{2}{3}, \frac{4}{9}, \frac{8}{13}$$

The value of a proper fraction is *less than 1.*

**Improper fraction:** The top number is greater than or equal to the bottom number:

$$\frac{3}{2}, \frac{5}{3}, \frac{14}{9}, \frac{12}{12}$$

The value of an improper fraction is *1 or more.*

**Mixed number:** A fraction written to the right of a whole number:

$$3\frac{1}{2}, 4\frac{2}{3}, 12\frac{3}{4}, 24\frac{3}{4}$$

The value of a mixed number is *more than 1.* It is the sum of the whole number plus the fraction.

## Changing Improper Fractions into Mixed or Whole Numbers

It's easier to add and subtract fractions that are mixed numbers rather than improper fractions. To change an improper fraction, say $\frac{13}{2}$, into a mixed number, follow these steps:

1. Divide the denominator (2) into the numerator (13) to get the whole number portion (6) of the mixed number:

$$\begin{array}{r} 6 \\ 2\overline{)13} \\ \underline{12} \\ 1 \end{array}$$

2. Write the remainder of the division (1) over the old denominator (2): $\quad 6\frac{1}{2}$

3. Check: Change the mixed number back into an improper fraction (see steps that follow).

## Changing Mixed Numbers into Improper Fractions

It's easier to multiply and divide fractions when you're working with improper fractions rather than mixed numbers. To change a mixed number, say $2\frac{3}{4}$, into an improper fraction, follow these steps:

1. Multiply the whole number (2) by the denominator (4):  $2 \times 4 = 8$
2. Add the result (8) to the numerator (3):  $8 + 3 = 11$
3. Put the total (11) over the denominator (4):  $\frac{11}{4}$
4. Check: Reverse the process by changing the improper fraction into a mixed number. If you get the number you started with, your answer is right.

## Reducing Fractions

Reducing a fraction means writing it in *lowest terms*, that is, with the smallest numbers possible. For instance, 50¢ is $\frac{50}{100}$ of a dollar, or $\frac{1}{2}$ of a dollar. Reducing a fraction does not change its value.

Follow these steps to reduce a fraction:

1. Find a whole number that divides *evenly* into both the numerator and the denominator.
2. Divide that number into the numerator and replace the numerator with the quotient (the answer you got when you divided).
3. Repeat the same division step for the denominator.
4. Repeat steps 1–3 until you can't find a number that divides evenly into both numbers of the fraction.

For example, let's reduce $\frac{8}{24}$. We could do it in two steps: $\frac{8 \div 4}{24 \div 4} = \frac{2}{6}$; then $\frac{2 \div 2}{6 \div 2} = \frac{1}{3}$. Or we could do it in a single step: $\frac{8 \div 8}{24 \div 8} = \frac{1}{3}$.

**Shortcut:** When the numerator and denominator both end in zeros, cross out the same number of zeros in both numbers to begin the reducing process. For example $\frac{300}{4,000}$ reduces to $\frac{3}{40}$ when you cross out two zeros in both numbers.

Whenever you do arithmetic with fractions, reduce your answer. On a multiple-choice test, don't panic if your answer isn't listed. Try to reduce it and then compare it to the choices.

Reduce these fractions to lowest terms:

_____ **5.** $\frac{3}{12}$

_____ **6.** $\frac{14}{35}$

_____ **7.** $\frac{27}{72}$

## Raising Fractions to Higher Terms

Sometimes before you can add and subtract fractions, you have to know how to raise a fraction to higher terms. This is actually the *opposite* of reducing a fraction.

Follow these steps to raise $\frac{2}{3}$ to 24ths:

1. Divide the old denominator (3) into the new one (24):  $3\overline{)24} = 8$
2. Multiply the answer (8) by the old numerator (2):  $2 \times 8 = 16$
3. Put the answer (16) over the new denominator (24):  $\frac{16}{24}$
4. Check: Reduce the new fraction to see if you get back the original one:  $\frac{16 \div 8}{24 \div 8} = \frac{2}{3}$

Raise these fractions to higher terms:

_____ **8.** $\frac{5}{12} = \frac{?}{24}$

_____ **9.** $\frac{2}{9} = \frac{?}{27}$

_____ **10.** $\frac{2}{5} = \frac{?}{500}$

## Adding Fractions

If the fractions have the same denominators, just add the numerators together and write the total over the denominator.

**Examples**

$\frac{2}{9} + \frac{4}{9} = \frac{2+4}{9} = \frac{6}{9}$  Reduce the sum: $\frac{2}{3}$.

$\frac{5}{8} + \frac{7}{8} = \frac{12}{8}$  Change the sum to a mixed number: $1\frac{4}{8}$; then reduce: $1\frac{1}{2}$.

There are a few extra steps to add mixed numbers with the same denominators, say $2\frac{3}{5} + 1\frac{4}{5}$:

**1.** Add the fractions: $\quad\quad\quad \frac{3}{5} + \frac{4}{5} = \frac{7}{5}$

**2.** Change the improper fraction into a mixed number: $\quad \frac{7}{5} = 1\frac{2}{5}$

**3.** Add the whole numbers: $\quad 2 + 1 = 3$

**4.** Add the results of steps 2 and 3: $\quad 1\frac{2}{5} + 3 = 4\frac{2}{5}$

### Finding the Least Common Denominator

If the fractions you want to add don't have the same denominator, you will have to raise some or all of the fractions to higher terms so that they do; this number is then called the **common denominator**. All of the original denominators divide evenly into the common denominator. If it is the smallest number that they all divide into evenly, it is called the **least common denominator (LCD)**.

Here are a few tips for finding the LCD, the smallest number into which all the denominators evenly divide:

- First, see if all the denominators divide evenly into the biggest one.
- Inspect multiples of the largest denominator until you find a number into which all the other ones evenly divide.
- When all else fails, multiply all the denominators together.

**Example:** $\frac{2}{3} + \frac{4}{5}$

**1.** Find the LCD. Multiply the denominators: $\quad\quad 3 \times 5 = 15$

**2.** Raise each fraction to 15ths:
$$\frac{2}{3} = \frac{10}{15}$$
$$+ \frac{4}{5} = \frac{12}{15}$$
$$\overline{\quad\quad \frac{22}{15}}$$

**3.** Add as usual:

Try these addition problems:

_____ **11.** $\frac{3}{4} + \frac{4}{6}$

_____ **12.** $\frac{7}{8} + \frac{2}{3} + \frac{3}{4}$

_____ **13.** $4\frac{1}{3} + 2\frac{3}{4} + \frac{1}{6}$

## Subtracting Fractions

If the fractions have the same denominators, just subtract the numerators and write the difference over the denominator.

**Example:** $\frac{4}{9} - \frac{3}{9} = \frac{4-3}{9} = \frac{1}{9}$

If the fractions you want to subtract don't have the same denominator, you will have to raise some or all of the fractions to higher terms so that they all have the same denominator, or LCD. If you forgot how to find the LCD, just reread the section on adding fractions with different denominators.

**Example:** $\frac{5}{6} - \frac{3}{4}$

1. Raise each fraction to 12ths because 12 is the LCD, the smallest number that both 6 and 4 divide into evenly:

$$\frac{5}{6} = \frac{10}{12}$$

$$-\frac{3}{4} = \frac{9}{12}$$

2. Subtract as usual:

$$\frac{1}{12}$$

Subtracting mixed numbers with the same denominator is similar to adding mixed numbers.

**Example:** $4\frac{3}{5} - 1\frac{2}{5}$

1. Subtract the fractions: $\frac{3}{5} - \frac{2}{5} = \frac{1}{5}$
2. Subtract the whole numbers: $4 - 1 = 3$
3. Add the results of steps 1 and 2: $\frac{1}{5} + 3 = 3\frac{1}{5}$

Sometimes, there is an extra "borrowing" step when you subtract mixed numbers with the same denominators, say $7\frac{3}{5} - 2\frac{4}{5}$:

1. You can't subtract the fractions the way they are because $\frac{4}{5}$ is bigger than $\frac{3}{5}$. So you borrow 1 from the 7, making it 6, and change that 1 to $\frac{5}{5}$ because 5 is the denominator: $7\frac{3}{5} = 6\frac{5}{5} + \frac{3}{5}$

2. Add the numbers from step 1: $6\frac{5}{5} + \frac{3}{5} = 6\frac{8}{5}$

3. Now you have a different version of the original problem: $6\frac{8}{5} - 2\frac{4}{5}$

4. Subtract the fractional parts of the two mixed numbers: $\frac{8}{5} - \frac{4}{5} = \frac{4}{5}$

5. Subtract the whole number parts of the two mixed numbers: $6 - 2 = 4$

6. Add the results of the last two steps together: $4 + \frac{4}{5} = 4\frac{4}{5}$

Try these subtraction problems:

_____ **14.** $\frac{4}{5} - \frac{2}{3}$

_____ **15.** $\frac{7}{8} - \frac{1}{4} - \frac{1}{2}$

_____ **16.** $4\frac{1}{3} - 2\frac{3}{4}$

Now, let's put what you have learned about adding and subtracting fractions to work in some real-life problems:

_____ **17.** Visiting nurse Alan drove $3\frac{1}{2}$ miles to the office to check his assignments for the day. Then he drove $4\frac{3}{4}$ miles to his first patient. When he left there, he drove 2 miles to his next patient. Then he drove $3\frac{2}{3}$ miles back to the office for a meeting. Finally, he drove $3\frac{1}{2}$ miles home. How many miles did he travel in total?
   a. $17\frac{5}{12}$
   b. $16\frac{5}{12}$
   c. $15\frac{7}{12}$
   d. $15\frac{5}{12}$
   e. $13\frac{11}{12}$

_____ **18.** Before leaving the hospital, the ambulance driver noted that the mileage gauge on Ambulance 2 registered $4{,}357\frac{4}{10}$ miles. When he arrived at the scene of the accident, the mileage gauge then registered $4{,}400\frac{1}{10}$ miles. How many miles did he drive from the hospital to the accident?

    **a.** $42\frac{3}{10}$

    **b.** $42\frac{7}{10}$

    **c.** $43\frac{7}{10}$

    **d.** $47\frac{2}{10}$

## Multiplying Fractions

Multiplying fractions is actually easier than adding them. All you do is multiply the numerators and then multiply the denominators. You do not need to find a common denominator.

**Examples:**

$\frac{2}{3} \times \frac{5}{7} = \frac{2 \times 5}{3 \times 7} = \frac{10}{21}$

$\frac{1}{2} \times \frac{3}{5} \times \frac{7}{4} = \frac{1 \times 3 \times 7}{2 \times 5 \times 4} = \frac{21}{40}$

Sometimes, you can *cancel* before multiplying. Canceling is a shortcut that makes the multiplication go faster because you're multiplying with smaller numbers. It's very similar to reducing: If there is a number that divides evenly into one numerator and its opposite denominator, do that division before multiplying. If you forget to cancel, you will still get the right answer, but you will have to reduce it.

**Example:** $\frac{5}{6} \times \frac{9}{20}$

**1.** Cancel the 6 and the 9 by dividing 3 into both of them: $6 \div 3 = 2$ and $9 \div 3 = 3$. Cross out the 6 and the 9 and replace with the reduced numbers: $\frac{5}{\overset{}{\underset{2}{6}}} \times \frac{\overset{3}{9}}{20}$

**2.** Cancel the 5 and the 20 by dividing 5 into both of them: $5 \div 5 = 1$ and $20 \div 5 = 4$. Cross out the 5 and the 20 and replace with the reduced numbers: $\frac{\overset{1}{5}}{\underset{2}{6}} \times \frac{\overset{3}{9}}{\underset{4}{20}}$

**3.** Multiply across the new numerators and the new denominators: $\frac{1 \times 3}{2 \times 4} = \frac{3}{8}$

Try these multiplication problems:

_____ **19.** $\frac{1}{5} \times \frac{2}{3}$

_____ **20.** $\frac{2}{3} \times \frac{4}{7} \times \frac{3}{5}$

_____ **21.** $\frac{3}{4} \times \frac{8}{9}$

To multiply a fraction by a whole number, first rewrite the whole number as a fraction with a denominator of 1.

**Example:** $5 \times \frac{2}{3} = \frac{5}{1} \times \frac{2}{3} = \frac{10}{3}$ (Optional: Convert $\frac{10}{3}$ to a mixed number: $3\frac{1}{3}$)

To multiply with mixed numbers, it's easier to change them to improper fractions before multiplying.

**Example:** $4\frac{2}{3} \times 5\frac{1}{2}$

**1.** Convert $4\frac{2}{3}$ to an improper fraction: $4\frac{2}{3} = \frac{4 \times 3 + 2}{3} = \frac{14}{3}$

**2.** Convert $5\frac{1}{2}$ to an improper fraction: $5\frac{1}{2} = \frac{5 \times 2 + 1}{2} = \frac{11}{2}$

**3.** Cancel and multiply the fractions: $\frac{\overset{7}{14}}{3} \times \frac{11}{\underset{1}{2}} = \frac{77}{3}$

**4.** Optional: Convert the improper fraction to a mixed number: $\frac{77}{3} = 25\frac{2}{3}$

Now, try these multiplication problems with mixed numbers and whole numbers:

_____ **22.** $4\frac{1}{3} \times \frac{2}{5}$

_____ **23.** $2\frac{1}{2} \times 6$

_____ **24.** $3\frac{3}{4} \times 4\frac{2}{5}$

Here are a few more real-life problems to test your skills:

_____ **25.** After driving $\frac{2}{3}$ of the 15 miles to work, Dr. Stone received an emergency call from the hospital. How many miles had he driven when he got the call?
   a. 5
   b. $7\frac{1}{2}$
   c. 10
   d. 12
   e. $15\frac{2}{3}$

_____ **26.** If Henry spent $\frac{3}{4}$ of a 40-hour week learning to use new laboratory equipment, how many hours did he spend in training?
   a. $7\frac{1}{2}$
   b. 10
   c. 20
   d. 25
   e. 30

_____ **27.** Technician Chin makes $14.00 an hour. When she works more than 8 hours a day, she gets overtime pay of $1\frac{1}{2}$ times her regular hourly wage for the extra hours. How much did she earn for working 11 hours in one day?
   a. $77
   b. $154
   c. $175
   d. $210
   e. $231

## Dividing Fractions

To divide one fraction by a second fraction, invert the second fraction (that is, flip the top and bottom numbers; this is called the *reciprocal*) and then multiply. That's all there is to it!

**Example:** $\frac{1}{2} \div \frac{3}{5}$

1. Invert the second fraction ($\frac{3}{5}$): $\qquad \frac{5}{3}$

2. Change the division sign ($\div$) to a multiplication sign ($\times$): $\qquad \frac{1}{2} \times \frac{5}{3}$

3. Multiply the first fraction by the new second fraction: $\qquad \frac{1}{2} \times \frac{5}{3} = \frac{1 \times 5}{2 \times 3} = \frac{5}{6}$

To divide a fraction by a whole number, first change the whole number to a fraction by putting it over 1. Then follow the division steps above.

**Example:** $\frac{3}{5} \div 2 = \frac{3}{5} \div \frac{2}{1} = \frac{3}{5} \times \frac{1}{2} = \frac{3 \times 1}{5 \times 2} = \frac{3}{10}$

When the division problem has a mixed number, convert it to an improper fraction and then divide as usual.

**Example:** $2\frac{3}{4} \div \frac{1}{6}$

1. Convert $2\frac{3}{4}$ to an improper fraction: $\qquad 2\frac{3}{4} = \frac{2 \times 4 + 3}{4} = \frac{11}{4}$

2. Rewrite the division problem and change $\div$ to $\times$: $\qquad \frac{11}{4} \div \frac{1}{6} = \frac{11}{4} \times \frac{6}{1}$

3. Cancel and multiply: $\qquad \frac{11}{\underset{2}{4}} \times \frac{\overset{3}{6}}{1} = \frac{11 \times 3}{2 \times 1} = \frac{33}{2}$

Here are a few division problems to try:

_____ **28.** $\frac{1}{3} \div \frac{2}{3}$

_____ **29.** $2\frac{3}{4} \div \frac{1}{2}$

_____ **30.** $\frac{3}{5} \div 3$

_____ **31.** $3\frac{3}{4} \div 2\frac{1}{3}$

Let's wrap this up with some real-life problems.

_____ **32.** If Dr. McCarthy's four assistants evenly divided $6\frac{1}{2}$ pounds of candy among themselves, how many pounds of candy did each assistant get?
   **a.** $\frac{8}{13}$
   **b.** $1\frac{5}{8}$
   **c.** $1\frac{1}{2}$
   **d.** $1\frac{5}{13}$
   **e.** 4

_____ **33.** How many $2\frac{1}{2}$-pound chunks of cheese can be cut from a single 20-pound piece of cheese?
   **a.** 2
   **b.** 4
   **c.** 6
   **d.** 8
   **e.** 10

_____ **34.** Ms. Goldbaum earned $36.75 for working $3\frac{1}{2}$ hours. What was her hourly wage?
   **a.** $10.00
   **b.** $10.50
   **c.** $10.75
   **d.** $12.00
   **e.** $12.25

# Decimals

## What Is a Decimal?

A decimal is another way to represent a fraction. You use decimals every day when you deal with money—$10.35 is a decimal that represents 10 dollars and 35 cents. The decimal point separates the dollars from the cents. Because there are 100 cents in one dollar, 1 cent is $\frac{1}{100}$ of a dollar, or $0.01.

Each decimal digit to the right of the decimal point has a name:

> **Examples:** $0.1 = 1$ tenth $= \frac{1}{10}$
> $0.02 = 2$ hundredths $= \frac{2}{100}$
> $0.003 = 3$ thousandths $= \frac{3}{1,000}$
> $0.0004 = 4$ ten-thousandths $= \frac{4}{10,000}$

When you add zeros after the rightmost decimal place, you don't change the value of the decimal. For example, 6.17 is the same as all of the following:

6.170
6.1700
6.17000000000000000

If there are digits on both sides of the decimal point (like 10.35), the number is called a **mixed decimal**. If there are digits only to the right of the decimal point (like 0.53), the number is called a **decimal**. A whole number (like 15) is understood to have a decimal point at its right (15.). Thus, 15 is the same as 15.0, 15.00, 15.000, and so on.

## Changing Fractions to Decimals

To change a fraction to a decimal, divide the denominator into the numerator after you put a decimal point and a few zeros to the right of the numerator. When you divide, bring the decimal point into your answer.

**Example:** Change $\frac{3}{4}$ to a decimal.

1. Add a decimal point and 2 zeros to the numerator (3):  3.00
2. Divide the denominator (4) into 3.00:

$$\begin{array}{r} 0.75 \\ 4)\overline{3.00} \\ \underline{-2\ 8} \\ 20 \\ \underline{-20} \\ 0 \end{array}$$

3. The quotient (result of the division) is the answer:  0.75

Some fractions may require you to add many decimal zeros in order for the division to come out evenly. In fact, when you convert a fraction like $\frac{2}{3}$ to a decimal, you can keep adding decimal zeros to the numerator forever because the division will never come out evenly. As you divide 3 into 2, you will keep getting 6s:

$$2 \div 3 = 0.6666666666 \text{ etc.}$$

This is called a *repeating decimal,* and it can be written as $0.\overline{666}$ or as $0.66\frac{2}{3}$. You can approximate it as 0.67, 0.667, 0.6667, and so on. When a bar is written above a digit or digits in a repeating decimal, those numbers are understood to repeat (for example, $0.\overline{42}$ means $0.42424242\dots$).

## Changing Decimals to Fractions

To change a decimal to a fraction, write the digits of the decimal as the numerator and write the decimal's name (the name of the farthest right non-zero digit after the decimal point) as the denominator. Then reduce the fraction, if possible.

**Example:** .018

1. Write 18 as the numerator:  $\frac{18}{}$
2. Three places to the right of the decimal means *thousandths,* so write 1,000 as the denominator:  $\frac{18}{1,000}$
3. Reduce by dividing 2 into the numerator and denominator:  $\frac{18 \div 2}{1,000 \div 2} = \frac{9}{500}$

Change these decimals or mixed decimals to fractions:

_____ **35.** 0.005

_____ **36.** 3.48

_____ **37.** 123.456

## Comparing Decimals

Because decimals are easier to compare when they have the same number of digits after the decimal point, you can tack zeros onto the end of the shorter decimals without affecting the number value. Then all you have to do is compare the numbers as if the decimal points weren't there:

**Example:** Compare 0.08 and 0.1.

1. Tack one zero at the end of 0.1:  0.10
2. To compare 0.10 to 0.08, just compare 10 to 8.
3. Since 10 is larger than 8, 0.1 is larger than 0.08.

## Adding and Subtracting Decimals

To add or subtract decimals, line them up so their decimal points are aligned. You may want to tack on zeros at the end of shorter decimals so that you can keep all your digits lined up evenly. Remember, if a number doesn't have a decimal point, then put one at the right end of the number and add zeros after it.

**Example:** $1.23 + 57 + 0.038$

1. Line up the numbers like this:

$$\begin{array}{r} 1.230 \\ 57.000 \\ +\ .038 \\ \hline \end{array}$$

2. Add:  58.268

**Example:** $1.23 - 0.038$

1. Line up the numbers like this:  $\begin{aligned}1.230\\-.038\end{aligned}$

2. Subtract:  $1.192$

Try these addition and subtraction problems:

_____ **38.** $0.905 + 0.02 + 3.075$

_____ **39.** $0.005 + 8 + 0.3$

_____ **40.** $3.48 - 2.573$

_____ **41.** $123.456 - 122$

_____ **42.** James drove 3.7 miles to his physical therapist's office. He then walked 1.6 miles on the treadmill to strengthen his legs. He got back into the car, drove 2.75 miles to his radiology appointment, and then drove 2 miles back home. How many miles did he drive in total?
   a. 8.05
   b. 8.45
   c. 8.8
   d. 10
   e. 10.05

_____ **43.** The average number of emergency room visits at City Hospital fell from 486.4 per week to 402.5 per week. By how many emergency room visits per week did the average fall?
   a. 73.9
   b. 83
   c. 83.1
   d. 83.9
   e. 84.9

## Multiplying Decimals

To multiply decimals, ignore the decimal points and just multiply the numbers. Then count the total number of decimal digits (the digits to the *right* of the decimal point) in all of the numbers you are multiplying. Count off that total number of digits in your answer beginning at the right side and put the decimal point to the *left* of those digits.

**Example:** $215.7 \times 2.4$

1. Multiply 2157 times 24:
$$\begin{aligned}2157\\\times 24\\\hline 8628\\+43140\\\hline 51768\end{aligned}$$

2. Because there are a total of two decimal digits in 215.7 and 2.4, count off two places from the right in 51768, placing the decimal point to the *left* of the last two digits:  $517.68$

If your answer doesn't have enough digits, tack zeros on to the left of the answer.

**Example:** $0.03 \times 0.006$

1. Multiply 3 times 6:  $3 \times 6 = 18$
2. You need 5 decimal digits in your answer, so tack on 3 zeros:  $00018$
3. Put the decimal point at the front of the number (which is 5 digits in from the right):  $0.00018$

You can practice multiplying decimals with these:

_____ **44.** $0.05 \times 0.6$

_____ **45.** $0.053 \times 6.4$

_____ **46.** $38.1 \times 0.0184$

**47.** Joe earns $14.50 per hour as an occupational therapist. Last week, he worked 37.5 hours. How much money did he earn that week?
  **a.** $518.00
  **b.** $518.50
  **c.** $525.00
  **d.** $536.50
  **e.** $543.75

**48.** Nuts cost $3.50 per pound. Approximately how much will 4.25 pounds of nuts cost?
  **a.** $12.25
  **b.** $12.50
  **c.** $12.88
  **d.** $14.50
  **e.** $14.88

## Dividing Decimals

To divide a decimal by a whole number, set up the division (8)$\overline{.256}$) and immediately bring the decimal point straight up into the answer (8)$\overline{.256}$). Then divide as you would normally divide whole numbers:

**Example:**
$$
\begin{array}{r}
.032 \\
8)\overline{.256} \\
-\underline{0} \\
25 \\
-\underline{24} \\
16 \\
-\underline{16} \\
0
\end{array}
$$

To divide any number by a decimal, there is an extra step to perform before you can divide. Move the decimal point to the very right of the number you're dividing by, counting the number of places you're moving it. Then move the decimal point the *same* number of places to the right in the number you're dividing into. In other words, first change the problem to one in which you're dividing by a whole number.

**Example:** .06)$\overline{1.218}$

1. Because there are 2 decimal digits in 0.06, move the decimal point 2 places to the right in both numbers and move the decimal point straight up into the answer:

.06)$\overline{1.21\,8}$

2. Divide using the new numbers:
$$
\begin{array}{r}
20.3 \\
6)\overline{121.8} \\
-\underline{12} \\
01 \\
-\underline{00} \\
18 \\
-\underline{18} \\
0
\end{array}
$$

Under certain conditions, you have to tack on zeros to the right of the last decimal digit in the number you are dividing into:

- If there aren't enough digits for you to move the decimal point to the right
- If you are dividing a whole number by a decimal. Then you will have to tack on the decimal point as well as some zeros.
- If the answer doesn't come out evenly when you do the division

Try your skills on these division problems:

**49.** 7)$\overline{9.8}$

**50.** 0.0004)$\overline{.0512}$

**51.** 0.05)$\overline{28.6}$

**52.** 0.14)$\overline{196}$

_____ **53.** If James Worthington drove the mobile blood bank unit 92.4 miles in 2.1 hours, what was his average speed in miles per hour?

   **a.** 41
   **b.** 44
   **c.** 90.3
   **d.** 94.5
   **e.** 194.04

_____ **54.** Mary Sanders walked a total of 18.6 miles in 4 days. On average, how many miles did she walk each day?

   **a.** 4.15
   **b.** 4.60
   **c.** 4.65
   **d.** 22.60
   **e.** 74.40

# Percents

## What Is a Percent?

A percent is another way to represent a fraction or a part of something. When you write percents as fractions, the denominator is always 100. For example, 17% is the same as $\frac{17}{100}$. Literally, the word _percent_ means _per 100 parts_. The root _cent_ means 100: A _century_ is 100 years; there are 100 _cents_ in a dollar, etc. Thus, 17% means 17 parts out of 100. Because fractions can also be expressed as decimals, 17% is also equivalent to 0.17, which is 17 hundredths.

You come into contact with percents every day. Sales tax, interest, and discounts are just a few common examples.

If you're shaky on fractions, you may want to review the fraction section before reading further.

## Changing a Decimal to a Percent and Vice Versa

To change a decimal to a percent, move the decimal point two places to the right and tack on a percent sign (%) at the end. If the decimal point moves to the very right of the number, you don't have to write the decimal point. If there aren't enough places to move the decimal point, add zeros on the right before moving the decimal point.

To change a percent to a decimal, drop off the percent sign and move the decimal point two places to the left. If there aren't enough places to move the decimal point, add zeros on the left before moving the decimal point.

Try changing these decimals to percents:

_____ **55.** 0.45

_____ **56.** 0.008

_____ **57.** $0.16\frac{2}{3}$

Now, change these percents to decimals:

_____ **58.** 12%

_____ **59.** $87\frac{1}{2}\%$

_____ **60.** 250%

| CONVERSION TABLE | | |
| --- | --- | --- |
| DECIMAL | % | FRACTION |
| 0.25 | 25% | $\frac{1}{4}$ |
| 0.50 | 50% | $\frac{1}{2}$ |
| 0.75 | 75% | $\frac{3}{4}$ |
| 0.10 | 10% | $\frac{1}{10}$ |
| 0.20 | 20% | $\frac{1}{5}$ |
| 0.40 | 40% | $\frac{2}{5}$ |
| 0.60 | 60% | $\frac{3}{5}$ |
| 0.80 | 80% | $\frac{4}{5}$ |
| $0.33\overline{3}$ | $33\frac{1}{3}\%$ | $\frac{1}{3}$ |
| $0.66\overline{6}$ | $66\frac{2}{3}\%$ | $\frac{2}{3}$ |

## Changing a Fraction to a Percent and Vice Versa

To change a fraction to a percent, there are two techniques.

Technique 1: Multiply the fraction by 100%.
Multiply $\frac{1}{4}$ by 100%:

$$\frac{1}{\overset{1}{\underset{}{4}}} \times \frac{\overset{25}{\cancel{100}}\%}{1} = 25\%$$

Technique 2: Divide the fraction's denominator into the numerator, then move the decimal point two places to the right and tack on a percent sign (%).
Divide 4 into 1 and move the decimal point two places to the right:

$$4\overline{)1.00} \quad .25$$

$$0.25 = 25\%$$

To change a percent to a fraction, remove the percent sign and write the number over 100. Then reduce if possible.

**Example:** Change 4% to a fraction.

1. Remove the % and write the fraction 4 over 100: $\frac{4}{100}$

2. Reduce: $\frac{4 \div 4}{100 \div 4} = \frac{1}{25}$

Here's a more complicated example: Change $16\frac{2}{3}\%$ to a fraction.

1. Remove the % and write the fraction $16\frac{2}{3}$ over 100: $\frac{16\frac{2}{3}}{100}$

2. Since a fraction means "numerator divided by denominator," rewrite the fraction as a division problem: $16\frac{2}{3} \div 100$

3. Change the mixed number ($16\frac{2}{3}$) to an improper fraction ($\frac{50}{3}$): $\frac{50}{3} \div \frac{100}{1}$

4. Flip the second fraction and multiply: $\frac{\overset{1}{\cancel{50}}}{3} \times \frac{1}{\underset{2}{\cancel{100}}} = \frac{1}{6}$

Try changing these fractions to percents:

_____ **61.** $\frac{1}{8}$

_____ **62.** $\frac{13}{25}$

_____ **63.** $\frac{7}{12}$

Now, change these percents to fractions:

_____ **64.** 95%

_____ **65.** $37\frac{1}{2}\%$

_____ **66.** 125%

Sometimes it is more convenient to work with a percentage as a fraction or a decimal. Rather than having to *calculate* the equivalent fraction or decimal, consider memorizing the above conversion table.

Not only will this increase your efficiency on the math test, but it will also be practical for real-life situations.

## Percent Word Problems

Word problems involving percents come in three main varieties:

- Find a percent of a whole.
  **Example:** What is 30% of 40?
- Find what percent one number is of another number.
  **Example:** 12 is what percent of 40?
- Find the whole when the percent of it is given.
  **Example:** 12 is 30% of what number?

While each variety has its own approach, there is a single shortcut formula you can use to solve each of these:

$$\frac{is}{of} = \frac{\%}{100}$$

The **is** is the number that usually follows or is just before the word *is* in the question.

The **of** is the number that usually follows the word *of* in the question.

The **%** is the number that is in front of the **%** or *percent* in the question.

Or you may think of the shortcut formula as:

$$\frac{part}{whole} = \frac{\%}{100}$$

To solve each of the three varieties, we're going to use the fact that the **cross products** of these two functions are always equal. The cross products are the products of the numbers diagonally across from each other. Remembering that *product* means *multiply*, here's how to create the cross products for the percent shortcut:

$$\frac{part}{whole} = \frac{\%}{100}$$
$$part \times 100 = whole \times \%$$

Here's how to use the shortcut with cross products:

- Find a percent of a whole.
  What is 30% of 40?
  30 is the % and 40 is the *of* number:
  Cross multiply and solve for *is*:

$$\frac{is}{40} = \frac{30}{100}$$
$$is \times 100 = 40 \times 30$$
$$is \times 100 = 1,200$$
$$is = \frac{1,200}{100} = 12$$

Thus, **12 is** 30% of 40.

- Find what percent one number is of another number.
  12 is what percent of 40?
  12 is the *is* number and 40 is the *of* number:
  Cross multiply and solve for %:

$$\frac{12}{40} = \frac{\%}{100}$$
$$12 \times 100 = 40 \times \%$$
$$1,200 = 40 \times \%$$
$$\% = \frac{1,200}{40} = 30$$

Thus, 12 is **30%** of 40.

- Find the whole when the percent of it is given.
  12 is 30% of what number?
  12 is the *is* number and 30 is the %:

$$\frac{12}{of} = \frac{30}{100}$$

Cross multiply and solve for *of*:

$$12 \times 100 = of \times 30$$
$$1,200 = of \times 30$$
$$of = \frac{1,200}{30} = 40$$

Thus, 12 is 30% *of* **40**.

You can use the same technique when asked to find a percent increase or decrease. The *is* number is the actual increase or decrease, and the *of* number is the original amount.

**Example:** If a merchant puts his $20 hats on sale for $15, by what percent does he decrease the selling price?

1. Calculate the actual decrease, the *is* number:  $20 − $15 = $5

2. The *of* number is the original amount, $20.

3. Set up the equation and solve for *of* by cross multiplying:

$$\frac{5}{20} = \frac{\%}{100}$$
$$5 \times 100 = 20 \times \%$$
$$500 = 20 \times \%$$
$$\% = \frac{500}{20} = 25$$

4. Thus, he decreased the selling price by **25%**.

If the merchant later raises the price of the hats from $15 back to $20, don't be fooled into thinking that the percent increase is also 25%! It's actually more, because the increase amount of $5 is now based on a lower original price of only $15: Thus, the selling price is increased by **33%**.

$$\frac{5}{15} = \frac{\%}{100}$$

$$5 \times 100 = 15 \times \%$$

$$500 = 15 \times \%$$
$$\% = \frac{500}{15} = 33\tfrac{1}{3}$$

Find a percent of a whole:

_____ **67.** 1% of 25

_____ **68.** 18.2% of 50

_____ **69.** $37\tfrac{1}{2}$% of 100

_____ **70.** 125% of 60

Find what percent one number *is* of another number:

_____ **71.** 10 is what % of 20?

_____ **72.** 4 is what % of 12?

_____ **73.** 12 is what % of 4?

Find the whole when the percent *of* it is given:

_____ **74.** 15% of what number is 15?

_____ **75.** $37\tfrac{1}{2}$% of what number is 3?

_____ **76.** 200% of what number is 20?

Now, try your percent skills on some real-life problems:

_____ **77.** Last Monday, 20% of the 140-member nursing staff was absent. How many nurses were absent that day?
a. 14
b. 20
c. 28
d. 112
e. 126

_____ **78.** Forty percent of General Hospital's medical technologists are women. If there are 80 female medical technologists, how many medical technologists are male?
a. 32
b. 112
c. 120
d. 160
e. 200

_____ **79.** Of the 840 biopsies performed last month, 42 were positive. What percent of the biopsies were positive?
- **a.** 0.5%
- **b.** 2%
- **c.** 5%
- **d.** 20%
- **e.** 50%

_____ **80.** Sam's Shoe Store put all of its merchandise on sale for 20% off. If Jason saved $10 by purchasing one pair of shoes during the sale, what was the original price of the shoes before the sale?
- **a.** $12
- **b.** $20
- **c.** $40
- **d.** $50
- **e.** $70

# Averages

An **average**, also called an arithmetic mean, is a number that *typifies* a group of numbers and functions as a measure of central tendency. You come into contact with averages on a regular basis: your bowling average, the average grade on a test, the average number of hours you work per week.

To calculate an average, add up the number of items being averaged and divide by the total number of items.

**Example:** What is the average of 6, 10, and 20?

**Solution:** Add the three numbers together and divide by 3: $\frac{6 + 10 + 20}{3} = 12$

## *Shortcut*

Here are a few neat shortcuts for average problems.

- Look at the numbers being averaged. If they are equally spaced when placed in ascending order, like 5, 10, 15, 20, and 25, then the average is the number in the middle, or 15 in this case.
- If there are an even number of such equally spaced numbers, say 10, 20, 30, and 40, then there is no middle number. In this case, the average is halfway between the two middle numbers. In this case, the average is halfway between 20 and 30, or 25.
- If the numbers are almost evenly spaced, you can probably estimate the average without going to the trouble of actually computing it. For example, the average of 10, 20, and 32 is just a little more than 20, the middle number.

Try these average questions:

_____ **81.** Bob's bowling scores for the last five games were 180, 182, 184, 186, and 188. What was his average bowling score?
- **a.** 182
- **b.** 183
- **c.** 184
- **d.** 185
- **e.** 186

_____ **82.** Ambulance Driver Conroy averaged 30 miles an hour for the two hours he drove in town and 60 miles an hour for the two hours he drove on the highway. What was his average speed in miles per hour?
- **a.** 18
- **b.** $22\frac{1}{2}$
- **c.** 45
- **d.** 60
- **e.** 90

**83.** There are ten females and 20 males in the first aid course. If the females achieved an average score of 85 and the males achieved an average score of 95, what was the class average? (Hint: Don't fall for the trap of taking the average of 85 and 95; there are more 95s being averaged than 85s, so the average is closer to 95.)
a. $90\frac{2}{3}$
b. $91\frac{2}{3}$
c. 92
d. $92\frac{2}{3}$
e. 95

# Working with Length and Time Units

The United States uses the *English system* to measure length; however, most other countries use the *metric system*, which is also prevalent in scientific use in the United States. The English system requires knowing many different equivalences, but you're probably used to dealing with these equivalences on a daily basis. Mathematically, however, it's simpler to work in metric units because their equivalences are all multiples of 10. The meter is the basic unit of length, with all other length units defined in terms of the meter.

## Length Conversions
Math questions on standardized tests, especially geometry word problems, may require conversions within a particular system. An easy way to convert from one unit of measurement to another is to multiply by an equivalence ratio.

| ENGLISH SYSTEM | |
|---|---|
| UNIT | EQUIVALENCE |
| foot (ft.) | 1 ft. 5 12 in. |
| yard (yd.) | 1 yd. 5 3 ft. <br> 1 yd. 5 36 in. |
| mile (mi.) | 1 mi. 5 5,280 ft. <br> 1 mi. 5 1,760 yds. |

| METRIC SYSTEM | |
|---|---|
| UNIT | EQUIVALENCE |
| meter (m) | Basic unit <br> A giant step is about 1 meter long. |
| centimeter (cm) | 100 cm 5 1 m <br> Your index finger is about 1 cm wide. |
| millimeter (mm) | 10 mm 5 1 cm; 1,000 mm 5 1 m <br> Your fingernail is about 1 mm thick. |
| kilometer (km) | 1 km 5 1,000 m <br> Five city blocks are about 1 km long. |

| ENGLISH SYSTEM | |
|---|---|
| TO CONVERT BETWEEN | MULTIPLY BY THIS RATIO |
| inches and feet | $\frac{12 \text{ in.}}{1 \text{ ft.}}$ or $\frac{1 \text{ ft.}}{12 \text{ in.}}$ |
| inches and yards | $\frac{36 \text{ in.}}{1 \text{ yd.}}$ or $\frac{1 \text{ yd.}}{36 \text{ in.}}$ |
| feet and yards | $\frac{3 \text{ ft.}}{1 \text{ yd.}}$ or $\frac{1 \text{ yd.}}{3 \text{ ft.}}$ |
| feet and miles | $\frac{5,280 \text{ ft.}}{1 \text{ mi.}}$ or $\frac{1 \text{ mi.}}{5,280 \text{ ft.}}$ |
| yards and miles | $\frac{1,760 \text{ yds.}}{1 \text{ mi.}}$ or $\frac{1 \text{ mi.}}{1,760 \text{ yds.}}$ |

| METRIC SYSTEM | |
|---|---|
| TO CONVERT BETWEEN | MULTIPLY BY THIS RATIO |
| millimeters and centimeters | $\frac{10 \text{ mm}}{1 \text{ cm}}$ or $\frac{1 \text{ cm}}{10 \text{ mm}}$ |
| meters and millimeters | $\frac{1,000 \text{ mm}}{1 \text{ m}}$ or $\frac{1 \text{ m}}{1,000 \text{ mm}}$ |
| meters and centimeters | $\frac{100 \text{ cm}}{1 \text{ m}}$ or $\frac{1 \text{ m}}{100 \text{ cm}}$ |
| meters and kilometers | $\frac{1,000 \text{ m}}{1 \text{ km}}$ or $\frac{1 \text{ km}}{1,000 \text{ m}}$ |

**Example:** Convert 3 yards to feet.

Multiply 3 yards by the ratio $\frac{3\,\text{ft.}}{1\,\text{yd.}}$. Notice that we chose $\frac{3\,\text{ft.}}{1\,\text{yd.}}$ rather than $\frac{1\,\text{yd.}}{3\,\text{ft.}}$ because the yards cancel during the multiplication:

$$3\text{ yds.} \times \frac{3\text{ ft.}}{1\text{ yd.}} = \frac{3\text{ yds.} \times 3\text{ ft.}}{1\text{ yd.}} = 9\text{ ft.}$$

**Example:** Convert 31 inches to feet and inches.

1. First, multiply 31 inches by the ratio $\frac{1\,\text{ft.}}{12\,\text{in.}}$:
$$31\text{ in.} \times \frac{1\text{ ft.}}{12\text{ in.}} = \frac{31\text{ in.} \times 1\text{ ft.}}{12\text{ in.}} = \frac{31}{12}\text{ ft.} = 2\frac{7}{12}\text{ ft.}$$

2. Then change the $\frac{7}{12}$ portion to inches:
$$\frac{7\text{ ft.}}{12} \times \frac{12\text{ in.}}{1\text{ ft.}} = \frac{7\text{ ft.} \times 12\text{ in.}}{12 \times 1\text{ ft.}} = 7\text{ in.}$$

3. Thus, 31 inches is equivalent to both $2\frac{7}{12}$ **ft.** and

   **2 feet 7 inches.**

Convert as indicated.

**84.** 2 ft. = _____ in.

**85.** 3 cm = _____ mm

**86.** 16 m = _____ cm

**87.** 294 cm = _____ m

## Addition and Subtraction with Length Units

Finding the perimeter of a figure may require adding lengths of different units.

**Example:** Find the perimeter of the figure at right.

To add the lengths, add each column of length units separately:

$$
\begin{array}{rr}
5\text{ ft.} & 7\text{ in.} \\
2\text{ ft.} & 6\text{ in.} \\
6\text{ ft.} & 9\text{ in.} \\
+\ 3\text{ ft.} & 5\text{ in.} \\
\hline
\mathbf{16\text{ ft.}} & \mathbf{27\text{ in.}}
\end{array}
$$

Since 27 inches is more than 1 foot, the total of **16 ft. 27 in.** must be simplified:

■ Convert 27 inches to feet and inches:
$$27\text{ in.} \times \frac{1\text{ ft.}}{12\text{ in.}} = \frac{27}{12}\text{ ft.} = 2\frac{3}{12}\text{ ft.} = 2\text{ ft. }3\text{ in.}$$

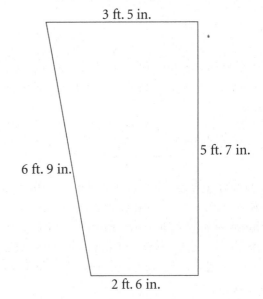

3 ft. 5 in.

5 ft. 7 in.

6 ft. 9 in.

2 ft. 6 in.

■ Add:
$$
\begin{array}{r}
16\text{ ft.} \\
+\ 2\ \text{ ft. }3\text{ in.} \\
\hline
\mathbf{18\text{ ft. }3\text{ in.}}
\end{array}
$$

Thus, the perimeter is **18 feet 3 inches.**

Finding the length of a line segment may require subtracting lengths of different units.

**Example:** Find the length of line segment *AB* below.

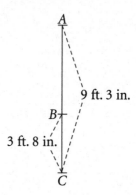

To subtract the lengths, subtract each column of length units separately, starting with the rightmost column.

$$9 \text{ ft. } 3 \text{ in.}$$
$$- \, 3 \text{ ft. } 8 \text{ in.}$$

*Warning*: You can't subtract 8 inches from 3 inches because 8 is larger than 3! As in regular subtraction, you have to *borrow* 1 from the column on the left. However, borrowing 1 ft. is the same as borrowing 12 inches; adding the borrowed 12 inches to the 3 inches gives 15 inches. Thus:

$$\begin{array}{r} \overset{8}{\cancel{9}} \overset{12}{\cancel{\phantom{0}}} \overset{15}{\cancel{3}} \text{ ft. } \cancel{3} \text{ in.} \\ - \, 3 \text{ ft. } 8 \text{ in.} \\ \hline \mathbf{5 \text{ ft. } 7 \text{ in.}} \end{array}$$

Thus, the length of $\overline{AB}$ is **5 feet 7 inches**.

Add and simplify.

**88.**  5 ft. 3 in.
  + 2 ft. 9 in.

**89.**  7 km 220 m
  4 km 180 m
  + 9 km 770 m

Subtract and simplify.

**90.**  4 ft. 1 in.
  − 2 ft. 9 in.

**91.**  14 cm 2 mm
  − 6 cm 4 mm

## Time Conversions

Word problems involving time typically ask you to determine how long something takes. You might have to add together the amount of time several activities take in order to determine the total amount of time the entire process takes or calculate the elapsed time from the start to the finish of a particular activity.

Adding and subtracting time units is a lot like adding and subtracting length units. You have to make sure that you are adding hours to hours, minutes to minutes, and seconds to seconds. If the given information is in different time units, then you'll have to convert to a common time unit before you can proceed. Use the following conversion ratios:

- **To convert minutes to hours:** $\frac{1 \text{ hour}}{60 \text{ minutes}}$
- **To convert hours to minutes:** $\frac{60 \text{ minutes}}{1 \text{ hour}}$
- **To convert seconds to minutes:** $\frac{1 \text{ minute}}{60 \text{ seconds}}$
- **To convert minutes to seconds:** $\frac{60 \text{ seconds}}{1 \text{ minute}}$
  **Example:** Convert $2\frac{1}{4}$ hours to seconds.

1. Convert hours to minutes: $\frac{2\frac{1}{4} \text{ hr.}}{1} \times \frac{60 \text{ min.}}{1 \text{ hr.}} = 135 \text{ min.}$

2. Convert minutes to seconds: $\frac{135 \text{ min.}}{1} \times \frac{60 \text{ sec.}}{1 \text{ min.}} = 8{,}100 \text{ sec.}$

The hours and minutes cancel, giving an answer in seconds.

## Calculating Elapsed Time

Calculating elapsed time when you're given the starting and ending time can be a bit tricky, depending on the starting and ending time. If the starting and ending times are both A.M. or both P.M. of the same day, you can calculate the elapsed time by simply subtracting the starting time from the ending time. However, you may have to "regroup," or "borrow."

**Example:** Radiology Associates opens at 6:45 A.M. and closes for lunch at 11:35 A.M. How long are they open in the morning?

1. Set up the subtraction:

$$\begin{array}{r} ^{10}\ ^{95} \\ \cancel{11{:}35} \\ -\ 6{:}45 \\ \hline 4{:}50 \end{array}$$

2. You can't subtract 45 minutes from 35 minutes, so you have to "borrow" 1 hour from the 11 hours. Borrowing 1 hour from 11 hours is equivalent to borrowing 60 minutes. Thus, you're actually subtracting 45 minutes from 95 minutes (that is, 35 + 60 minutes).

Radiology Associates is open for 4 hours 50 minutes in the morning.

If the starting time is A.M. and ending time is P.M. of the same day, you have to calculate the elapsed time in two steps and then add the results together. Calculate the elapsed morning time by subtracting the starting time from noon. The elapsed afternoon time is equivalent to the ending time. So you add the elapsed morning time and the elapsed afternoon time to get the total elapsed time.

**Example:** If Radiology Associates opens at 7:15 A.M. and closes at 5:30 P.M., how long are they open?

1. Subtract the starting time from noon:
(You'll have to "borrow" 60 minutes from 12.)
Radiology Associates is open for 4 hours 45 minutes in the morning.

$$\begin{array}{r} ^{11}\ ^{60} \\ \cancel{12{:}00} \\ -\ 7{:}15 \\ \hline 4{:}45 \end{array}$$

2. Radiology Associates closes at 5:30 P.M. Thus, they're open for 5 hours 30 minutes in the afternoon.

3. Add the results together:

$$\begin{array}{r} 4{:}45 \\ +\ 5{:}30 \\ \hline 9{:}75 \end{array}$$

4. The sum of 9 hours 75 minutes needs to be adjusted because 75 minutes is more than an hour. There's a "carry" of 1 hour: the 75 minutes is equivalent to 1 hour 15 minutes. Thus, 9 hours 75 minutes is the same as 10 hours 15 minutes.

You follow the same procedure when the starting time is P.M. of one day and the ending time is A.M. of the next day. Calculate the elapsed P.M. time by subtracting the starting time from midnight. Then add the elapsed A.M. time, which is equivalent to the ending time.

If the starting and ending times are on different days, you calculate the elapsed time in three steps: elapsed time on the starting day, elapsed time on the ending day, and the time of the intervening days. Then you add the results of the three steps together.

**Example:** Each week, employees of Radiology Associates turn their computers on at 6:45 A.M. on Monday and turn them off for the weekend at 5:30 P.M. on Friday. How long are the computers on, in hours?

**1.** Starting day, Monday

  **a.** For the A.M. hours, subtract the starting time from noon:

$$\begin{array}{r}{}^{11}\;{}^{60}\\ \cancel{12{:}00}\\ -\;6{:}45\\ \hline 5{:}15\end{array}$$

  **b.** For the P.M. hours, there are 12 hours from noon until midnight.   12

  **c.** Add the A.M. and P.M. hours to get the total hours on the starting day:

$$\begin{array}{r}5{:}15\\ +\;12{:}00\\ \hline 17{:}15\end{array}$$

On Monday, 17 hours 15 minutes elapse.

**2.** Ending day, Friday

  **a.** For the A.M. hours, there are 12 hours from midnight until noon:   12:00

  **b.** For the P.M. hours, the ending time is the elapsed time:   + 5:30

  **c.** Add the A.M. and P.M. hours to get the total hours on the ending day:   17:30

On Friday, 17 hours 30 minutes elapse.

**3.** The intervening days: Tuesday, Wednesday, and Thursday

3 days × 24 hours per day = 72 hours

**4.** Add the results of steps 1–3 together:

$$\begin{array}{r}17{:}15\\ 17{:}30\\ +\;72{:}00\\ \hline 106{:}45\end{array}$$

The total elapsed time is 106 hours 45 minutes.

**5.** Since the question asks for the amount of time the computers are on in hours, the 45 minutes

portion of the answer must be converted to a fraction of an hour:

$$45 \text{ minutes} \times \frac{1 \text{ hour}}{60 \text{ minutes}} = \frac{3}{4} \text{ hour}$$

Thus, the computers were on for a total of $106\frac{3}{4}$ hours.

Now, try these time problems:

**92.** Jan ran three tests in the lab that each required 45 minutes. If she then ran a final test and all four tests required a total of $3\frac{1}{4}$ hours, how long did the final test take?

  **a.** $\frac{1}{2}$ hour

  **b.** $\frac{2}{3}$ hour

  **c.** $\frac{3}{4}$ hour

  **d.** 1 hour

  **e.** $1\frac{1}{4}$ hours

**93.** If each of eight radiology rooms is in use for 5 hours 15 minutes per day, and a total of 84 procedures are performed, how long does each procedure take on average?

  **a.** 20 minutes

  **b.** 30 minutes

  **c.** 40 minutes

  **d.** 50 minutes

  **e.** 1 hour

**94.** Clara cultured a particular virus at 2:30 P.M. on Monday and stored the culture in the refrigerator until 11:30 A.M. on Wednesday. How long was the culture in the refrigerator?

  **a.** 3 hours

  **b.** 21 hours

  **c.** 27 hours

  **d.** 45 hours

  **e.** 69 hours

## Algebra

Popular topics for algebra questions on nursing school exams include:

- Solving equations
- Positive and negative numbers
- Algebraic expressions

### What Is Algebra?

**Algebra** is a way to express and solve problems using numbers and symbols. These symbols, called *unknowns* or *variables*, are letters of the alphabet that are used to represent numbers.

For example, let's say you are asked to find out what number, when added to 3, gives you a total of 5. Using algebra, you could express the problem as $x + 3 = 5$. The variable $x$ represents the number you are trying to find.

Here's another example, but this one uses only variables. To find the distance traveled, multiply the rate of travel (speed) by the amount of time traveled: $d = r \times t$. The variable $d$ stands for *distance*, $r$ stands for *rate*, and $t$ stands for *time*.

In algebra, the variables may take on different values. In other words, they *vary*, and that's why they're called *variables*.

### Operations

Algebra uses the same operations as arithmetic: addition, subtraction, multiplication, and division. In arithmetic, we might say $3 + 4 = 7$, while in algebra, we would talk about two numbers whose values we don't know that add up to 7, or $x + y = 7$. Here's how each operation translates to algebra:

| ALGEBRAIC OPERATIONS | |
|---|---|
| The sum of 2 numbers | $a + b$ |
| The difference of 2 numbers | $a - b$ |
| The product of 2 numbers | $a \times b$ or $a \cdot b$ or $ab$ |
| The quotient of 2 numbers | $\frac{a}{b}$ |

### Equations

An equation is a mathematical sentence stating that two quantities are equal. For example:

$$2x = 10$$
$$x + 5 = 8$$

The idea is to find a replacement for the unknown that will make the sentence true. That's called solving the equation. Thus, in the first example, $x = 5$ because $2 \times 5 = 10$. In the second example, $x = 3$ because $3 + 5 = 8$.

Sometimes you can solve an equation by inspection, as with the above examples. Other equations may be more complicated and require a step-by-step solution, for example:

$$\frac{n+2}{4} + 1 = 3$$

The general approach is to consider an equation like a balance scale, with both sides equally balanced. Essentially, whatever you do to one side, you *must* also do to the other side to maintain the balance. Thus, if you were to add 2 to the left side, you would also have to add 2 to the right side.

Let's apply this *balance* concept to our previous complicated equation. We want to solve for $n$, which means we must somehow rearrange the equation so the $n$ is isolated on one side of it. Its value will then be on the other side. Looking at the equation, you can see that $n$ has been increased by 2 and then divided by 4 and ultimately added to 1. Therefore, we will undo these operations to isolate $n$.

Begin by subtracting 1 from both sides of the equation:

Next, multiply both sides by 4:

Finally, subtract 2 from both sides:

This isolates $n$ and solves the equation:

$$\frac{n+2}{4} + 1 = 3$$

$$\frac{-1 \quad -1}{\frac{n+2}{4} \quad = \quad 2}$$

$$4 \times \frac{n+2}{4} = 2 \times 4$$

$$n + 2 = 8$$

$$\frac{-2 \quad -2}{n \quad = 6}$$

Notice that each operation in the original equation was undone by using its inverse operation. That is, addition was undone by subtraction, and division was undone by multiplication. In general, each operation can be undone by its *inverse*.

| ALGEBRAIC INVERSES | | | |
|---|---|---|---|
| **OPERATION** | **INVERSE** | **OPERATION** | **INVERSE** |
| Addition | Subtraction | Subtraction | Addition |
| Multiplication | Division | Division | Multiplication |
| Square | Square Root | Square Root | Square |

After you solve an equation, check your work by plugging the answer back into the original equation to make sure it balances. Let's see what happens when we plug 6 in for $n$:

$$\frac{6+2}{4} + 1 = 3 \quad ?$$

$$\frac{8}{4} + 1 = 3 \quad ?$$

$$2 + 1 = 3 \quad ?$$

$$3 = 3 \quad \checkmark$$

Solve each equation:

_____ **95.** $x + 5 = 12$

_____ **96.** $3x + 6 = 18$

_____ **97.** $\frac{1}{4}x = 7$

## *Positive and Negative Numbers*

Positive and negative numbers, also known as *signed* numbers, are best shown as points along the number line:

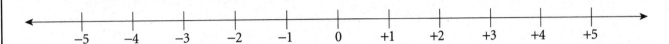

Numbers to the left of (smaller than) 0 are *negative* and those to the right of (greater than) 0 are *positive*. Zero is neither negative nor positive. If a number is written without a sign, it is assumed to be *positive*. Notice that when you are on the negative side of the number line, bigger numbers have smaller values. For example, –5 is *less than* –2. You come into contact with negative numbers more often than you might think; for example, very cold temperatures are recorded as negative numbers.

As you move to the right along the number line, the numbers get larger. Mathematically, to indicate that one number, say 4, is *greater than* another number, say –2, the *greater than* sign (>) is used:

$$4 > -2$$

1. Parentheses
2. Exponents
3. Multiplication or Division
   (whichever comes first when reading left to right)
4. Addition or Subtraction
   (whichever comes first when reading left to right)

Even when signed numbers appear in an equation, the step-by-step process works exactly as it does for positive numbers. You just have to remember the

On the other hand, to say that –2 is *less than* 4, we use the *less than* sign (<):

$$-2 < 4$$

## Arithmetic with Positive and Negative Numbers

The table on the next page illustrates the rules for doing arithmetic with signed numbers. Notice that when a negative number follows an operation, it is often enclosed in parentheses to avoid confusion.

When more than one arithmetic operation appears, you must know the correct sequence in which to perform the operations. For example, do you know what to do first when calculating $2 + 3 \times 4$? You're right if you said, "Multiply first." The correct answer is 14. If you add first, you'll get the wrong answer of 20! The correct sequence of operations is:

If you remember this saying, you'll know the order of operations: **P**lease **E**xcuse **M**y **D**ear **A**unt **S**ally.

arithmetic rules for negative numbers. For example, let's solve $-14x + 2 = -5$.

**1.** Subtract 2 from both sides:

**2.** Divide both sides by $-14$:

$$-14x + 2 = -5$$
$$\phantom{-14x} -2 \quad -2$$
$$\frac{-14x}{-14} = \frac{-7}{-14}$$
$$x = \frac{1}{2}$$

| RULE | EXAMPLE |
|------|---------|
| **ADDITION** | |
| If both numbers have the same sign, just add them. The answer has the same sign as the numbers being added. | $3 + 5 = 8$ <br> $-3 + (-5) = -8$ |
| If both numbers have different signs, drop the signs and subtract the smaller number from the larger. The answer has the same sign as the larger number. | $-3 + 5 = 2$ <br> $3 + (-5) = -2$ |
| If both numbers are the same but have opposite signs, the sum is zero. | $3 + (-3) = 0$ |
| **SUBTRACTION** | |
| Change the subtraction sign to addition. Then change the sign of the second number. Add as above. | $3 - 5 = 3 + (-5) = -2$ <br> $-3 - 5 = -3 + (-5) = -8$ <br> $-3 - (-5) = -3 + 5 = 2$ |
| **MULTIPLICATION** | |
| Multiply the numbers together. If both numbers have the same sign, the answer is positive; otherwise, it is negative. | $3 \times 5 = 15$ <br> $-3 \times (-5) = 15$ <br> $-3 \times 5 = -15$ <br> $3 \times (-5) = -15$ |
| If one number (or both) is zero, the answer is zero. | $3 \times 0 = 0$ |
| **DIVISION** | |
| Divide the numbers. If both numbers have the same sign, the answer is positive; otherwise, it is negative. | $15 \div 3 = 5$ <br> $-15 \div (-3) = 5$ <br> $15 \div (-3) = -5$ <br> $-15 \div 3 = -5$ |
| If the number to be divided (or the numerator of a fraction) is zero, the answer is zero. But you cannot divide by zero; thus, the denominator of a fraction cannot be zero. | $3 \div 0$ is meaningless |

## Algebraic Expressions

An algebraic expression is a group of numbers, unknowns, and arithmetic operations, like $3x - 2y$. This one may be translated as "3 times some number minus 2 times another number." To *evaluate* an algebraic expression, replace each variable with its value. For example, if $x = 5$ and $y = 4$, we would evaluate $3x - 2y$ as follows:

$$3(5) - 2(4) = 15 - 8 = 7$$

Now, solve these problems with signed numbers.

_____ **98.** $1 - 3(-4) = x$

_____ **99.** $-3x + 6 = -18$

_____ **100.** $-\frac{x}{4} + 3 = -7$

Evaluate these expressions.

_____ **101.** $4a + 3b$; $a = 2$ and $b = -1$

_____ **102.** $3mn - 4m + 2n$; $m = 3$ and $n = -3$

_____ **103.** $-2x - \frac{1}{2}y + 4z$; $x = 5$, $y = -4$, and $z = 6$

_____ **104.** The volume of a cylinder is given by the formula $V = \pi r^2 h$, where $r$ is the radius of the base and $h$ is the height of the cylinder. What is the volume of a cylinder with a base radius of 3 and height of 4? (Leave $\pi$ in your answer.)

## Squares and Square Roots

It's not uncommon to see squares and square roots on standardized math tests, especially in questions that involve right triangles.

To find the **square** of a number, multiply that number by itself. For example, the square of 4 is 16, because $4 \times 4 = 16$. Mathematically, this is expressed as:

$$4^2 = 16$$
4 squared equals 16.

To find the **square root** of a number, ask yourself, "What number times itself equals the given number?" For example, the square root of 16 is 4 because $4 \times 4 = 16$. Mathematically, this is expressed as:

$$\sqrt{16} = 4$$
The square root of 16 is 4.

Because certain squares and square roots tend to appear more often than others on standardized tests, the best course is to memorize the most common ones.

| COMMON SQUARES AND SQUARE ROOTS | | | | | |
| --- | --- | --- | --- | --- | --- |
| **SQUARES** | | | **SQUARE ROOTS** | | |
| $1^2 = 1$ | $7^2 = 49$ | $13^2 = 169$ | $\sqrt{1} = 1$ | $\sqrt{49} = 7$ | $\sqrt{169} = 13$ |
| $2^2 = 4$ | $8^2 = 64$ | $14^2 = 196$ | $\sqrt{4} = 2$ | $\sqrt{64} = 8$ | $\sqrt{196} = 14$ |
| $3^2 = 9$ | $9^2 = 81$ | $15^2 = 225$ | $\sqrt{9} = 3$ | $\sqrt{81} = 9$ | $\sqrt{225} = 15$ |
| $4^2 = 16$ | $10^2 = 100$ | $16^2 = 256$ | $\sqrt{16} = 4$ | $\sqrt{100} = 10$ | $\sqrt{256} = 16$ |
| $5^2 = 25$ | $11^2 = 121$ | $20^2 = 400$ | $\sqrt{25} = 5$ | $\sqrt{121} = 11$ | $\sqrt{400} = 20$ |
| $6^2 = 36$ | $12^2 = 144$ | $25^2 = 625$ | $\sqrt{36} = 6$ | $\sqrt{144} = 12$ | $\sqrt{625} = 25$ |

You can multiply and divide square roots, but you cannot add or subtract them:

$$\sqrt{a} + \sqrt{b} = \sqrt{a+b} \qquad \sqrt{a} \times \sqrt{b} = \sqrt{a \times b}$$

$$\sqrt{a} - \sqrt{b} = \sqrt{a-b} \qquad \sqrt{\tfrac{a}{b}} = \frac{\sqrt{a}}{\sqrt{b}}$$

Use the previous rules to solve these problems in squares and square roots.

_____**105.** $\sqrt{4} \times \sqrt{9} = ?$

_____**106.** $\sqrt{\tfrac{1}{4}} = ?$

_____**107.** $\sqrt{9} + \sqrt{16} = ?$

### How to Solve an Equation

**Example:** $5 - 2(3x + 1) = 7x - 8$

**1.** Remove parentheses by distributing the value outside to both values within:

$$5 - 6x - 2 = 7x - 8$$

**2.** If there are like terms on the same side of the equal sign, combine them:

$$3 - 6x = 7x - 8$$

**3.** Decide where you want all of the $x$ terms. Put all the $x$ terms on one side by addition and subtraction:

$$\begin{aligned} +6x &= +6x \\ 3 &= 13x - 8 \end{aligned}$$

**4.** Get all the constants on the other side by addition and subtraction:

$$\begin{aligned} 3 &= 13x - 8 \\ +8 &= +8 \\ \hline 11 &= 13x \end{aligned}$$

**5.** Isolate the $x$ by performing the opposite operation:

$$\frac{11}{13} = \frac{\cancel{13}x}{\cancel{13}}$$
$$\frac{11}{13} = x$$

_____**108.** $\sqrt{9 + x} = 5$

_____**109.** $(3 + x)^2 = 49$

## Geometry

Geometry questions cover points, lines, planes, angles, triangles, rectangles, squares, and circles. You may be asked to determine the area or perimeter of a particular shape, the size of an angle, the length of a line, and so forth. Some word problems may also involve geometry.

## *Points, Lines, and Planes*
### What Is a Point?

A point has position but no size or dimension. It is usually represented by a dot named with an uppercase letter:

•A

### What Is a Line?

A line consists of an infinite number of points that extend endlessly in both directions.

A line can be named in two ways:

1. By a letter at one end (typically in lowercase): $l$

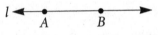

2. By two points on the line: $\overleftrightarrow{AB}$ or $\overleftrightarrow{BA}$

The following terminology is frequently used on math tests:

■ Points are collinear if they lie on the same line. Points J, U, D, and I are collinear.

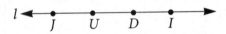

■ A **line segment** is a section of a line with two endpoints. The line segment at right is indicated as $\overline{AB}$.

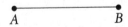

■ The **midpoint** is a point on a line segment that divides it into two line segments of equal length. $M$ is the midpoint of line segment $AB$. Two line segments of the same length are said to be **congruent**. Congruent line segments are indicated by the same mark on each line segment(like the double marks shown on $\overline{AB}$).

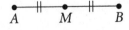

■ A line segment (or line) that divides another line segment into two congruent line segments is said to **bisect** it. $\overline{XY}$ bisects $\overline{AB}$.

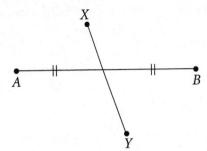

■ A **ray** is a section of a line that has one endpoint. The ray below is indicated as $\overrightarrow{AB}$.

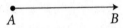

### What Is a Plane?

A plane is like a flat surface with no thickness. Although a plane extends endlessly in all directions, it is usually represented by a four-sided figure and named by an uppercase letter in a corner of the plane: *K*.

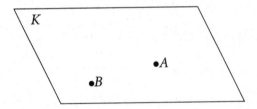

Points are *coplanar* if they lie on the same plane. Points *A* and *B* are coplanar.

### Angles

An angle is formed when two rays meet at a point: The lines are called the **sides** of the angle, and the point where they meet is called the **vertex** of the angle.

The symbol used to indicate an angle is $\angle$.

There are three ways to name an angle:

- By the letter that labels the vertex: $\angle B$
- By the three letters that label the angle: $\angle ABC$ or $\angle CBA$, with the vertex letter in the middle
- By the number inside the vertex: $\angle 1$

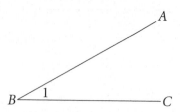

An angle's size is based on the opening between its sides. Size is measured in **degrees** (°). The smaller the angle, the fewer degrees it has. Angles are classified by size. Notice how the arc ( ⌒ ) shows which of the two angles is indicated:

**Acute angle:** less than 90°

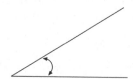

**Right angle:** exactly 90°

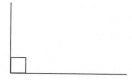

A little box indicates a right angle. A right angle is formed by two *perpendicular* lines.

**Straight angle:** exactly 180°

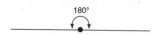

**Obtuse angle:** more than 90° and less than 180°

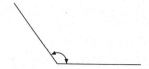

## Special Angle Pairs

- **Congruent angles:** Two angles that have the same degree measure.

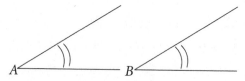

Congruent angles are indicated by identical markings. The symbol $\cong$ is used to indicate that two angles are congruent: $\angle A \cong \angle B$.

- **Complementary angles:** Two angles whose sum is 90°.

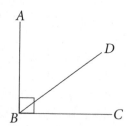

$\angle ABD$ and $\angle DBC$ are **complementary** angles.

$\angle ABD$ is the **complement** of $\angle DBC$, and vice versa.

- **Supplementary angles:** Two angles whose sum is 180°.

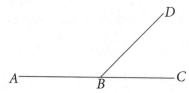

$\angle ABD$ and $\angle DBC$ are **supplementary** angles.

$\angle ABD$ is the **supplement** of $\angle DBC$, and vice versa.

**Hint:** To avoid confusion between complementary and supplementary:

C comes before **S** in the alphabet, and 90 comes before 180.

Complementary: 90°

Supplementary: 180°

- **Vertical angles:** Two angles that are opposite each other when two lines cross.

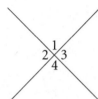

Two sets of vertical angles are formed:

∠1 and ∠4

∠2 and ∠3

Vertical angles are congruent.

When two lines cross, the **adjacent** angles are supplementary and the sum of all four angles is 360°.

Angle-pair problems tend to ask for an angle's complement or supplement.

**Example:** If the measure of ∠2 = 70°, what are the measures of the other three angles?

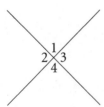

1. ∠2 ≅ ∠3 because they're vertical angles.
   Therefore, ∠3 = **70°**.
2. ∠1 and ∠2 are adjacent angles and therefore supplementary.
   Thus, ∠1 = **110°** (180° − 70° = 110°).
3. ∠1 ≅ ∠4 because they're also vertical angles.
   Therefore, ∠4 = **110°**.
   **Check:** Add the angles to be sure their sum is 360°: 70° + 70° + 110° + 110° = 360° ✔

To solve geometry problems more easily, draw a picture if one is not provided. Try to draw the picture to scale. As the problem presents information about the size of an angle or line segment, label the corresponding part of your picture to reflect the given information. As you begin to find the missing information, label your picture accordingly.

These word problems require you to find the measures of angles.

_____ **110.** In order to paint the second story of his house, Alex leaned a ladder against the side of his house, making an acute angle of 58° with the ground. Find the size of the supplementary obtuse angle the ladder made with the ground.

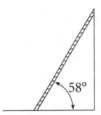

_____ **111.** Confusion Corner is an appropriately named intersection that confuses drivers who are unfamiliar with the area.
Referring to the street plan on the right, find the size of the marked angle.

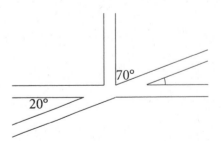

## Special Line Pairs
### Parallel Lines

Parallel lines lie in the same plane and never cross at any point.

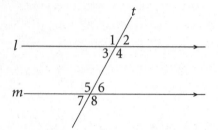

The arrowheads on the lines indicate that they are parallel. The symbol ∥ is used to indicate that two lines are parallel: $l \parallel m$.

When two parallel lines are crossed by another line, two groups of four angles each are formed. One group consists of ∠1, ∠2, ∠3, and ∠4; the other group contains ∠5, ∠6, ∠7, and ∠8.

These angles have special relationships:

- The four obtuse angles are always congruent: ∠1 ≅ ∠4 ≅ ∠5 ≅ ∠8.
- The four acute angles are always congruent: ∠2 ≅ ∠3 ≅ ∠6 ≅ ∠7.
- The sum of any one acute angle and any one obtuse angle is always 180° because the acute angles lie on the same line as the obtuse angles.

Don't be fooled into thinking two lines are parallel just because they look parallel. Either the lines *must* be marked with similar arrowheads or there *must* be an angle pair as just described.

### Perpendicular Lines

Perpendicular lines lie in the same plane and intersect to form four right angles.

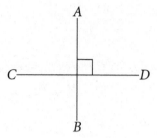

The little box where the lines cross indicates a right angle. Because vertical angles are equal and the sum of all four angles is 360°, each of the four angles is a right angle and 90°. However, only one little box is needed to indicate this.

The symbol ⊥ is used to indicate that two lines are perpendicular: $\overleftrightarrow{AB} \perp \overleftrightarrow{CD}$.

Don't be fooled into thinking two lines are perpendicular just because they look perpendicular. The problem *must* indicate the presence of a right angle (by stating that an angle measures 90° or by the little right angle box in a corresponding diagram), or you *must* be able to prove the presence of a 90° angle.

Determine the measure of the marked angles.

_____ **112.**

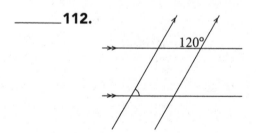

_____ **113.**

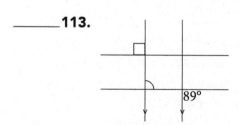

## Polygons

A polygon is a closed, plane (flat) figure formed by three or more connected line segments that don't cross each other. Familiarize yourself with the following polygons; they are the four most common polygons appearing on standardized tests—and in life.

### Triangle

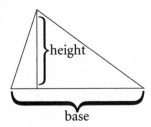

Three-sided polygon

### Square

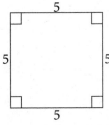

Four-sided polygon with four right angles; all sides are congruent (equal), and each pair of opposite sides is parallel.

### Rectangle

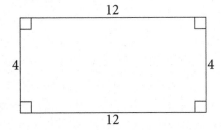

Four-sided polygon with four right angles; each pair of opposite sides is parallel and congruent.

### Parallelogram

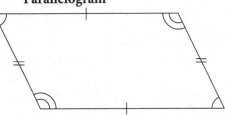

Four-sided polygon; each pair of opposite sides is parallel and congruent.

### Perimeter

**Perimeter** is the distance around a polygon. The word *perimeter* is derived from *peri*, which means around (as in *peri*scope and *peri*pheral vision), and *meter*, which means *measure*. Thus, *perimeter* is the *measure around* something. There are many everyday applications of perimeter. For instance, a carpenter measures the perimeter of a room to determine how many feet of ceiling molding she needs. A farmer measures the perimeter of a field to determine how many feet of fencing he needs to surround it.

Perimeter is measured in length units, like feet, yards, inches, meters, etc.

> To find the perimeter of a polygon, add the lengths of the sides.

**Example:** Find the perimeter of the following polygon:

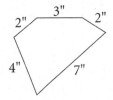

Write down the length of each side and add:

3 inches  
2 inches  
7 inches  
4 inches  
+ 2 inches  
18 inches  

**Note:** The notion of perimeter also applies to a circle; however, the perimeter of a circle is referred to as its **circumference**. We will take a closer look at circles and circumference later in this chapter.

Find the perimeters for these word problems:

_____**114.** Maryellen has cleared a 10-foot-by-6-foot rectangular plot of ground for her herb garden. She must completely enclose it with a chain-link fence to keep her dog out. How many feet of fencing does she need, excluding the 3-foot gate at the south end of the garden?

_____**115.** Terri plans to hang a wallpaper border along the top of each wall in her square dressing room. Wallpaper border is sold only in 12-foot strips. If each wall is 8 feet long, how many strips should she buy?

## Area

*Area* is the total amount of space taken by a figure's surface. Area is measured in square units.

For instance, a square that is 1 unit on all sides covers *1 square unit*. If the unit of measurement for each side is feet, for example, then the area is measured in *square feet*. Other possibilities are units like square inches, square miles, square meters, and so on.

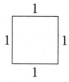

You could measure the area of any figure by counting the number of square units the figure occupies. The first two figures are easy to measure because the square units fit into them evenly, while the following two figures are more difficult to measure because the square units don't fit into them evenly.

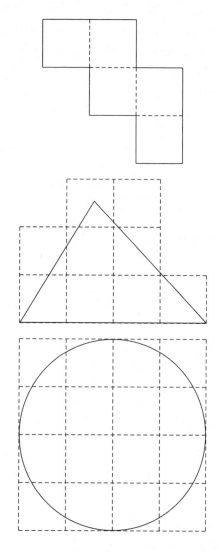

Because it's not always practical to measure a particular figure's area by counting the number of square units it occupies, an area formula is used. As each figure is discussed, you'll learn its area formula. Although there are perimeter formulas as well, you don't really need them (except for circles) if you understand the perimeter concept: It is merely the sum of the lengths of the sides.

## Triangles

A triangle is a polygon with three sides, like those shown here:

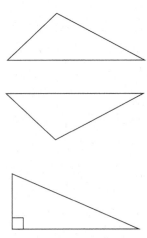

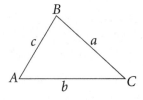

The symbol used to indicate a triangle is △. Each vertex—the point at which two lines meet—is named by a capital letter. The triangle is named by the three letters at the vertices, usually in clockwise order: △*ABC*.

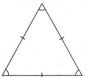

There are two ways to refer to a side of a triangle:

- By the letters at each end of the side: *AB*
- By the letter—typically a lowercase letter—next to the side: *c*

  Notice that the name of the side is the same as the name of the angle opposite it, except the angle's name is a capital letter.

There are two ways to refer to an angle of a triangle:

- By the letter at the vertex: ∠*A*
- By the triangle's three letters, with that angle's vertex letter in the middle: ∠*BAC* or ∠*CAB*

## Types of Triangles

A triangle can be classified by the size of its angles and sides.

### Equilateral Triangle

- three congruent angles, each 60°
- three congruent sides

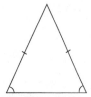

**Hint to help you remember:** The word *equilateral* comes from *equi*, meaning *equal*, and *lat*, meaning *side*. Thus, *all equal sides*.

### Isosceles Triangle

- two congruent angles, called *base angles*; the third angle is the *vertex angle.*
- Sides opposite the base angles are also congruent.
- An equilateral triangle is also isosceles, since it always has two congruent base angles.

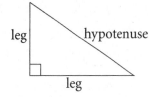

### Right Triangle

- one right (90°) angle, which is the largest angle in the triangle
- The side opposite the right angle is the *hypotenuse*, which is the longest side of the triangle. (**Hint:** The word *hypotenuse* reminds us of *hippopotamus*, a very large animal.)
- The other two sides are called *legs.*

## Area of a Triangle

To find the area of a triangle, use this formula:

$$Area = \frac{1}{2}(base \times height)$$

Although any side of a triangle may be called its **base**, it's often easiest to use the side on the bottom. To use another side, rotate the page and view the triangle from another perspective.

A triangle's **height** is represented by a perpendicular line drawn from the angle opposite the base down to the base. Depending on the triangle, the height may be inside, outside, or on the triangle. Notice the height of the second triangle: We extended the base to draw the height perpendicular to the base. The third triangle is a **right** triangle: One leg may be its base and the other its height.

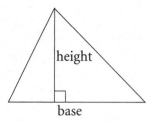

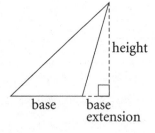

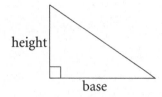

**Hint:** Think of a triangle as being half a rectangle. The area of that triangle is half the area of the rectangle.

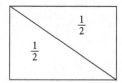

**Example:** Find the area of a triangle with a 2-inch base and a 3-inch height.

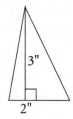

1. Draw the triangle as close to scale as you can.
2. Label the size of the base and height.
3. Write the area formula; then substitute the base and height numbers into it: $Area = \frac{1}{2}(base \times height)$
4. The area of the triangle is **3 square inches**. $Area = \frac{1}{2}(2 \times 3) = \frac{1}{2} \times 6$; $Area = 3$

Find the area of the following triangles:

_____ **116.**

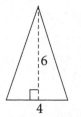

_____ **117.**

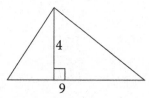

## Triangle Rules

The following rules tend to appear more frequently on standardized tests than other rules. A typical test question follows each rule.

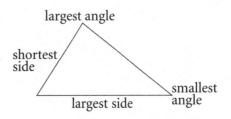

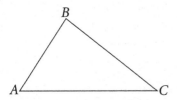

The sum of the angles in a triangle is 180°:
$\angle A + \angle B + \angle C = 180°$

The longest side of a triangle is opposite the largest angle. This rule implies that the second-longest side is opposite the second-largest angle, and the shortest side is opposite the shortest angle.

**Example:** One base angle of an isosceles triangle is 30°. Find the vertex angle.

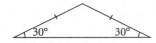

1. Draw a picture of an isosceles triangle. Drawing it to scale helps: Since it is an isosceles triangle, draw both base angles the same size (as close to 30° as you can) and make sure the sides opposite them are the same length. Label one base angle as 30°.

2. Since the base angles are congruent, label the other base angle as 30°.

3. There are two steps needed to find the vertex angle:
   - Add the two base angles together: 30° + 30° = 60°
   - The sum of all three angles is 180°. To find the vertex angle, subtract the sum of the two base angles (60°) from 180°: 180° − 60° = **120°**

Thus, the vertex angle is **120°**.

> **Check:** Add all three angles together to make sure their sum is 180°:
> 30° + 30° + 120° = 180° ✔

**Example:** In the triangle shown below, which side is the shortest?

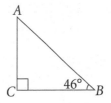

1. Determine the size of $\angle A$, the missing angle, by adding the two known angles and then subtracting their sum from 180°: 90° + 46° = 136°; 180° − 136° = 44°. Thus, $\angle A$ is 44°.

2. Since $\angle A$ is the smallest angle, side $BC$, which is opposite $\angle A$, is the shortest side.

Find the missing angles:

_____**118.**

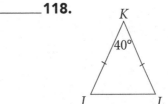

**119.**

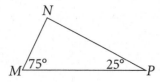

## Right Triangles

> To find the missing side of a RIGHT triangle,
> use the *Pythagorean theorem*:
> $$a^2 + b^2 = c^2$$
> (*c* is the hypotenuse)

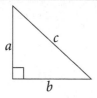

**Example:** What is the perimeter of the triangle shown below?

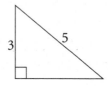

1. Since the perimeter is the sum of the lengths of the sides, we must first find the missing side. Use the Pythagorean theorem since you know this is a right triangle.

   $$a^2 + b^2 = c^2$$

2. Substitute the given sides for two of the letters. Remember: Side *c* is always the hypotenuse.

   $$3^2 + b^2 = 5^2$$
   $$9 + b^2 = 25$$

3. To solve this equation, subtract 9 from both sides:

   $$\begin{array}{rcr} -9 & & -9 \\ b^2 & = & 16 \end{array}$$

4. Then, take the square root of both sides. Thus, the missing side has a length of **4** units:

   $$\sqrt{b^2} = \sqrt{16}$$
   $$b = 4$$

5. Adding the three sides yields a perimeter of **12**: $3 + 4 + 5 = 12$

## Simplifying Radicals

Index $\overset{\text{Radical sign}}{\sqrt[3]{48}}$

Radicand

A radical is **simplified** if there is no perfect square factor of the radicand. For example, $\sqrt{10}$ is simplified because 10 has no perfect square factors. But, $\sqrt{20}$ is not simplified because 20 has a perfect square factor of 4.

In order to simplify a radical, rewrite the radical as the product of two radicals, one of which is the largest perfect square factor of the radicand. The square root of a perfect square always simplifies to a rational number. Simplify the perfect square radical to get your final answer.

**Example:** Simplify $\sqrt{50}$.

$$\sqrt{50} = \sqrt{25 \times 2} = \sqrt{25} \times \sqrt{2} = 5\sqrt{2}$$

Find the perimeter and area of each triangle (**Hint:** Use the Pythagorean theorem):

_____ **120.**

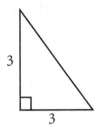

_____ **121.**

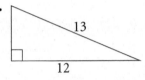

_____ **122.** Irene is fishing at the edge of a 40-foot-wide river, directly across from her friend Sam, who is fishing at the edge of the other side. Sam's friend Arthur is fishing 30 feet down the river from Sam. How far is Irene from Arthur?

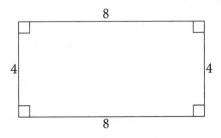

## Quadrilaterals

A quadrilateral is a four-sided polygon. Following are examples of quadrilaterals that are most likely to appear on standardized tests (and in everyday life):

**Rectangle**

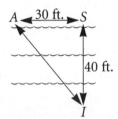

**Square**

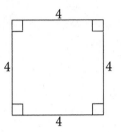

**Parallelogram**

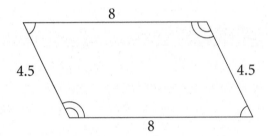

**Rhombus**

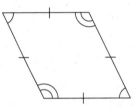

Four-sided polygon with each pair of opposite sides parallel and *all* sides congruent. A square is an example of a rhombus.

**Trapezoid**

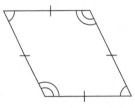

Four-sided polygon with exactly one pair of opposite sides parallel.

**Isosceles Trapezoid**

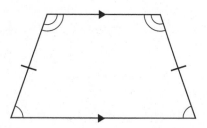

Trapezoid whose nonparallel sides are congruent. Base angles are ≅.

The quadrilaterals in the table below have something in common besides having four sides:

- Opposite sides are the same size and parallel.
- Opposite angles are the same size.

However, each quadrilateral has its own distinguishing characteristics:

| QUADRILATERALS | | | |
|---|---|---|---|
| | **RECTANGLE** | **SQUARE** | **PARALLELOGRAM** |
| **SIDES** | Adjacent sides are not necessarily the same length. | All four sides are the same length. | Adjacent sides are not necessarily the same length. |
| **ANGLES** | All the angles are right angles. | All the angles are right angles. | The opposite angles are the same size, but they don't have to be right angles. (A rectangle leaning to one side is a parallelogram.) |

The naming conventions for quadrilaterals are similar to those for triangles:

- The figure is named by the letters at its four consecutive corners, usually in clockwise order: rectangle ABCD.
- A side is named by the letters at its ends: side *AB*.
- An angle is named by its vertex letter: ∠*A*.

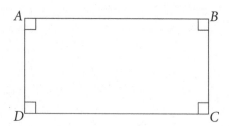

The sum of the angles of a quadrilateral is 360°:
∠*A* + ∠*B* + ∠*C* + ∠*D* = 360°

**Perimeter**

To find the perimeter of a quadrilateral, follow this simple rule:

*Perimeter = sum of all four sides*

**Shortcut:** Take advantage of the fact that the opposite sides of a rectangle and a parallelogram are equal: Just add two adjacent sides and double the sum. Similarly, multiply one side of a square by four.

Following are two word problems involving perimeters of quadrilaterals:

_____ **123.** What is the length of a side of a square
room whose perimeter is 58 feet?
- **a.** 8 ft.
- **b.** 14 ft.
- **c.** 14.5 ft.
- **d.** 29 ft.
- **e.** 232 ft.

_____ **124.** Find the dimensions of a rectangle
with perimeter of 16 feet and whose
long side is three times the length of its
short side.
- **a.** 4 ft. by 4 ft.
- **b.** 4 ft. by 12 ft.
- **c.** 3 ft. by 5 ft.
- **d.** 2 ft. by 6 ft.
- **e.** 2 ft. by 8 ft.

## Area

To find the area of a rectangle, square, or parallelogram, use this formula:

$$Area = base \times height$$

The **base** is the length of one of the sides. It is easiest if you call the side on the bottom the base, but any side can be a base. The **height** (or **altitude**) is the length of a perpendicular line drawn from the base up to the side opposite it. The height of a rectangle and a square is the same as the length of its non-base side.

### Rectangle

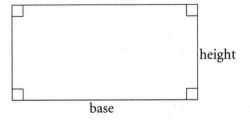

### Square

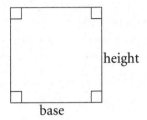

**Caution:** A parallelogram's height is not usually the same as the length of the side connecting the base to its opposite side (called the *slant height*), but the length of a perpendicular line drawn from the base to the side opposite it.

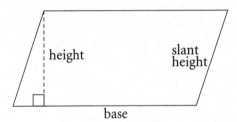

**Example:** Find the area of a rectangle with a base of 4 meters and a height of 3 meters.

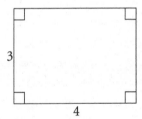

1. Draw the rectangle as close to scale as possible.
2. Label the length of the base and height.
3. Write the area formula; then substitute the base and height numbers into it:

$$A = b \times h$$
$$A = 4 \times 3 = 12$$

Thus, the area is **12 square meters.**

Now, try some area word problems:

_____ **125.** Tristan is laying 12-inch by 18-inch tiles on the laboratory floor. If the lab measures 15 feet by 18 feet, how many tiles does Tristan need, assuming there's no waste? (Hint: Do *all* your work in either feet or inches.)
   **a.** 12
   **b.** 120
   **c.** 180
   **d.** 216
   **e.** 270

_____ **126.** What is the length in feet of a rectangular parking lot that has an area of 8,400 square feet and a width of 70 feet?
   **a.** 12
   **b.** 120
   **c.** 1,200
   **d.** 4,000
   **e.** 4,130

## Circles

We can all recognize a circle when we see one, but its definition is a bit technical. A **circle** is a set of points that are all the same distance from a given point called the **center**. That distance is called the **radius**. The **diameter** is twice the length of the radius; it passes through the center of the circle.

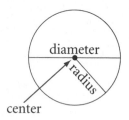

## Circumference

The **circumference** of a circle is the distance around the circle (it is the *perimeter* of the circle). To determine the circumference of a circle, use either of these two equivalent formulas:

$$Circumference = 2\pi r$$
$$or$$
$$Circumference = \pi d$$

- *r* is the radius
- *d* is the diameter (which is the same as 2*x* the radius)
- *p* is approximately equal (denoted by the symbol ≈) to 3.14 or $\frac{22}{7}$

   **Note:** Math often uses letters of the Greek alphabet, like π (pi). Perhaps that's what makes math seem like Greek to some people! In the case of the circle, you can use π as a hint to recognize a circle question: A *pie* is shaped like a circle.

   **Example:** Find the circumference of a circle whose radius is 7 inches.

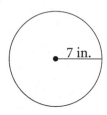

**1.** Draw this circle and write the radius version of the circumference formula (because you're given the radius):   $C = 2\pi r$
**2.** Substitute 7 for the radius:   $C = 2 \times \pi \times 7$
**3.** On a multiple-choice test, look at the answer choices o determine whether to leave π in your answer or substitute the *value of* π in the formula.

If the answer choices don't include π, substitute $\frac{22}{7}$ or 3.14 for π and multiply:

$$C = 2 \times \frac{22}{7} \times 7;$$
$$C \approx \mathbf{44}$$
$$C = 2 \times 3.14 \times 7;$$
$$C \approx \mathbf{43.96}$$

If the answer choices include π, just multiply:

$$C = 2 \times \pi \times 7;$$
$$C = \mathbf{14\pi}$$

All the answers—**44 inches, 43.96 inches,** and **14π inches**—are considered correct.

**Example:** What is the diameter of a circle with a circumference of 62.8 centimeters? Use 3.14 for π.

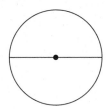

1. Draw a circle with its diameter and write the diameter version of the circumference formula (because you're asked to find the diameter): $C = \pi d$

2. Substitute 62.8 for the circumference, 3.14 for π, and solve the equation: $62.8 = 3.14 \times d$
   The diameter is **20 centimeters**. $d = \frac{62.8}{3.14} = \mathbf{20}$

These word problems require you to find the circumference:

_____ **127.** What is the circumference of a circular room whose diameter is 15 feet?
   **a.** 7.5π ft.
   **b.** 15π ft.
   **c.** 30π ft.
   **d.** 45π ft.
   **e.** 225π ft.

_____ **128.** What is the approximate circumference of a round tower whose radius is $3\frac{2}{11}$ feet?
   **a.** 10 ft.
   **b.** 20 ft.
   **c.** 33 ft.
   **d.** 40 ft.
   **e.** 48 ft.

_____ **129.** Find the circumference of a water pipe whose radius is 1.2 inches.
   **a.** 1.2π in.
   **b.** 1.44π in.
   **c.** 2.4π in.
   **d.** 12π in.
   **e.** 24π in.

## Area

The **area** of a circle is the space its surface occupies. To determine the area of a circle, use this formula:

$$\text{Area} = \pi r^2$$

**Hint:** To avoid confusing the area and circumference formulas, just remember that *area* is always measured in *square* units, like 12 *square yards* of carpeting. Thus, the *area* formula is the one with the *squared* term in it.

**Example:** Find the area of the circle at right, rounded to the nearest tenth:

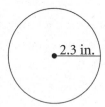

.2.3 in.

1. Write the area formula: $A = \pi r^2$
2. Substitute 2.3 for the radius: $A = \pi \times 2.3^2$
3. On a multiple-choice test, look at the answer choices to determine whether to use $\pi$ or an approximate *value* of $\pi$ (decimal or fraction) in the formula.
   If the answers don't include $\pi$, use 3.14 for $\pi$ (because the radius is a decimal):
   $A = 3.14 \times 2.3 \times 2.3$
   $\mathbf{A = 16.6}$
   If the answers include $\pi$, multiply and round:
   $A = \pi \times 2.3 \times 2.3$
   $\mathbf{A = 5.3\pi}$

Both answers—**16.6 square inches** and **5.3π square inches**—are correct.

**Example:** What is the diameter of a circle with an area of 9π square centimeters?

1. Draw a circle with its diameter (to help you remember that the question asks for the diameter); then write the area formula: $A = \pi r^2$
2. Substitute 9π for the area and solve the equation:
   $9\pi = \pi r^2$
   $9 = r^2$

Since the radius is 3 centimeters, the diameter is **6 centimeters.**   $3 = r$

Try these word problems on the area of a circle:

_____ **130.** What is the area in square inches of the bottom of a beaker with a diameter of 6 inches?
   **a.** 6π
   **b.** 9π
   **c.** 12π
   **d.** 18π
   **e.** 36π

_____ **131.** James Band is believed to be hiding within a 5-mile radius of his home. What is the approximate area, in square miles, of the region in which he may be hiding?
   **a.** 15.7
   **b.** 25
   **c.** 31.4
   **d.** 78.5
   **e.** 157

_____ **132.** If a circular parking lot covers an area of 2,826 square feet, what is the size of its radius? (Use 3.14 for π.)
   **a.** 30 ft.
   **b.** 60 ft.
   **c.** 90 ft.
   **d.** 450 ft.
   **e.** 900 ft.

# Answers to Math Practice Problems

## Word Problems

**1.** a.

**2.** e.

**3.** d.

**4.** e.

## Fractions

**5.** $\frac{1}{4}$

**6.** $\frac{2}{5}$

**7.** $\frac{3}{8}$

**8.** 10

**9.** 6

**10.** 200

**11.** $\frac{17}{12}$ or $1\frac{5}{12}$

**12.** $\frac{55}{24}$ or $2\frac{7}{24}$

**13.** $7\frac{1}{4}$

**14.** $\frac{2}{15}$

**15.** $\frac{1}{8}$

**16.** $\frac{19}{12}$ or $1\frac{7}{12}$

**17.** a.

**18.** b.

**19.** $\frac{2}{15}$

**20.** $\frac{8}{35}$

**21.** $\frac{2}{3}$

**22.** $\frac{26}{15}$ or $1\frac{11}{15}$

**23.** 15

**24.** $\frac{33}{2}$ or $16\frac{1}{2}$

**25.** c.

**26.** e.

**27.** c.

**28.** $\frac{1}{2}$

**29.** $\frac{11}{2}$ or $5\frac{1}{2}$

**30.** $\frac{1}{5}$

**31.** $\frac{45}{28}$ or $1\frac{17}{28}$

**32.** b.

**33.** d.

**34.** b.

## Decimals

**35.** $\frac{5}{1,000}$ or $\frac{1}{200}$

**36.** $3\frac{48}{100}$ or $3\frac{12}{25}$

**37.** $123\frac{456}{1,000}$ or $123\frac{57}{125}$

**38.** 4

**39.** 8.305

**40.** 0.907

**41.** 1.456

**42.** b.

**43.** d.

**44.** 0.03

**45.** 0.3392

**46.** 0.70104

**47.** e.

**48.** e.

**49.** 1.4

**50.** 128

**51.** 572

**52.** 1,400

**53.** b.

**54.** c.

## Percents

**55.** 45%

**56.** 0.8%

**57.** $16.\overline{6}$% or $16\frac{2}{3}$%

**58.** 0.12

**59.** 0.875

**60.** 2.5

**61.** 12.5% or $12\frac{1}{2}$%

**62.** 52%

**63.** $58.\overline{3}$% or $58\frac{1}{3}$%

**64.** $\frac{19}{20}$

**65.** $\frac{3}{8}$

**66.** $\frac{5}{4}$ or $1\frac{1}{4}$

**67.** $\frac{1}{4}$ or 0.25

**68.** 9.1

**69.** $37\frac{1}{2}$ or 37.5

**70.** 75

**71.** 50%

**72.** $33\frac{1}{3}$%

**73.** 300%

**74.** 100

**75.** 8

**76.** 10

**77.** c.

**78.** c.

**79.** c.

**80.** d.

## Averages
**81.** c.
**82.** c.
**83.** b.

## Length and Time
**84.** 24
**85.** 30
**86.** 1,600
**87.** 2.94
**88.** 8 ft.
**89.** 21 km 170 m
**90.** 1 ft. 4 in.
**91.** 7 cm 8 mm
**92.** d.
**93.** b.
**94.** d.

## Algebra
**95.** 7
**96.** 4
**97.** 28
**98.** 13
**99.** 8
**100.** 40
**101.** 5
**102.** −45
**103.** 16
**104.** $36\pi$
**105.** 6
**106.** $\frac{1}{2}$
**107.** 7
**108.** 16
**109.** 4

## Geometry
**110.** 122°
**111.** 20°
**112.** 60°
**113.** 91° (The horizontal lines are not parallel.)
**114.** 29 feet
**115.** 3 strips (She will have some extra.)
**116.** 12 square units
**117.** 18 square units
**118.** $\angle J = \angle L = 70°$
**119.** $\angle N = 80°$
**120.** Perimeter = $6 + 3\sqrt{2}$ units
Area = 4.5 square units
**121.** Perimeter = 30 units
Area = 30 square units
**122.** 50 feet
**123.** c.
**124.** d.
**125.** c.
**126.** b.
**127.** b.
**128.** b.
**129.** c.
**130.** b.
**131.** d.
**132.** a.

# 7 ▶ BIOLOGY REVIEW

### CHAPTER SUMMARY
This chapter reviews the key biology concepts tested by nursing school entrance exams. After surveying the important concepts and testing yourself with the sample questions in this chapter, you will know where to concentrate your studies.

## Biology Review: Important Concepts

## I. General Introduction

### A. Description of How Nursing School Entrance Exams Test Biology
All nursing school entrance exams do not measure scientific knowledge in the same way. The natural sciences section (which is comprised of chemistry, biology, and health) of the Registered Nursing School Aptitude Exam (RNSAE) and the Aptitude for Practical Nursing Exam (APNE) is made up of approximately 90 multiple-choice questions. The Nurse Entrance Test (NET) has reading comprehension questions that focus on the sciences.

### B. How to Use This Chapter
This chapter includes major biology concepts you will encounter on the exam. There is also a section on other content areas that will be helpful to you in taking the test: the scientific method, the origin of life, a brief description of taxonomic classification systems, and the social behavior of animals. The general discussions in this chapter, lists of terms and concepts, and "You Should Review" sections are meant to guide you in your studies—*they are not exhaustive* and must be supplemented with a good college textbook, a reliable medical dictionary and dictionary of biology, and a fair amount of general reading on the subject. Suggested sources of study materials are found at the end of this chapter.

After each main subject heading in this chapter, you will find several sample questions that represent the content and level of difficulty of the questions that will appear on the test. You should first read through the outline and try to answer the sample questions, and then make notes on those areas in which you need more work. After that, you will want to go to your source material and review all subject areas, with special emphasis on those areas where you feel least confident.

Allow yourself plenty of time to prepare before the exam. Remember that thorough preparation is the most important factor in test-taking success. By studying and taking practice tests, you become familiar with subject areas and typical test questions, boosting your ability to do your best on the exam.

# II. Main Topics

## A. Cell Biology

### 1. Definition of a Cell

The cell is the structural and functional unit of life. **The Cell Doctrine**, generally credited to Schleiden (1838) and Schwann (1839), maintains that:

- All living things are made up of cells and the products formed by cells.
- Cells are units of structure and function.
- All cells arise from preexisting cells.

### 2. Two Types of Cells
#### a. Prokaryotic Cells
**Prokaryotic cells:** cells found only in bacteria and archaea. These cells lack a true nucleus and organelles and have a cell wall and a cell membrane.

#### b. Eukaryotic Cells
**Eukaryotic cells:** cells found in all organisms except bacteria and archaea. These cells contain subcellular structures called organelles, including a nucleus.

### 3. Organization of a Cell
Cells contain specialized structures that each serve a specific purpose. Eukaryotes possess a nucleus and membrane-bound organelles, while prokaryotes do not.

**Nucleus:** the membrane-enclosed organelle that houses the genetic material in eukaryotic cells. Prokaryotic cells do not have a nucleus.

**Organelle:** a specialized compartment within a cell that is designed to perform a specific function. Only eukaryotes possess organelles.

**Cell membrane:** a boundary layer, made up primarily of phospholipids, that separates the cell interior from its exterior. Found in all types of cells.

**Chromosome:** a long threadlike structure, consisting of DNA and protein, that carries genes in a linear sequence and is found in the nucleus of eukaryotic cells. Humans possess 46 chromosomes. The chromosome in prokaryotes forms a circular coil known as a plasmid.

**Ribosomes:** responsible for protein assembly. The ribosome receives messenger RNA (mRNA) and translates it into proteins. Found in all types of cells.

**Cell wall:** a semi-rigid outer layer that lies outside the cell membrane and gives structural support and protection to the cell. Cell walls are found in plant, bacterial, fungal, and algal cells.

**Mitochondria:** the "power plant" of the cell. The mitochondria are responsible for generating most of the cell's energy through ATP synthesis. Found in eukaryotes.

**Chloroplasts:** the organelle responsible for photosynthesis. Chloroplasts contain machinery that allows them to extract energy from light and convert it to ATP. They also convert carbon dioxide to sugars, releasing oxygen.

**Endoplasmic reticulum:** this organelle, which creates a network of phospholipid membranes that run across a cell, can be either smooth or rough. Rough endoplasmic reticula, which have ribosomes attached to its membranes, synthesize proteins. Smooth endoplasmic reticula aid in several metabolic functions, including the synthesis of lipids and steroids, metabolism of carbohydrates, and detoxification of drugs.

**Golgi apparatus:** the organelle responsible for packaging and processing complex macro-molecules before they are transported to other parts of the cell. Found in eukaryotes.

**Lysosomes:** organelles found primarily in ani-mal cells and in some plant cells. Lysosomes are compartments that envelop and destroy waste materials within the cell.

**Vacuoles:** compartments in the cell which store and isolate various items depending on a cell's needs. These organelles are found pri-marily in plant cells but may also be observed in other organisms.

**Cilia:** finger-like projections founds in eukary-otes that primarily serve as sensors for the cell. In more complex organisms, cilia along multiple cells can also be used to transport

small particles —for example, to sweep par-ticles out of the trachea.

**Flagella:** similar to cilia, flagella are tail-like structures that protrude from the cell and are used to control the motion of the cell. Found in prokaryotes and eukaryotes.

**Centrioles:** found in animal cells, these organelles aid the process of cell division.

## 4. Energy Transformation in a Cell
### a. General Discussion of Energy

The two concepts most basic to science are **matter** and **energy**.

**Matter:** anything that has mass and takes up space (volume).

**Energy:** the capacity to do work.

There are two types of energy: **kinetic** and **potential**.

**Kinetic energy:** The energy an object possess due to its motion.

| | PROKARYOTES | EUKARYOTES | |
| --- | --- | --- | --- |
| | BACTERIA AND ARCHAEA | PLANTS | ANIMALS |
| Nucleus | | ✔ | ✔ |
| Cell Membrane | ✔ | ✔ | ✔ |
| Chromosome(s) | ✔ | ✔ | ✔ |
| Ribosomes | ✔ | ✔ | ✔ |
| Cell Wall | ✔ | ✔ | |
| Mitochondria | | ✔ | ✔ |
| Chloroplasts | | ✔ | |
| Endoplasmic reticulum | | ✔ | ✔ |
| Golgi Apparatus | | ✔ | ✔ |
| Lysosomes | | ✔ | ✔ |
| Vacuoles | | ✔ | ✔ |
| Cilia | | | ✔ |
| Flagella | ✔ | | ✔ |
| Centrioles | | ✔ | ✔ |

**Potential energy:** The energy stored in a system (e.g., in the chemical bonds of ATP or in a compressed spring).

### b. Thermodynamics

**Thermodynamics:** the physics of what is and is not possible with regard to energy.

**First law of thermodynamics:** Energy can be transferred and transformed, but it cannot be created or destroyed (conservation of energy).

**Second law of thermodynamics:** Every energy transfer or transformation results in the release of heat from the system to the rest of the universe.

### c. Cell Metabolism

**Cell metabolism:** energy management by a cell. The complex structure of a cell includes pathways along which metabolism proceeds, aided by enzymes.

**Bioenergetics:** the study of how organisms manage energy, including heat production and transfer and regulation of body temperature (endothermy and ectothermy).

**Metabolism:** the totality of chemical reactions that take place in an organism.

**Anabolism:** the metabolic synthesis of proteins, fats, etc., from simpler molecules; requires energy in the form of adenosine triphosphate (ATP).

**Catabolism:** the metabolic breakdown of molecules.

**Cellular respiration:** a catabolic pathway for the production of ATP, in which oxygen is sometimes consumed along with an organic fuel (food). At other times, the process proceeds without atmospheric oxygen, but this is less efficient.

- **Anaerobic pathway of cellular respiration:** Food (especially carbohydrates) is partially oxidized, and chemical energy is released; however, atmospheric oxygen is not involved in the process.

- **Aerobic pathway of cellular respiration:** Food is completely oxidized to carbon dioxide and water, and chemical energy is released; atmospheric oxygen is involved in the process. The Krebs cycle, electron-transport chain, and oxidative phosphorylation are important concepts here.

**Photosynthesis:** conversion of light energy into chemical energy on which, directly or indirectly, all living things depend. Photosynthesis occurs in plants, algae, and certain prokaryotes.

### d. Enzymology

**Enzymology:** the study of the speed of the process of transformation of energy in a cell; enzymes are biological catalysts that accelerate the rate of a reaction without themselves being consumed by that reaction.

### e. Movement of Molecules

Small molecules are steadily transported across the cell membrane. Types of transport include **diffusion** and **passive transport**; **osmosis** (a special case of passive transport); and **active transport**.

## 5. Cell Reproduction

### a. General Discussion of Cell Reproduction

All cells arise from other cells. The basis of all biological reproduction is cell division. A single, intact chain of life extends backward from today to the first bacteria on Earth.

Prokaryotes often reproduce by binary fission, or division into identical halves. Eukaryotes have much more complicated genomes, and therefore, their process of reproduction is more complex.

### b. The Cell Cycle

The cell cycle describes the entire reproductive life cycle of a cell and occurs in an orderly sequence. The cell cycle can be divided into interphase—

where most time is spent—and M phase—where mitosis (cell division) occurs. Each of these phases can be divided into smaller components. When not dividing or preparing to divide, the cell exists in a resting state, known as G0 phase. G0 phase follows cell division.

### c. Interphase

Interphase describes the time when the cell grows, takes in nutrients, and copies its DNA. It can be divided into three shorter phases:

- **G1 phase:** the point in the cell life cycle where most cell growth occurs, organelles are synthesized, and nutrients are collected. Only when certain safeguards are met will the cell move on to the next phase.
- **S phase:** chromosomes are replicated. During this phase, minimal RNA transcription takes place.
- **G2 phase:** the last phase before mitosis. Critical machinery is manufactured within the cell to enable cell division to occur. At the end of G2 phase, M phase begins.

### d. M phase

During M phase, the division of the nucleus and cytoplasm occurs—replication of the chromosomes is completed during the S phase of interphase.

**Mitosis:** division of the nucleus and distribution of nuclear materials, particularly chromosomes, occurs. For descriptive purposes, mitosis is divided into five phases:

- **Prophase:** DNA fibers (chromatids) condense into chromosomes, the nuclear envelope breaks down, and spindles begin to form at the poles of the cell.
- **Prometaphase:** the nuclear envelope completely dissolves; kinetochores develop on each chromosome, and microtubules spread outward from the spindles

and begin attaching to the kinetochores.

- **Metaphase:** chromosomes align at the center of the cell.
- **Anaphase:** chromosomes split, and sister chromatids separate to opposite poles of the cell.
- **Telophase:** nuclear envelope re-forms around separated sister chromatids.

**Cytokinesis:** division of the cytoplasm into two identical, separate daughter cells.

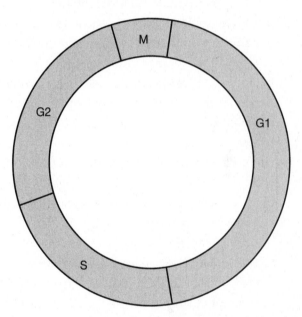

The cell cycle. The size of each segment approximates the length of time the cell spends in each phase.

### e. Control of Cell Division

A certain timing and rate of division are necessary to normal growth. Cell division can be interfered with by lack of nutrients, poisons, lack of growth factors (for example, platelet-derived growth factor, or PDGF), cell size, and density.

### f. When Things Go Wrong

In abnormal cell division (e.g., cancer), cells do not heed the restriction point in the G1 phase; they may divide excessively, invading surrounding tissue. If given enough nutrients, they may divide "forever" (see "immortal," or HeLa, cells); or abnormal cells may stop dividing at any point in the cell cycle, not just at the restriction point.

### You Should Review

- the structure and function of prokaryotic and eukaryotic cells; comparison of the two
- the composition, structure, and function of organelles: nucleus and chromosomes; ribosomes; rough endoplasmic reticulum; smooth endoplasmic reticulum; Golgi apparatus; lysosomes; vacuoles; mitochondria; chloroplasts in plants and some protists; cell wall in plants, fungi, and some protists; cilia; flagella; and centrioles.
- cell membrane structure and function
- major features of bioorganic molecules (carbohydrates, proteins, lipids, DNA, and RNA); makeup of amino acids; RNA genetic code showing base sequence
- why compartmental organization is important in eukaryotic cells, and an understanding of the way in which the various compartments interrelate— i.e., how organelles "cooperate"
- biological membranes and the importance of their selective permeability; the fluid mosaic model of cell membrane structure; structure and function of lipids, proteins, and carbohydrates
- differences between organelles of cells found in organisms in the various kingdoms
- properties of energy
- heat production and transfer mechanisms in various species; regulation of body temperature
- ATP: structure and hydrolysis; how it performs; regeneration from ADP and phosphate; metabolic disequilibrium; ATP syntheses
- metabolic map: the catabolic and anabolic pathways
- control of metabolism: feedback inhibition
- how body size affects metabolic rate
- enzymes (most of which are proteins): six major groups (oxidoreductases, transferases, hydrolases, lyases, isomerases, ligases) and the ways in which the various classes work; molecular structure;

how enzymes function as biological catalysts; types and shapes of active sites; response to environmental conditions; enzyme inhibitors
- coenzymes, especially vitamins: classifications and functions
- cellular respiration
- basic mechanisms of prokaryotic and eukaryotic cell reproduction
- the cell cycle
- how cell division is controlled
- main features of abnormal cell division
- the following terms and concepts (among others): genome, haploid nucleus, diploid nucleus, chromatin, chromosome, centriole, atrophy, karyolysis, nucleic acid (especially DNA and RNA), pyrimidines (cytosine, thymine, uracil), purines (guanine and adenine), nucleotide, transcription, translation, meiosis (not to be confused with mitosis), basal metabolic rate

## Questions

1. Most of a cell membrane's specific functions are controlled by
   a. lipids.
   b. proteins.
   c. plasma.
   d. nitrogen.

2. The basic method by which chloroplasts and mitochondria generate ATP is
   a. oxidation.
   b. photorespiration.
   c. respiration.
   d. chemiosmosis.

**3.** Which of the following regions exists just outside the nuclear membrane of most animal cells?
  **a.** the centrosome
  **b.** the equatorial plane
  **c.** the organelle
  **d.** the pellicle

**4.** The decay of a leaf after it falls from a tree indicates an increase in its
  **a.** ecological efficiency.
  **b.** entropy.
  **c.** metabolic disequilibrium.
  **d.** estivation.

**5.** Alcoholic fermentation is a form of
  **a.** anaerobic respiration.
  **b.** aerobic respiration.
  **c.** cation exchange.
  **d.** absorption.

**6.** Phagocytosis is a form of
  **a.** hydrolysis.
  **b.** exocytosis.
  **c.** glycolysis.
  **d.** endocytosis.

**7.** In the structure of cells, in which of the following organisms would one find a cell wall?
  **a.** a dog
  **b.** a fruit fly
  **c.** a tulip
  **d.** a mackerel

**8.** Which of the following is the electron acceptor in fermentation?
  **a.** pyridoxine
  **b.** pyruvate
  **c.** pyrimidine
  **d.** pyrrole

**9.** The small spherical bodies within a cell where proteins are assembled according to genetic instructions are called
  **a.** mitochondria.
  **b.** ribosomes.
  **c.** Golgi apparatus.
  **d.** lysosomes.

**10.** Metastasis refers to the
  **a.** uncontrolled division of cancer cells.
  **b.** irregularity in shape of a cancer cell.
  **c.** spread of cancer cells to sites beyond their origin.
  **d.** transformation of a normal cell into a cancer cell.

## Answers

**1. b.** Although a cell membrane's main fabric is made of lipids, its specific functions are largely determined by proteins.

**2. d.** Chemiosmosis is the term used for this process. It is important to cellular work, including ATP synthesis.

**3. a.** The centrosome (also called the microtubule-organizing center) is found in all eukaryotic cells and is important during cell division.

**4. b.** Entropy (symbol S) is the quantitative measure of a system's disorder or randomness. As systems—whether houses, people, leaves, or stars—break down and undergo irreversible changes, making less energy available to them, their entropy increases.

**5. a.** Alcoholic fermentation is the anaerobic catabolism of organic nutrients; one of its end products is ethanol.

**6. d.** Phagocytosis and pinocytosis are both forms of endocytosis, the process by which materials enter a cell without passing through the cell membrane.

**7. c.** The cell wall is one of the cell structures that helps differentiate plants and animals.

**8. b.** Pyruvate is the correct answer. Under anaerobic conditions, like fermentation, it is converted to lactate or ethanol.

**9. b.** The ribosome is the site of protein synthesis.

**10. c.** Metastasis refers to the spread of cancer cells to areas beyond their original site.

## B. Heredity

### 1. Pre-Mendelian Concepts
Before Mendel's discoveries, theories included averages or blending of colors like the mixing of paints; physical characteristics carried only by the male; characteristics carried by blood; small human grown large; pangenesis; and others.

### 2. Mendelian Inheritance
#### a. Mendel's Experiments
Gregor Mendel, the father of classical genetics, was an Austrian monk who, in a small monastery, tended a little garden and did experiments on garden peas, which have great variety. He allowed pure strains (one with purple flowers, one with white) to either self-pollinate or cross-pollinate, strictly controlling the parentage. Cross-pollinated breeds (hybrids) of purple and white flowers showed all purple flowers in the first generation. But when the second generation self-pollinated, the white trait reappeared. Through his work, the theory of dominant and recessive traits was formed.

#### b. Mendel's Major Discoveries
Mendel found that no averages or blendings took place; instead, particular characteristics, which are either dominant or recessive, were retained. Today, we know the mechanisms: genes, chromosomes, and DNA.

### 3. Chromosomal Genetics
Not all of a eukaryotic cell's genes are located on nuclear chromosomes—some are found in cytoplasmic organelles.

#### a. Genes and Chromosomes
**Gene:** a discrete heritable unit of information located on the chromosomes and made up of DNA

**Chromosome:** a long threadlike structure carrying genes in a linear sequence, found in the nucleus of eukaryotic cells and consisting of DNA (which stores or contains genetic information) and protein. Humans possess 46 chromosomes; the ovum and sperm each contain 23, of which 22 are autosomes and one is a sex chromosome.

**Chromatin:** the substance of which eukaryotic chromosomes are composed, consisting mostly of proteins, DNA, and RNA

**Chromatid:** a threadlike strand formed as a chromosome condenses during the early stages of cell division

**Character (or trait):** a heritable feature; for each character, an organism inherits two genes

**Genome:** all the genes contained in a single set of chromosomes; an organism's complete genetic material

**Autosome:** a chromosome not directly involved in determining sex

**Alleles:** alternative versions of a gene, one from each parent. The existence of alleles explains why there is variation in inherited traits. An expressed trait is determined by two alleles. A **dominant** allele is fully expressed in the organism's appearance; a **recessive** allele has no noticeable effect unless two recessive alleles are inherited, in which case, the recessive trait will be expressed. For some traits, there is incomplete dominance.

**Phenotype:** an organism's appearance; its observable, physical, and physiological traits; often depends on environment as well as genes

**Genotype:** an organism's genetic makeup (which is not always apparent); the combination of alleles it possesses

## b. Punnett Square

A **Punnett Square** is a convenient tool for determining possible genotypes and phenotypes when two organisms with known genotypes are crossed. For example, if two blue flowers with a heterozygous genotype—one dominant blue allele (B) and one recessive white allele (b)—are crossed, the offspring can have one of three genotypes with the following probabilities—BB (25%), Bb (50%), or bb (25%). There is a 75% chance the offspring will exhibit a blue phenotype.

|   | B | b |
|---|---|---|
| **B** | BB | Bb |
| **b** | Bb | bb |

## c. DNA and RNA

**DNA (deoxyribonucleic acid):** a double-stranded, helical nucleic acid molecule capable of replicating. DNA makes up the genetic material of most living organisms and plays a central role in determining heredity.

**RNA (ribonucleic acid):** a single-stranded nucleic acid molecule involved in protein synthesis, the structure of which is specified by DNA. Messenger RNA (mRNA) is responsible for carrying the genetic code transcribed from DNA to specialized sites within a cell (ribosomes) where the information is translated into a protein.

## 4. Molecular and Human Genetics
### a. Molecular Genetics

Molecular genetics is a specialized type of molecular biology that is concerned with the analysis of genes. Perhaps the most famous molecule in the world is the double-stranded helix, DNA, the substance of genes.

### b. Human Genetics

Because humans are much more complex organisms than the ones Mendel studied, and because experimental breeding of humans is socially unacceptable, study of human genetics must be done by analyzing the results of matings that have already occurred. This is done by examining the pedigree of the subjects involved—the interrelationships of parents and children across generations—and constructing a pedigree chart to study both past and future. Through the study of pedigrees, one can analyze genetic traits, from harmless (such as eye color and texture of hair) to harmful or lethal (such as the diseases discussed below). Various tests for genetic defects are also useful in the study of human genetics.

## 5. Treatment of Genetic Diseases and Genetic Engineering
### a. Genetic Diseases

Although most harmful alleles are recessive, some genetic combinations can lead to lethal conditions. Examples are Huntington's disease, Tay-Sachs disease, sickle-cell anemia, and cystic fibrosis, as well as sex-linked disorders such as hemophilia. The likelihood of two carriers of the same harmful allele mating is increased in consanguineous ("same blood") mating—i.e., mating between two close relatives (for example, siblings or first cousins). However, consanguineous mating can also lead to a concentration of favorable alleles.

In addition to simple Mendelian disorders, there are multifactorial disorders that result from effects of harmful alleles along with environmental factors—for example, heart disease, diabetes, cancer, alcoholism, schizophrenia, and bipolar disorder.

Genetic engineering (discussed next) may be important in the treatment of some genetic diseases. Already, genetic screening and counseling is being undertaken in many hospitals, using tests along with family history to compute the odds. Trait recognition is now possible through various tests, such as amniocentesis and chorionic villi sampling. Likewise, newborns can be screened for genetic disorders, most of which are untreatable, but a few of which—for example, phenylketonuria—can be treated.

### b. Genetic Engineering

Begun in the 1970s, genetic engineering is the manipulation of genes—i.e., inserting new genes into DNA, removing existing genes, or changing part of a gene. Examples are:

- The gene for human insulin has been added to a common bacterium so that the bacterium produces insulin; bacteria is grown in tanks, and the insulin is then removed for treatment of diabetes.
- Human proteins (hormones, enzymes, and other biological chemicals) made in the same manner can be used to treat hemophilia, multiple sclerosis, and other diseases that were previously untreatable.
- New genes can be introduced into farm animals to make them larger, or into plants to make them disease- or insect-resistant.

Scientists have set up regulating and ethics committees to regulate genetic engineering because of the worry that the process might set up dangerous new life forms.

## You Should Review

- Mendel's experiments with garden peas—self-pollination and cross-pollination; dominant and recessive characteristics
- meiosis versus mitosis
- the genetic basis of variation among individuals in a population
- genetic probability determined from a Punnett square
- how to use probability to determine inherited characteristics; the statistical nature of inheritance or inheritance as a game of chance; the rule of multiplication and the rule of addition
- the testcross: breeding of a recessive homozygote with an organism of dominant phenotype but unknown genotype
- inheritance patterns based on dominant and recessive alleles
- the "particulate model"—i.e., parents pass on discrete heritable units
- aneuploidy (chromosomal aberration); also, polyploidy (triploidy and tetraploidy), deletion, duplication, inversion, and translocation
- genomic imprinting
- mutation

- the Punnett square: a grid representing all possible genotypic combinations in the second generation produced by a male (gametes listed horizontally) and a female (gametes listed vertically) of the first generation
- the process of hybridization
- Mendel's Law of Segregation (named after the sorting of alleles into separate gametes)
- Mendel's Law of Independent Assortment
- segregation of genes during gamete production
- recessively inherited disorders and dominantly inherited disorders; multifactorial disorders
- Thomas Hunt Morgan's experiments with *Drosophila melanogaster* (the fruit fly)
- genetic mapping
- the process of transcribing DNA to mRNA
- discovery of the double helix by James Watson and Francis Crick and what the discovery has meant to the study of genetics
- processes of DNA replication and DNA repair
- process of protein synthesis
- the genetic code
- the basics of genetic engineering
- recombinant DNA and gene cloning
- the following terms and concepts (among others): homozygous and heterozygous; genotypic ratio; protein synthesis; transcription; translation; linked genes; crossing over; Barr body; karyotype; complete dominance, incomplete dominance, and codominance; pleiotropy; epistasis; quantitative characters; polygenetic inheritance; norm of reaction; gene sequencing; pedigree chart

## Questions

**11.** The probabilities for all possible outcomes of an event must add up to
   a. 0.1
   b. 1
   c. 10
   d. 100

**12.** When a red snapdragon is crossed with a white one, all the F1 hybrids have pink flowers. This is an example of
   a. inheritance of acquired characteristics.
   b. the blending theory of inheritance.
   c. incomplete dominance.
   d. codominance.

**13.** While doing his experiments on garden peas, Gregor Mendel was unaware of the
   a. laws of probability.
   b. statistical nature of inheritance.
   c. existence of particulate inheritance.
   d. role of chromosomes in inheritance.

**14.** Which of the following is NOT a feature of Mendel's Law of Segregation?
   a. The variation in inherited characters is caused by alternative versions of heritable factors.
   b. For each character, an organism inherits two heritable factors, one from each parent.
   c. The two heritable factors for each character segregate during gamete production.
   d. When heritable factors cannot segregate, they must be linked together and then passed on.

**15.** Sometimes, a gene at one locus on the chromosome suppresses the phenotypic expression of a gene at a different locus. This is called
   a. epistasis.
   b. meiosis.
   c. carrier recognition.
   d. consanguinity.

**16.** Traits that are alternatives to the wild type (for example, white eyes in a fruit fly as opposed to the usual red) are called
   a. point mutations.
   b. mutant phenotypes.
   c. missense mutations.
   d. frameshift mutations.

**17.** When, in the 1960s, molecular biologists performed a series of experiments that showed the amino acid translations of each of the codons of nucleic acids, they
   **a.** created a model for most later genetic studies.
   **b.** called into question an important Mendelian law.
   **c.** cracked the code of life.
   **d.** established the first link between practical and applied genetics.

**18.** Lethal recessive mutations are perpetuated by the reproduction of carriers with normal
   **a.** genotypes.
   **b.** Barr bodies.
   **c.** linked genes.
   **d.** phenotypes.

**19.** In helping determine whether a genetic disorder is present in a fetus, which of the following is an alternative to amniocentesis?
   **a.** chorionic villi sampling
   **b.** carrier recognition testing
   **c.** RFLP analysis
   **d.** use of labeled DNA probes

**20.** Which of the following is NOT a sex-linked genetic disorder?
   **a.** color-blindness
   **b.** Duchenne's muscular dystrophy
   **c.** syphilis
   **d.** hemophilia

## Answers

**11. b.** The probabilities for all possible outcomes of an event, added together, must equal 1. For example, in the toss of a two-headed coin, the probability of tossing tails is $\frac{1}{2}$ and of tossing heads $\frac{1}{2}$; in the throw of a six-sided die, the probability of rolling the number 3 is $\frac{1}{6}$, and the probability of rolling a number other than 3 is $\frac{5}{6}$.

**12. c.** Incomplete dominance is the correct answer. Characteristics acquired during an individual's lifetime (choice **a**)—for example, increased muscle mass in a runner's legs due to running—are not genetically controlled and are therefore not heritable. The blending theory of inheritance (choice **b**) was discredited by Mendel's experiments with garden peas. The blending theory would predict only pink offspring from this crossing, whereas the reality is that the red or white traits can appear in the next generation—that is, one can predict a phenotypic ratio of 1 red to 2 pink to 1 white. Codominance (choice **d**) arises when both alleles in a heterozygous organism are dominant and shown in the phenotype.

**13. d.** Until 1918, most biologists dismissed the importance of chromosomes in inheritance. Mendel died in 1884.

**14. d.** The discovery of linked heritable factors (now called genes) did not occur until after Mendel's death. The discovery was made by Bateson and Punnett of Cambridge University in 1906.

**15. a.** Epistasis (Greek for *standing still on*) is the correct answer.

**16. b.** Phenotypes are the observable physical and physiological traits of an organism. A trait alternative to the normal phenotypic character (the "wild type") is a mutant phenotype.

**17. c.** Cracking the genetic code was one of the most important steps taken in the field of molecular biology. Marshall Nirenberg, of the National Institutes of Health, deciphered the first codon in 1961.

**18. d.** Unlike lethal dominant alleles, lethal recessive alleles are masked under "normal" phenotypes in their heterozygous carriers.

**19. a.** Chorionic villi sampling is the suctioning off of a small amount of fetal tissue from the villi of the embryonic membrane. It yields more rapid results than amniocentesis, but its risks have not yet been fully assessed.

**20. c.** Syphilis is caused by infection by the bacterium *Treponema pallidum*.

## C. Structure and Function of Human Systems

### 1. Integumentary System
#### a. Definition and Structure
The integument is the outermost covering of the body and is its largest organ. It consists of the epidermis (thinner, outermost layer) and dermis (thicker, innermost layer). It also includes specialized structures, the hair and nails. Within the layers, there are also other structures. Beneath the skin is the subcutaneous tissue.

#### b. Function
The integumentary system has the following functions:

- In cooperation with the immune system, it provides protection for the body from injury, dehydration, and invasion by harmful agents such as bacteria.
- As a sense organ, it provides sensitivity to pain, temperature, and pressure.
- It aids in the regulation of body temperature.

### 2. Skeletal System
#### a. Definition and Structure
The skeleton is the chief structural system which, along with the skin, provides form and shape to the body. Comprised of 206 bones in adults, along with cartilage and ligaments, the skeletal system is rigid, yet flexible because of joints; the bones form levers that are moved by muscles. There are two types of tissue that make up bone:

- **Cortical, or compact, bone:** strong and dense skeletal tissue. It makes up the hard outer portion of bone that supports the skeletal system.
- **Cancellous, or trabecular, bone:** spongy skeletal tissue. It has a high surface area and contains many blood vessels.

There are five types of bone:

- **Long:** bones are longer than they are wide—for example, the femur, humerus, tibia, and fibia.
- **Flat:** bones form long flat plates—for example, the cranium and pelvis.
- **Short:** bones are cube-shaped, with a hard exterior and spongy interior—for example, the bones of the wrist and ankle.
- **Sesamoid:** bones are embedded in the tendons—for example, the patella (kneecap).
- **Irregular:** bones which do not fit into the aforementioned types—for example, the spine.

#### b. Function
The skeletal system has the following functions:

- It provides mechanical support.
- It protects vulnerable organs within the body.

- Along with the muscular system, it makes body movement possible.
- It stores calcium in the bones, which contain marrow for production of red and white blood cells and platelets.

## 3. Muscular System
### a. Definition and Structure

The muscular system is made up of muscle tissue in sheets or bundles of cells. Muscles can only actively contract—expansion is passive—and are attached to the skeleton, generally in pairs that work against each other. There are three major types of muscle:

- **voluntary (skeletal):** can be controlled by conscious thought—for example, the biceps.
- **involuntary (visceral, smooth):** cannot be controlled by the will—for example, the esophagus.
- **cardiac (heart muscles, striated, and smooth):** specialized and particular to the heart, contract spontaneously, and are regulated by nervous system intervention.

### b. Function

Along with the skeletal system, the muscular system is responsible for flexibility, movement, and tension.

## 4. Circulatory System
### a. Definition and Structure

The circulatory system consists of the cardiovascular and lymphatic systems: the heart; blood vessels (tubes through which blood is carried to and from the heart, including arteries, arterioles, capillaries, venules, and veins); blood; lymphatic vessels and sinuses; and lymph nodes.

### b. Function

The circulatory system distributes blood and associated chemicals throughout the body and underlies all aspects of function within the human body.

## 5. Immune System
### a. Definition and Structure

The immune system is the body's protective mechanism. It consists of the lymphatic system; the white cells of the blood and bone marrow; the thymus gland; and the outer fortress, the skin. There are two types of immunity: inherited (natural or innate) and acquired (active and passive).

The basic characteristics of the immune system include the concepts of:

- **Specificity:** the immune system's capacity to recognize and get rid of antigens—harmful pathogens and molecules—by producing lymphocytes and antibodies (specific proteins). An antigen (literally meaning "antibody-generating") can include anything "foreign" to the body, such as the molecules of viruses, bacteria, fungi, protozoans, parasitic worms, pollen, insect poison, and, unfortunately, tissue that has been transplanted from another person.
- **Diversity:** the immune system's capacity to respond to literally millions of invaders, which is due to the great variety of lymphocytes keyed to particular antigen markers.
- **Self/nonself recognition:** the immune system's ability to distinguish its own body's molecules ("self") from antigens ("nonself").
- **Memory:** the immunological system's capacity to remember formerly encountered antigens and react more quickly when exposed again—called acquired immunity. There are two kinds of acquired immunity: active, as a response by the individual's own immune system, either naturally or artificially acquired as through vaccines; and passive, as a response by antibodies transferred from one person to another—for example, a mother's passing antibodies to the fetus or the artificial introduction of antibodies from an immune animal or human.

### b. Function

The immune system protects the body from infection (invasion by pathological agents—microorganisms or viruses), diseases, and injury-causing agents.

## 6. Respiratory System
### a. Definition and Structure

The respiratory system consists of the organs responsible for the interchange of gases between body and atmosphere—the lungs (its center), the nose, pharynx, larynx, trachea, bronchi, and diaphragm.

### b. Function

The respiratory system functions to take in oxygen and eliminate carbon dioxide.

## 7. Digestive (or Gastrointestinal) System
### a. Definition and Structure

The digestive system includes the gastrointestinal tract (or alimentary canal), which is a tube with two openings, the mouth and anus, for intake of food and elimination of waste; as well as accessory structures and organs such as the teeth, tongue, liver, pancreas, and gallbladder.

### b. Function

The digestive system's function is to break down food for energy, reabsorb water and nutrients, and eliminate waste.

## 8. Renal System
### a. Definition and Structure

The renal system consists of:

- two kidneys: compact, bean-shaped organs through which blood is cycled for removal of nitrogenous waste and other substances
- the nephrons or excretory tubules contained within the kidneys
- the blood vessels that serve the kidneys
- the structures that carry waste, in the form of urine, out of the body. Urine is 95% water and 5% solids in solution, including organic constituents (urea, hippuric acid, uric acid, creatinine) and inorganic constituents (mainly salts of sodium and potassium)

### b. Function

The kidneys remove nitrogenous waste or toxic byproducts from the blood and maintain the homeostasis of blood and body fluids.

## 9. Nervous System
### a. Definition and Structure

The nervous system is one of two coordinating systems. (The other is the endocrine system, with which the nervous system interacts and cooperates.) It is made up of the nerves, brain, and sense organs for sight, sound, smell, taste, and touch. The nervous system is divided into two parts:

- the **central nervous system:** the brain and spinal cord
- the **peripheral nervous system:** the rest of the neural network—the cervical, thoracic, lumbar, and sacral nerves that branch from the spine

The brain is the nervous system's main control center and consists of three parts:

- the cerebral hemispheres, which are responsible for the higher functions, such as speech and hearing
- the cerebellum, which is responsible for subconscious activities and some balance functions
- the brain stem, which is responsible for necessary functions such as breathing and circulation

The cells of the nervous system consist of neurons and supporting cells.

### b. Function

The nervous system controls the flow of information in the body between the sensory and motor cells and organs.

## 10. Endocrine System
### a. Definition and Structure

The endocrine system is the internal system of chemical communication, involving:

- **Hormones:** substances that regulate the growth or functioning of a specific tissue or organ in a distant part of the body—for example, insulin, sex hormones, corticosteroids, adrenaline, thyroxine, and growth hormone
- the ductless glands that secrete hormones directly into the interstitial spaces: the pituitary, adrenal, thyroid, parathyroid, ovary, testis, placenta, and part of the pancreas
- the molecular receptors on or in target cells that respond to hormones

### b. Function

In concert with the nervous system, the endocrine system affects internal regulation and maintains homeostasis. Hormones affect the overall rate of metabolism and the metabolism of specific substances, growth and developmental processes, development and functioning of reproductive organs and sexual characteristics, development of higher nervous functions (for example, personality), and the ability of the body to handle stress and resist disease.

## 11. Reproductive System
### a. Definition and Structure

Reproduction is the method by which new individuals are created from existing ones. In humans, this involves two sets of organs: the internal reproductive organs and the external genitalia. Reproduction involves the fusion of two haploid gametes—the female ovum and the male spermatozoon—to form a diploid zygote.

The male reproductive system is made up of:

- the external genitalia: the scrotum and penis
- the internal reproductive organs: the gonads (testes) and hormones, accessory glands, and a set of ducts that carry sperm and glandular secretions

The female reproductive system is made up of:

- the external genitalia: the clitoris and two sets of labia
- the internal system: the fallopian tubes, ovaries, uterus, vagina, and related organs. The ovaries contain thousands of eggs. During a female's fertile years, an egg is released by one of the ovaries into the fallopian tube about once a month. If fertilization occurs, the egg attaches to the wall of the uterus and grows into a fetus.

### b. Function

The reproductive system functions to create new individuals from existing ones and propagate the species.

### c. Fertilization, Descriptive Embryology, and Developmental Mechanics

**Fertilization (syngamy):** the union of male and female gametes to form a zygote. Each gamete contains half the correct number of chromosomes; together, they form a full complement.

**Embryology:** the science that studies the development of the embryo.

The development of the human embryo occurs roughly in the second through eighth week after fertilization. During the first week, the zygote is formed and enters the uterus, where implantation occurs. In the second through eighth weeks, the embryo develops and begins to show human form. The development of the embryo occurs in the following stages:

- **Cleavage:** zygote divides to form the blastula
- **Gastrulation:** cells become arranged into three primary germ layers

■ **Organogenesis or organogeny:** further cell division and differentiation results in the formation of organs

At this point, we refer to the growing organism as a fetus. Over nine months, the human fetus develops until it comprises all the organs necessary for life outside the womb.

## You Should Review

- the structure of the skin, including sweat pores, high and low temperature receptors, pain receptors, papillary region, hair and hair follicles, sebaceous glands, arrector pili, Meissner's corpuscle, stratum corneum, stratum granulosum, Malpighian layer, sweat glands and sweat ducts, blood capillaries, the Pacinian corpuscles (pressure receptors), sensory nerves, adipose (fat) tissue
- the way the skin functions in the immune system
- the main parts of the skeleton and a little about their individual functions, including the cranium and its parts, and the mandible, sternum, clavicle, rib cage, vertebrae, carpals, metacarpals, phalanges, femur, patella, tibia, fibula, metatarsals, tarsals, phalanges, scapula, humerus, iliac crest, ulna, radius, pelvis, coccyx, ischium
- the synovial joints and their structure and function: the ball-and-socket, ellipsoidal, gliding, hinged, pivot, saddle, sutures/immovable joints
- the way bones, muscle, and cartilage work together to support weight and enable movement
- axial versus appendicular skeletal components
- the location, size, and shape of the main muscle groups, their action, origin, insertion, and innervation (You needn't memorize all—there are about 700 of them!)
- the structure and action of a voluntary muscle: the tendon, epimysium, bundle of muscle fibers, nucleus, single muscle fiber, and myofibril (light band, dark band, sarcomere unit containing contractile proteins); flexor versus extensor muscles

- the structure and action of an involuntary muscle; location is in the skin, around hair follicles, and in the internal organs (digestive tract, respiratory tract, urogenital tract, and circulatory system); the way an involuntary muscle is supplied by the autonomic nervous system; its composition of fusiform or spindle-shaped cells without striations
- the structure and function of the cardiac muscle: for example, Purkinje fibers; intercalated discs; pacemaker channels; action of the vagus nerve to produce bradycardia; action of cholinergic stimulation to increase blood pressure and heart rate
- the structures of the heart; how the cardiac muscle works; how blood circulates; and names of major blood vessels and lymphatic vessels
- the makeup of blood: (1) plasma—90% water; also contains fibrinogen (plasma protein to help clotting), inorganic ions, dissolved gases (for example, oxygen and carbon dioxide), organic nutrients (amino acids and fats), hormones, antibodies, enzymes, and waste materials (for example, uric acid and urea); (2) erythrocytes (red blood cells); (3) leukocytes and phagocytes (white blood cells); and (4) platelets. You should become familiar with what each type of blood cell does.
- the makeup of lymph (called tissue fluid in the intercellular spaces): alkaline, colorless (or yellowish or milky), and consisting mostly of water; also contains (1) proteins (serum albumin, serum globulin, serum fibrinogen); (2) salts; and (3) organic substances (urea, creatinine, neutral fats, glucose). You should become familiar with what each component contributes.
- general facts about blood groups, blood banks, tissue and organ transplants
- general facts about blood types/antigens (for example, ABO, Rh factor) and blood transfusion; why blood typing is important
- some common blood disorders: for example, various kinds of anemia, hemophilia, leukemia, polycythemia, or thrombosis

- basics of homeostasis: acids, bases, normal blood pH, fluid and electrolyte balance
- the basic characteristics of the immune system
- characteristics and importance of B cells and T cells (the two main classes of lymphocytes) and their antigen receptors; the central role of T cells—cytotoxic or killer T cells and helper T cells
- the molecular basis of antigen-antibody specificity
- the nature of antibodies (a class of proteins called immunoglobulins or Igs—includes IgM, IgG, IgA, IgD, and IgE) and how they work in the human body
- the cellular basis for specificity and diversity
- the humoral response and activation of B cells; T-dependent and T-independent antigens
- the main immune disorders—autoimmune diseases, immunodeficiency, especially AIDS (acquired immunodeficiency syndrome) and HIV—and their treatment
- the following terms and concepts related to the immune system (among others): humoral immunity, cell-mediated immunity, effector cells, plasma cells, clonal selection, primary and secondary immune responses, memory cells, self-tolerance, cytokines (for example, interleukin-1 and -2), interferon
- the organs of respiration (especially the lungs) and their specific structures and functions
- how breathing is controlled (nerves in the breathing center)
- gas exchange in humans
- the following terms and concepts related to the respiratory system (among others): oxygen transport and carbon dioxide transport, negative pressure breathing, tidal volume, volume capacity, residual volume
- major structures of the digestive system and the function of each: oral cavity, esophagus, diaphragm, liver, gallbladder, stomach, pancreas, spleen, large intestine (colon), small intestine, cecum, sigmoid colon, appendix, rectum, anus. The alimentary canal and accessory organs—the salivary glands (saliva, salivary amylase), pancreas, liver, and gallbladder—and their functions
- the various sphincters and the mechanism of peristalsis
- the function and composition of gastric juices (for example, pepsin/pepsinogen, hydrochloric acid), zymogens, gastrin, acid chyme
- hormones and enzymes involved in the digestive process
- how digestive secretions are regulated
- absorption and distribution of nutrients—the villi, microvilli, lacteal, chylomicrons, lipoproteins, capillaries, and hepatic portal vein leading to the liver
- the process of elimination of waste
- the structure and function of the renal system, especially the kidneys (collecting duct, cortex, medulla, glomeruli, Bowman's capsule, loop of Henle, and others) and the renin-angiotensin-aldosterone axis
- renal fluid composition
- concepts of pressure gradients, diffusion, osmosis, active transport, filtration, concentration, diuresis
- the nervous system and functions of its main parts—for example, the spinal cord and its regions (cervical, thoracic, lumbar, sacral); and nerves (ulnar, median, radial, cauda equina, sciatic, femoral, saphenous, vagus)
- the brain and functions of main parts—frontal lobe, temporal lobe, parietal lobe, occipital lobe, cerebellum, brain stem
- the various areas of control in the brain—for example, the voluntary motor area, frontal lobe, speech center, olfactory area, somatic sensory area, visual area, cerebellum, auditory area
- the cells of the nervous system, i.e., the neurons and supporting cells
- neurons—cell body, dendrites, axons, Schwann's cells, myelin sheath (covers the axons of nerve cells, composed of lipids and proteins), synaptic terminals, synapses. The three kinds of neurons: sensory neurons, motor neurons, and interneurons

- supporting cells (glial cells—meaning "glue cells")—for example, in the central nervous system, astrocytes (which contribute to the blood-brain barrier) and oligodendrocytes; in the peripheral nervous system, Schwann cells
- how electrical signals are transmitted along a neuron
- the origin of electrical membrane potential
- the endocrine glands: hypophysis/pituitary, parathyroid, thyroid, suprarenal/adrenal glands, islet of Langerhans in the pancreas, and gonads (ovaries/testes)
- the hormones (chemical signals transmitted throughout the body via the circulatory system; act upon body structures more or less distant) and their target cells
- the three general classes of hormones based on chemical structure: (1) steroid hormones, including sex hormones; (2) amino acid derivatives, generally from tyrosine, which include epinephrine/adrenaline, the "fight or flight" hormone; and (3) peptides, the most diverse class, which includes insulin
- the hormone receptors
- the male and female reproductive structures and functions
- the hormonal control of human reproduction: (1) in males, androgens, especially testosterone; (2) in females, the menstrual cycle, consisting of menstrual flow phase, proliferative phase, secretory phase; and the ovarian cycle, consisting of the follicular phase/ovulation and the luteal phase, hormones, in particular, estrogen, progesterone, and oxytocin
- spermatogenesis and oogenesis
- the main aspects of fertilization, embryo formation, and development from zygote to fetus
- the three trimesters of pregnancy

# Questions

21. Which of the following is one of the functions of Meissner's corpuscles?
    a. to detect light touch
    b. to detect pain
    c. to detect heat
    d. to detect cold

22. Which of the following structures is part of the axial skeleton?
    a. the bones of the limbs
    b. the pectoral girdle
    c. the pelvic girdle
    d. the skull

23. Repetitive muscle contraction depends upon a phosphate group being added to ADP by
    a. phosphagens.
    b. phosphorylases.
    c. phospholipids.
    d. phosphokinase.

24. The inner layer of squamous cells that lines the blood vessels is called the
    a. endoderm.
    b. endothelium.
    c. endometrium.
    d. endomembrane.

25. Which of the following aspects of the immune system is responsible for the rejection of organ transplants?
    a. phagocytosis
    b. the formation of antibodies
    c. the major histocompatibility complex
    d. the activation of B cells

**26.** The enzyme that hydrolyzes protein in the digestive system is called
   **a.** erepsin.
   **b.** steapsin.
   **c.** ptyalin.
   **d.** pepsin.

**27.** The process of inhaling air begins with stimulation of the diaphragm by the
   **a.** phrenic nerve.
   **b.** trigeminal nerve.
   **c.** pressor nerve.
   **d.** splanchnic nerve.

**28.** Which of the following is a disorder of body fluids common in renal disease?
   **a.** acidocytosis
   **b.** phagocytosis
   **c.** acidosis
   **d.** polyposis

**29.** Much of typically human emotion is thought to rely on interactions between the cerebral cortex and the
   **a.** hindbrain.
   **b.** R-complex.
   **c.** corpus callosum.
   **d.** limbic system.

**30.** The area of the brain that integrates endocrine and neural functions is the
   **a.** hippocampus.
   **b.** gyrus.
   **c.** hypothalamus.
   **d.** pons.

**31.** LH and FSH are both
   **a.** pituitary gonadotropins.
   **b.** placental hormones.
   **c.** steroids.
   **d.** androgens.

**32.** Which of the following structures is partially responsible for the fact that a mother does not reject the embryo as a foreign body, as she would a tissue or organ graft?
   **a.** the endometrium
   **b.** the erythroblast
   **c.** the placenta
   **d.** the trophoblast

# Answers

**21. a.** Meissner's corpuscles, which lie relatively close to the surface of the skin, detect light touch.

**22. d.** The vertebrate frame has two parts, the axial skeleton and the appendicular skeleton. The skull, vertebral column, and rib cage make up the axial skeleton. The other answer choices make up the appendicular skeleton.

**23. a.** Phosphagens are high-energy phosphate compounds found in animal tissues that supply a phosphate group to ADP to make ATP.

**24. b.** Endothelium is the correct answer. The other choices relate to systems other than the human circulatory system.

**25. c.** The major histocompatibility complex is part of the cell-mediated response system. Choice **a**, phagocytosis, is involved in the inflammatory response; choices **b** and **d** are part of the humoral immune response system.

**26. d.** Pepsin is the chief enzyme found in gastric juice and is responsible for hydrolyzing protein. Choices **a**, **b**, and **c** are enzymes present in intestinal juice, pancreatic juice, and saliva, respectively.

**27. a.** The phrenic nerve arises in the cervical plexus, enters the thorax, and passes into the diaphragm. Choices **b**, **c**, and **d** are involved in processes of nonrespiratory organs.

**28. c.** Acidosis is the excess acidity of body fluids found in renal disease and diabetes.

**29. d.** The limbic system is that area of the human brain midway between the R-complex and the neocortex in both locale and evolutionary age. It is thought to play a major role in the generation of strong, vivid emotions. Some scientists believe that the beginnings of altruistic behavior are to be found in the limbic system.

**30. c.** The hypothalamus initiates endocrine signals after receiving information about the environment from the peripheral nerves and other parts of the brain.

**31. a.** LH (luteinizing hormone) and FSH (follicle-stimulating hormone) are pituitary gonadotropins, which are hormones whose levels affect oogenesis and spermatogenesis.

**32. d.** The trophoblast is a barrier that prevents the embryo from coming into contact with maternal tissue.

## D. Bacteria and Viruses

### 1. Definitions
#### a. Viruses

**Viruses:** the simplest of all genetic systems, infectious particles the largest of which can barely be seen with a light microscope

Viruses hover between life and nonlife, being either very complex molecules or very simple life forms. They lack the structure and most of the equipment of cells and enzymes for metabolism; they are merely aggregates of nucleic acids and proteins—cores of nucleic acid packaged in protein coats called *capsids*. Some also bear an outer envelope of proteins and lipids. Viruses are parasites of animals, plants, and some bacteria, and can only metabolize and reproduce within a living host cell. The discovery of viruses began with the German scientist Adolf Mayer in 1883; however, most of the research conducted with viruses has been done in the last twenty years.

**Structure:** nucleic acid coated with a shell of protein called a capsid, and sometimes a membranous envelope (shell of protein and lipids) coating the capsid. The envelope may help the virus enter the host cell. Whereas other genes are made of double-stranded DNA, genomes of a virus may consist of double-stranded DNA or single-stranded DNA (in DNA viruses), or double-stranded RNA or single-stranded RNA (in RNA viruses).

### b. Bacteria

**Bacteria:** unicellular organisms—prokaryotes—with no true nucleus

Bacteria are classified into two groups, gram-positive and gram-negative, based on differences in cell wall composition detected by Gram's staining. Gram-negative bacteria are more dangerous to other life forms than Gram-positive bacteria due to endotoxins in the outer membrane of the Gram-negative cell wall. Bacteria are extremely adaptable with regard to their physiological adjustment to changes in the environment. They are the principal decomposers of most ecosystems. Bacteria were discovered by the Dutch inventor of the microscope, Antoni van Leeuwenhoek (1632–1723).

### 2. Structure, Shapes, Metabolism, and Life Cycle of Bacteria
#### a. Structure
The bacterial genome is mainly a single double-stranded DNA molecule (plasmid). Prokaryotes lack membrane-enclosed organelles. (See Section A of this chapter for more detail.)

### b. Shapes and Metabolic Requirements
Bacteria are initially grouped according to:

- **Shape:** Bacteria can be placed into three groups: cocci, with a spherical shape; bacilli, with a rod-like shape; and spirilla, with a spiral shape.

- **Metabolic requirements:** Bacteria are further classified as to, for example, whether they require oxygen.
  - **Aerobic bacteria** require oxygen.
  - **Anaerobic bacteria** do not require oxygen

Bacteria have greater metabolic diversity than all eukaryotes combined. With regard to procurement of energy and carbon, they fall into four categories:

- **Photoautotrophs** harness light energy for the synthesis of organic compounds from carbon dioxide—for example, cyanobacteria (formerly called blue-green algae).
- **Photoheterotrophs** use light to generate ATP but can get carbon only in organic form (i.e., not from $CO_2$).
- **Chemoautotrophs** obtain energy by oxidizing inorganic substances, although they need only $CO_2$ as source of carbon—for example, *Sulfolobus*, which oxidizes sulfur.
- **Chemoheterotrophs** use organic molecules for both energy and carbon—the majority of bacteria are in this category.

Bacteria also vary in the effect oxygen has on metabolism (obligate aerobes, facultative anaerobes, obligate anaerobes) and in nitrogen metabolism.

### c. Life Cycle
In their life cycle, bacteria do not undergo mitosis or meiosis, although they may undergo genetic recombination by three mechanisms: transformation, conjugation, and transduction. Instead, they reproduce by binary fission, with each daughter cell receiving a copy of the single parental chromosome. Bacteria are exceptionally resistant to environmental destruction; some cannot even be killed by boiling water, and endospores may remain dormant for centuries. Unchecked by unfavorable environmental conditions, their growth is geometric. Generation times are usually one to three hours, but some species may double every 20 minutes.

### 3. Classification of Bacteria

Bacteria used to be classified as plants; however, prokaryotes and plants have a completely different molecular composition. Instead of cellulose, bacterial walls are composed of peptidoglycan, which consists of polymers of modified sugars cross linked by short polypeptides that vary according to species. Classification of bacteria is still in flux.

#### a. Kingdom Archaea

Archaebacteria may be descendants of the earliest forms of life. They include methanogens, extreme halophiles, and thermoacidophiles.

#### b. Kingdom Bacteria

Eubacteria (or "true" bacteria) are sometimes said to belong to the order Schizomycetes, although, as noted previously, classification of bacteria is in flux. Eubacteria include, among others, actinomycetes (e.g., *Mycobacterium*), chemoautotrophic bacteria (e.g., *Nitrobacter*), cyanobacteria (e.g., *Chroococcus*), endospore-forming bacteria (e.g., *Bacillus*), enteric bacteria (e.g., *Escherichia*), mycoplasmas (e.g., *Mycoplasma*), myxobacteria (e.g., *Myxococcus*), nitrogen-fixing aerobic bacteria (e.g., *Azotobacter*), pseudomonads (e.g., *Pseudomonas*), rickettsias and chlamydias (e.g., *Rickettsia* and *Chlamydia*), and spirochetes (e.g., *Borrelia*).

### 4. Diseases
#### a. Viral Diseases

Not all viruses are disease-causing; many viruses do no apparent harm. Diseases caused by viruses include the common cold, influenza, AIDS, herpes, viral pneumonia, meningitis, hepatitis, polio, rabies in animals, and tobacco mosaic disease in plants. Types of viruses include adenovirus, arbovirus, herpesvirus, human immunodeficiency virus (HIV, the retrovirus that causes AIDS), myxovirus, papillomavirus, picornavirus, poxvirus, retrovirus, and (in plants) the tobacco mosaic virus.

Bacterial viruses are called *bacteriophages*, or simply *phages*, and include, among many others, seven that infect *Escherichia coli*.

#### b. Bacterial Diseases

Approximately half of all human diseases are caused by bacteria; they may be intruders from outside or opportunistic—that is, they live inside the body of a healthy host, becoming destructive only when the host's defenses are weakened. Pathogenic bacteria can disrupt the physiology of the host by growing inside and invading the tissues. Others exude poisons that are one of two types: exotoxins or endotoxins. (See Mechanisms of Infection/*Bacteria*.)

Examples of diseases caused by bacteria include pneumonia, caused by the bacterium *Streptococcus pneumoniae*; tuberculosis, caused by the bacterium *Mycobacterium tuberculosis*, which destroys parts of the lung tissue and is spread through inhalation and exhalation; syphilis, caused by the bacterium *Treponema pallidum*; and many others.

*Escherichia coli* is a well-known bacterium. Most *E. coli* are harmless, while some can cause serious food poisoning. *E. coli* is widely used in laboratory experiments and biotechnology.

### 5. Mechanisms of Infection
#### a. Viruses

Lock-and-key fit is the method by which viruses identify their host. Some viruses can infect several species, like the swine flu virus and the rabies virus, and some can infect only a single species, like the human cold virus and HIV. Some viruses depend on coinfection by other viruses. The host range is the range of host cells a particular type of virus can infect.

- **Lytic cycle:** the reproductive cycle of virulent viruses that ends in the death of the host
- **Lysogenic cycle:** the reproductive cycle of temperate viruses, which coexist with the host rather than killing it
- **Vaccines:** variants or derivatives of pathogenic microbes that help the cell defend against

infection (e.g., polio, rubella, measles, and mumps). There is little that can be done to cure a viral infection once it begins, as antibiotics are powerless; however, many new antiviral agents have been developed in recent years.

### b. Bacteria

One mechanism of infection is growing and invading tissues. Bacteria that use this mechanism include rickettsias that cause Rocky Mountain spotted fever and typhus, and actinomycetes that cause tuberculosis and leprosy. Others produce toxins of two types:

- **Exotoxins:** proteins secreted by the bacterial cell; examples are *Clostridium botulinum*, which causes the often fatal disease botulism, and *Vibrio cholerae*, which causes cholera.
- **Endotoxins:** not secreted by the bacterium, but are merely components of its outer membrane; examples are the various species of *Salmonella*, which cause food poisoning, and *Salmonella typhi*, which causes typhoid fever.

Many bacteria are harmless or even beneficial; they have certainly had wide-ranging benefits to humankind. From bacteria, we have learned much about metabolism and molecular biology. Methanogens are used for sewage treatment by aerating sewage. Some soil species of pseudomonads are used to decompose pesticides and certain harmful synthetic substances. Bacteria are used to make vitamins, antibiotics, and certain foods—e.g., to convert milk to yogurt and some types of cheese.

Whether destructive or beneficial, bacteria do not act alone but often form relationships with other bacteria species and organisms from other kingdoms through symbiosis, which means "living together"—if one symbiont is larger than another, it is known as the host. There are three categories of symbiotic relationships:

- **Mutualism:** both symbionts benefit
- **Commensalism:** one symbiont receives benefits while neither harming nor helping the other
- **Parasitism:** one symbiont benefits but harms the host

### You Should Review

- the structure and evolutionary origin of viruses
- reproduction mechanism of viruses
- plant viruses and viroids (even simpler pathogens than viruses)
- characteristics of the two kinds of virus, DNA and RNA
- Gram's staining
- metabolic processes of prokaryotes
- nutritional needs of prokaryotes: Some are very specific in their needs (for example, *Lactobacillus* needs all 20 amino acids, several vitamins, and various organic compounds); some are not specific (for example, *E. coli* can grow on a medium containing glucose or a substitute for glucose as the only organic component).
- process of nitrogen fixation
- kinds of chemoheterotrophic bacteria—for example, saprophytes (decomposers) and parasites; there are no known present-day phagotrophic bacteria
- life cycle of bacteria
- reproductive process of binary fission
- the various diseases caused by viruses and bacteria
- Koch's postulates
- the reproductive cycle of the HIV virus
- the lytic cycle and defense mechanisms of certain bacteria against certain phages (e.g., restriction enzymes)
- the many variations of viral infection among animal viruses, especially viruses with envelopes and viruses with RNA genomes, and the reproductive cycle of each
- retroviruses; reverse transcriptase

- viruses and cancer; tumor viruses: HIV (the AIDS-causing virus)
- the main groups of bacteria and kinds of bacteria in these groups
- sizes of various bacteria, along with motility; capsules; spores; reproduction; colony formation; food, oxygen, and temperature requirements; and activities (enzyme production, toxin production, etc.)

# Questions

**33.** Which of the following is NOT a reason gram-negative bacteria are more threatening to other life forms than gram-positive bacteria are?
   **a.** The lipopolysaccharides on the walls of gram-negative bacteria are often toxic.
   **b.** The outer membrane provides protection for gram-negative bacteria against the defenses of their hosts.
   **c.** Gram-negative bacteria are more resistant to antibiotics than are gram-positive bacteria.
   **d.** Gram-negative bacteria cause hemolysis of blood, whereas gram-positive bacteria do not.

**34.** Which of the following is NOT a factor differentiating bacteria and viruses?
   **a.** Bacteria are susceptible to antibiotics, whereas viruses are not.
   **b.** The mechanism of replication is different in bacteria than in viruses.
   **c.** Unlike viruses, bacteria are true cells.
   **d.** Bacteria are often parasitic, whereas viruses cannot be.

**35.** The resistant cells some bacteria form to resist environmental destruction are called
   **a.** endospores.
   **b.** coenocytes.
   **c.** coenobia.
   **d.** endosomes.

**36.** If one member of an isolated bacterial colony is found to be genetically different from the rest, which of the following is the most likely explanation?
   **a.** Mitosis has taken place.
   **b.** Mutation has taken place.
   **c.** Sexual reproduction has taken place.
   **d.** Cloning has taken place.

**37.** Which of the following groups of microorganisms is an example of an obligate anaerobe?
   **a.** methanogens
   **b.** cyanobacteria
   **c.** chemoautotrophs
   **d.** chemoheterotrophs

**38.** The ability, possessed by certain bacteria, to assimilate atmospheric nitrogen into nitrogenous compounds that can be used by plants is called nitrogen
   **a.** production.
   **b.** fixation.
   **c.** cycling.
   **d.** equilibrium.

**39.** Which of the following microorganisms encodes the enzyme reverse transcriptase?
   **a.** the ECHO virus
   **b.** the masked virus
   **c.** the HIV virus
   **d.** the attenuated virus

**40.** Which of the following is a kind of movement of which certain bacteria are capable?
   **a.** chemotaxis
   **b.** chemosmosis
   **c.** chemosynthesis
   **d.** chemylosis

**41.** Destruction of bacteria by a lytic agent is called
   **a.** bacteriogenesis.
   **b.** bacteriophagia.
   **c.** bacteremia.
   **d.** bacteriostasis.

**42.** The discovery of the virus began with German scientist Adolf Mayer and occurred while he was seeking the cause of
   **a.** Rocky Mountain spotted fever.
   **b.** rabies.
   **c.** tobacco mosaic disease.
   **d.** fungal blight.

## Answers

**33. d.** Some gram-positive bacteria do cause hemolysis—for example, the very common *Streptococcus*.

**34. d.** Viruses are parasites, often even of bacteria.

**35. a.** The resistant cells, called endospores, can survive almost anything, including boiling water, lack of nutrients or water, and most poisons.

**36. b.** Since bacteria reproduce asexually by binary fission, generally in an isolated colony all will be genetically identical. Differences in offspring in an isolated colony can, however, be caused by mutation. Neither mitosis nor sexual reproduction (choices **a** and **c**) take place in bacteria; cloning (choice **d**) produces genetically identical individuals.

**37. a.** Methanogens produce methane and are obligate, or strict, anaerobes found in oxygen-deficient environments such as marshes, swamps, sludge, and the digestive systems of ruminants (such as cows).

**38. b.** Nitrogen fixation is important to the nutrition of plants and can only be performed by certain bacteria. In terms of nutrition, this ability makes cyanobacteria the most self-sufficient organisms on Earth.

**39. c.** The retrovirus HIV encodes the enzyme reverse transcriptase, which uses RNA as a template for DNA synthesis.

**40. a.** The word *chemotaxis* is derived from the Greek *chemeia* (chemistry) + *taxis* (arrangement). Positive chemotaxis is the moving toward a chemical; negative chemotaxis is the moving away from a chemical.

**41. b.** Bacteriophages are viruses that are parasitic to bacteria. The lytic cycle of a bacteriophage culminates in the death of the host.

**42.** **c.** Mayer noted that tobacco mosaic disease was contagious, but he could find no microbe in the infectious sap. He concluded that the causal agent was a bacterium too small to be seen with a microscope. Only later were scientists able to discern the characteristics that set viruses apart from bacteria.

## E. Plants

### 1. Distinction between Plants and Animals

Plants are multicellular eukaryotes that are nearly all terrestrial in origin, though some have evolved so that they can live in water. They differ from animals in structure, life cycle, and modes of nutrition and are the mainstay of most ecosystems on Earth. They draw their energy directly from sunlight and directly or indirectly feed the rest of the creatures on Earth, including animals; without them, most ecosystems would simply die. They are autotrophic in nutrition, making food by photosynthesis, or the conversion of light energy into chemical energy, a property they share with algae and certain prokaryotes.

### 2. Photosynthesis
#### a. Definition

**Photosynthesis:** the process by which light energy, captured by the chloroplasts of plants, is converted to chemical energy.

#### b. Process

Plants are equipped with the light-absorbing molecules chlorophyll a and chlorophyll b and certain carotenoid pigments that are necessary in order to collect maximum energy from the sun.

### 3. Cellular Anatomy

The cell walls of plants consist mostly of cellulose, and they store food in the form of starch. See Section A of this chapter for more on the structure of plant cells.

### 4. Nutritional Requirements

In order to live, plants require both macronutrients (nutrients required in large quantities), including carbon, oxygen, hydrogen, nitrogen, sulfur, phosphorus, calcium, potassium, and magnesium; and micronutrients (nutrients required in smaller quantities), including iron, chlorine, copper, manganese, zinc, molybdenum, boron, and nickel. Fixed nitrogen is important to all aspects of a plant's life cycle.

### 5. Structure and Function

Plants are classified as either nonvascular or vascular.

#### a. Nonvascular Plants

Nonvascular plants have simpler tissues than vascular plants. They are covered by a waxy cuticle to prevent dehydration, require water to reproduce, and lack woody tissue and so do not grow tall but rather grow in mats low to the ground. The nonvascular plants include mosses, liverworts, and hornworts.

#### b. Vascular Plants

Vascular plants have much more elaborate tissues, including vascular tissue; cells are joined into tubes for transport of nutrients and water throughout the plant. There are two types of vascular tissue: phloem, which transports sugars from leaves to other parts of the plant, and xylem, which transports water and dissolved mineral nutrients from roots to other parts of the plant. Vascular plants are of two types: seedless, including horsetails and ferns, and seed plants. Seed plants in turn fall into two categories:

- **Gymnosperms:** seeds are uncovered; plants achieve fertilization mainly through wind-borne pollen. This category includes conifers like pines, firs, and spruce; and cycads.
- **Angiosperms:** flowering plants such as garden and wild flowers and hardwood trees; the dominant plant form today (about 235,000 species). Angiosperms have the most advanced structural form; seeds are enclosed

in carpels; animals and insects are employed for transfer of pollen in order to achieve fertilization. Important structures of flowering plants include its flower, which is the reproductive structure (includes the stamen, with filament and anthers, petals, pistil with its stigma, style, ovary, and sepal); and the fruit, which is the structure formed from the ovary of a flower, usually after ovules have been fertilized, and which protects dormant seeds and aids dispersal.

## 6. Reproduction and Development

Some plants reproduce sexually; seeded plants hold an egg, which, after the plant matures, is fertilized by pollen from itself or another plant. Others reproduce asexually by cloning; bulbs, feelers, and rhizomes require only one plant; there is no change in the chromosome number, and the offspring is exactly the same genetically as the parent.

### You Should Review
- the process of photosynthesis
- plant cellular anatomy
- main characteristics of nonvascular and vascular plants
- plant morphology and anatomy, especially of flowering plants
- the processes of sexual and asexual reproduction in plants
- division of plants into monoecious plants (have both male and female reproductive organs in the same flower) and dioecious plants (have either male or female reproductive organs in separate flowers)
- symbiotic relationships that exist between certain plants and animals
- the various types of plants cells—for example, parenchyma cells, collenchyma cells, sclerenchyma cells, water-conducting cells, food-conducting cells

- the transport systems of plants
- plant hormones
- the following concepts and terms (among others): autotrophic nutrition; photoautotrophy; light reactions; the Calvin cycle; nitrogen fixation; dermal, vascular, and ground tissue systems; sporophyte and gametophyte

## Questions

**43.** The sticky tip of the carpel of a flower, which receives the pollen, is called the
a. stigma.
b. filament.
c. anther.
d. style.

**44.** The Calvin cycle is one of the two stages of plant
a. germination.
b. photoperiodism.
c. photosynthesis.
d. flowering.

**45.** A representation of the most recent evolutionary stage of plants is
a. the cypress tree.
b. the orchid.
c. the ostrich fern.
d. the liverwort.

**46.** The European butterwort, sundew, and pitcher plant are examples of plants that are
a. medicinal.
b. poisonous.
c. parasitic.
d. carnivorous.

**47.** The term *morphogenesis*, an area particularly important in plant development, refers to the development of an organism's
   **a.** external form.
   **b.** reproductive organs.
   **c.** cytoskeleton.
   **d.** nutritional uptake system.

**48.** The orientation of a plant toward or away from light is called
   **a.** photogenesis.
   **b.** phototropism.
   **c.** photosynthesis.
   **d.** photoautotrophism.

**49.** Which of the following could be called a plant "antiaging hormone"?
   **a.** cytokinin
   **b.** gibberellin
   **c.** auxin
   **d.** florigen

**50.** The major sites of photosynthesis in most plants are the
   **a.** stems.
   **b.** seeds.
   **c.** leaves.
   **d.** taproots.

**51.** The least specialized of all plant cells are the
   **a.** sclerenchyma cells.
   **b.** water-conducting cells.
   **c.** food-conducting cells.
   **d.** parenchyma cells.

**52.** Angiosperms respond physiologically to day length by flowering. This response is called
   **a.** the circadian rhythm.
   **b.** day-neutrality.
   **c.** photoperiodism.
   **d.** vernalization.

## Answers

**43. a.** The stigma, located on the carpel, is the reproductive organ of a flower that receives pollen.

**44. c.** Photosynthesis consists of two stages: light reactions and the Calvin cycle.

**45. b.** The orchid is an angiosperm, a type of flowering plant. Flowering plants came into existence about 140 to 125 million years ago. The other choices are all considerably older.

**46. d.** All these plants are carnivorous, supplementing their nutrition (usually in nutrient-poor habitats such as acid bogs) by feeding on insects.

**47. a.** The term *morphogenesis* is related to the term morphology, which is the study of the external structure of an organism.

**48. b.** Phototropism (*photo* means light and *tropos* means turning) is the correct answer. Positive phototropism is the turning of a plant shoot toward light, and negative phototropism the turning away from light.

**49. a.** Cytokinins inhibit protein breakdown, stimulate RNA and protein synthesis, and mobilize nutrients. These attributes are thought to be involved in the retardation of aging in some plant organs.

**50. c.** Although green stems do perform photosynthesis, the leaves are the most important photosynthetic organs in most plants.

**51. d.** Parenchyma cells, relatively unspecialized and usually lacking secondary walls, carry on most of the plant's metabolic functions.

**52. c.** Photoperiodism is the physiological response of any organism to day length.

## III. Other Concepts You Should Be Familiar With

The following are not formal divisions of your nursing school entrance exam; however, concepts within them overlap with the subjects mentioned previously and may find their way into some of the questions.

### A. The Scientific Method

#### 1. General

The scientific method is employed by all scientists to study the natural world, regardless of the particular subject matter.

#### 2. Steps

Ideally, the scientific method involves the following steps, though the process is never as smooth as that outlined here, and some steps may be taken out of order:

- Formulate the problem, the solution to which explains an order or process in nature.
- Collect data via observations, measurements, and review of the past—look for regularity and relationships between the data.
- Form a hypothesis, or an educated guess as to what is going on, using inductive logic (specific to general) to infer a general or universal premise. The hypothesis must be logical and testable. Then formulate the hypothesis using deductive logic (general to specific—If . . . , then . . . ).
- Test the hypothesis by experimentation and gathering new data. A hypothesis can be disproved, but never absolutely proved—it may change with tomorrow's evidence. Experiments must be free of bias and sampling error, with control and experimental groups. An adequate amount of data and/or adequate numbers of individuals must be tested, and

experiments must be reproducible by other scientists.
- Decide whether the hypothesis is to be accepted, modified, or denied.
- Formulate a new hypothesis and start again, if necessary.

#### 3. The Science of Biology

Biology applies the scientific method to living organisms in order to attempt to arrive at an understanding of them. It looks at life using chemical and physical approaches, mainly those processes that involve transformation of matter and energy. There are vast numbers of kinds of living entities and therefore many branches of biology.

### B. The Origin of Life

#### 1. The Mechanistic View

Held by most scientists, the mechanistic view of the origin of life holds that Earth is billions of years old and that life occurred at a point in time along a continuum of increasingly complex matter. Biologists postulate a natural origin for life.

#### 2. Distinction between Living and Nonliving Entities

Many biologists regard the distinction between living and nonliving entities as arbitrary, believing instead that there is a continuum, generally involving complexity.

Overall, however, there is a difference, in that living entities ordinarily are capable of self-regulation, metabolism, movement, irritability (response to stimuli in its internal and external environments), growth (increase in mass through use of materials from the environment), adaptation (a tendency to change, resulting in improved capacity to survive), and reproduction (production of new individuals like themselves).

## C. Classification of Living Entities

### 1. Systems of Classification

The classification of living entities is an artificial construct. There are various systems, ranging from 2- to 13-kingdom classifications. Following are three examples:

- 5-kingdom classification: Monera, Protista, Fungi, Plantae, Animalia
- 6-kingdom classification: Bacteria, Archaea, Protista, Fungi, Plantae, Animalia
- Ecological classification: Autotrophs, including green plants and some bacteria; heterotrophs, including herbivores, carnivores, omnivores, scavengers, decomposers, and parasites

### 2. Linnaean System

The hierarchical system most widely used is the Linnaean system, devised by Swedish botonist Carolus Linnaeus (Carl Linné, 1707–1778). This system consists of Kingdom, Phylum, Class, Order, Family, Genus, and Species.

### 3. Binomial Nomenclature

A system also devised by Linnaeus, binomial nomenclature is still used for naming the genus and species of an organism. The first part is the generic name, the second the specific—the creature's genus (capitalized) and species (lowercase) are reflected in the name. For example, the common house cat is *Felis silvestris;* a bacterium that causes one type of streptococcal pneumonia is *Streptococcus pneumoniae.*

## D. Social Behavior of Animals

### 1. Humans

A heated debate continues to rage over the distinction termed "nature versus nurture." Some scientists, particularly sociobiologists, believe that aspects of human behavior shared across cultures, such as avoidance of incest, can be viewed as innate, or somehow evolutionarily programmed. Others insist that such cultural features as taboos would be unnecessary if behavior were truly innate; therefore, they say, much of what we view as particularly human behavior is learned. Those on the "nurture" side of the debate often point to altruistic behavior, which exists to a much greater extent in humans than in any other species. Those on the "nature" side of the debate insist that most altruistic behavior, if carefully looked at, does in some way enhance the individual's fitness, even when it causes that individual's death.

### 2. Other Species

Although much of the social behavior between members of a species involves cooperation, it is still the case that individuals act in their own best interest and that a good deal of competitive behavior arises in all animal populations. Important aspects of social interaction include:

- agnostic behavior/competitive behavior—for example, for food or a mate—involving a contest in which individuals threaten one another until one backs down. Often such behavior is ritualistic, as natural selection would favor individuals able to settle a contest without injury.
- dominance hierarchies
- territoriality
- courtship rituals
- communication among individuals
- altruistic behavior, though to a lesser extent than in humans

# Questions

**53.** In science, which of the following is most nearly synonymous with the word "theory"?
   **a.** a proven fact
   **b.** a hypothesis that has withstood repeated testing
   **c.** an untested supposition
   **d.** a body of published data

**54.** A distinguishing feature of the Kingdom Monera is that the cells of the organisms in that kingdom
   **a.** contain many specialized parts.
   **b.** contain mitochondria.
   **c.** obtain food through photosynthesis.
   **d.** lack nuclei.

**55.** The majority of primary producers in an ecosystem are
   **a.** autotrophs.
   **b.** carnivores.
   **c.** detrivores.
   **d.** herbivores.

**56.** When rattlesnakes engage in "combat" in which one tries to pin the other to the ground, but neither uses its deadly fangs, such behavior is called
   **a.** survival of the fittest.
   **b.** territoriality.
   **c.** ritualistic agonistic behavior.
   **d.** a mating dance.

**57.** An alternative view of the mechanistic origin of life holds that at least some organic compounds, including amino acids, originated in the hundreds of thousands of meteorites and comets that hit the earth during its early formation—that is, that life had extraterrestrial origins. This idea is called
   **a.** abiotic synthesis.
   **b.** panspermia.
   **c.** protobiotic aggregation.
   **d.** the Oparin hypothesis.

**58.** From the point of view of the scientific method, the most important requirement for a sound hypothesis is that it be
   **a.** able to be confirmed.
   **b.** intuitively possible.
   **c.** useful in a practical sense.
   **d.** testable through experimentation.

**59.** The category of classification of organisms that contains one or several similar or closely related families is the
   **a.** phylum.
   **b.** class.
   **c.** order.
   **d.** genus.

**60.** The primary feature that distinguishes life from nonlife is that living organisms are capable of
   **a.** reproduction.
   **b.** entropy.
   **c.** chemical evolution.
   **d.** atomic bonding.

## Answers

**53. b.** A theory has undergone testing. The word is often mistakenly used to mean "just a guess." This misuse is seen in such a statement as "Evolution is just a theory." In fact, evolution is regarded in the scientific community as a hypothesis that is so well-supported by data as to be fact.

**54. d.** The Kingdom Monera consists of simple, single-celled prokaryotic organisms whose cells lack nuclei and certain other specialized parts.

**55. a.** The primary producers of an ecosystem are autotrophs, most of which are photosynthetic organisms that synthesize organic compounds directly from light energy. All the other choices are consumers, directly or indirectly dependent on photosynthetic products for nutrition.

**56. c.** This kind of ritualistic or symbolic combat has an advantage, in that even the loser lives to reproduce.

**57. b.** The theory of panspermia gained strength in 1986 when spacecraft flying near Halley's Comet showed that the comet contained far more organic material than had been previously thought.

**58. d.** A hypothesis that is not testable is useless from a scientific point of view. Hypotheses can never be absolutely confirmed (choice **a**). Hypotheses frequently fly in the face of intuition (choice **b**); for instance, a flat Earth probably seems more intuitively right than a spherical one. Many scientific hypotheses have no immediately recognizable practical applications (choice **c**); an example might be David Reznik's hypotheses concerning guppy populations in Trinidad.

**59. c.** Order is the category that holds one or several similar or closely related families of organisms. Order names typically end in *-ales* for botany, *-a* for zoology (for example, Rosales and Carnivora).

**60. a.** All the other choices are properties of both living and nonliving entities.

## IV. Suggested Sources for Further Study

All of the following are available in bookstores, as well as through the Internet from Amazon Books (www.amazon.com).

### Textbooks

Reece, Jane B., et al. *Campbell Biology, 9th Edition.* (San Francisco: Pearson Benjamin Cummings, 2011). This is an excellent 1,200-page basic college textbook: authoritative, thorough, clear, and readable (even enjoyable). It will be an excellent main source for you to study. Older editions are still a good reference and less expensive.

Gould, James L., and William T. Keeton with Carol Grant Gould. *Biological Science, 6th Edition.* (New York: Norton, 1996). This is a very fine textbook, well organized, thorough, and authoritative.

### Reference Works

Fargis, Paul. *The New York Public Library Desk Reference, 4th Edition.* (New York: Hyperion, 2002). The sections on "Biology" and "The Human Body and Biomedical Science" will make good supplements to more detailed works and will help you create an organized outline of subject areas.

Hine, Robert, ed. *Oxford Dictionary of Biology, 6th Edition.* (New York: Oxford University Press, 2008). This is an up-to-date and well-respected dictionary of biology—though by no means the only one—which contains the majority of the terms you will need to be familiar with on your nursing school entrance exam.

Stedman, Thomas. *Stedman's Medical Dictionary for the Health Professions and Nursing, 7th Edition*. (Philadelphia: Lippincott Williams & Wilkins, 2011). Stedman's is an excellent, user-friendly medical dictionary, illustrated and with a CD-ROM.

## Study Guides

Fried, George, and George Hademenos. *Schaum's Outline of Biology, 3rd Edition*. (New York: McGraw-Hill, 2009). As part of a popular college course series, this book contains a detailed overview of the subject of biology. It is well organized and readable.

## Supplemental Works

Gould, Stephen Jay. *Dinosaur in a Haystack: Reflections in Natural History*. (New York: Crown, 1996).

Gould, Stephen Jay. *The Panda's Thumb: More Reflections in Natural History*. (New York: Norton, 1992). Stephen Jay Gould is known for his provocative and authoritative essays on biology and natural history. Both this collection and the previous one will make good supplements to the more detailed textbooks mentioned.

Sagan, Carl. *Broca's Brain: Reflections on the Romance of Science*. (New York: Ballantine, 1993). Both works by Sagan contain knowledgeable, readable essays that make biology and natural history topics accessible to the layperson but never talk down. Like Stephen Jay Gould's books, these collections will be good additions to the other more complete, technical works in this list.

# CHAPTER

# 8 ▶ CHEMISTRY REVIEW

## CHAPTER SUMMARY
This chapter is a general outline and review of the important chemistry concepts that are tested by many nursing school entrance exams.

# Chemistry Review: Important Concepts

## I. General Introduction

### A. Description of How Nursing School Entrance Exams Test Chemistry

This chapter reviews essential concepts in chemistry that are covered in many nursing school entrance exams. Some tests contain specific chemistry or science sections; others ask you to be able to recognize important ideas and terms.

Some of these key concepts are atomic structure, the periodic table, chemical bonds, chemical equations, stoichiometry, energy and states of matter, reaction rates, equilibrium, acids, bases, oxidation-reduction, nuclear chemistry, and organic compounds.

## B. How to Use This Chapter

This chapter is presented in outline format as a systematic presentation of important chemistry topics to help you review for your exam. This does not constitute a comprehensive chemistry review—use it as an aid to help you recall concepts you have studied and to identify areas in which you need more study. At the end of this chapter, you will find a list of references and resources for a more complete review.

Read each topic and answer the questions that follow. After answering the sample test questions, you can pinpoint where you want to concentrate your efforts. If a question poses particular difficulty for you, study more problems of this type. The more you hone your problem-solving skills, understand basic principles, and recognize core terms, the more relaxed and confident you will feel on test day.

## STUDY TIPS FOR CHEMISTRY

- Review the topics covered in this chapter carefully. Keep a copy of one or more of the suggested resource books handy for more extensive review.
- Don't try to review all topics in one or two study sessions. Tackle a couple of topics at a time. Focus more in-depth study on the items within a topic about which you feel least confident first.
- Complete each group of practice questions after you study each topic, and check your answers. If you experience particular difficulty with one type of question, choose similar questions from the other resources listed to practice some more.
- Review all the answer choices carefully before making your selection. The wrong answers often give you hints at the correct one and help you confirm that you really do know the correct answer. Remember that recognition is not necessarily understanding.
- When checking your answers to practice questions with the answer key, be sure you understand why the identified choice is the correct one. Practice writing out your reasoning for choosing a particular answer and checking it against the reasoning given in the answer key.
- Practice pronouncing chemical terminology aloud. If you can pronounce a term with ease, you are more likely to remember the term and its meaning when reading it.
- Review carefully the visual aspects of chemistry, such as the use of symbols, arrows, and sub- and superscripts. If you know the circumstances under which particular symbols are used, you will have immediate clues to right and wrong answers.
- Focus on developing problem-solving skills. Almost all chemical problems require the analysis, sorting, and understanding of details.

## II. Main Topics

### A. Atoms

#### 1. Atomic Structure

An **atom** is the basic unit of an element that retains all of the element's chemical properties. An atom is composed of a nucleus (which contains one or more protons and neutrons) and one or more electrons in motion around it.

An **electron** is of negligible mass compared to the mass of the nucleus and has a negative charge of −1.

A **proton** has a mass of 1 amu (atomic mass unit) and a positive charge of +1.

A **neutron** has a mass of 1 amu also but no charge.

Atoms are electrically neutral because they are made up of equal numbers of protons and electrons.

#### 2. Dalton's Atomic Theory

In 1808, John Dalton proposed his hypotheses about the nature of matter that became the basis of Dalton's atomic theory:

- All elements are made of tiny, indivisible particles called atoms (from the Greek *atomos*, meaning indivisible).
- Atoms of one element are identical in size, mass, and chemical properties.
- Atoms of different elements have different sizes, masses, and chemical properties.
- Chemical compounds are made up of atoms of different elements in a ratio that is an integer (a whole number) or a simple fraction.
- Atoms cannot be created or destroyed. They can be combined or rearranged in a **chemical reaction**.

Later experiments completed the understanding of atoms:

- **J. J. Thomson** discovered the electron.
- **E. Rutherford** established that the atom is composed of negatively charged electrons

moving in the empty space surrounding a dense, positively charged nucleus.

- **A. Becquerel** and **Marie Curie** discovered that the decay of radioactive (unstable) nuclei resulted in the release of particles and energy.

#### 3. Mass Number

**Mass number** is the sum of protons and neutrons in the nucleus of an atom. It varies with the isotopes of each element. The mass number is indicated by the number to the upper left of the element symbol: $^{23}$Na.

#### 4. Atomic Number

**Atomic number** is the number of protons in the atom and is specific for each element. The atomic number is indicated by the number to the lower left of the element symbol: $_{11}$Na.

#### 5. Isotopes

**Isotopes** are atoms of the same element that have the same number of protons (same atomic number) but different number of neutrons (different mass number). Isotopes have identical chemical properties (same reactivity) but different physical properties (for example, some decay while others are stable).

| ISOTOPES OF HYDROGEN | |
| --- | --- |
| $^1$H | protium |
| $^2$H (or D) | deuterium |
| $^3$H (or T) | tritium |

The **atomic weight** (or mass) of an element is given by the weighted average of the isotopes' masses.

## 6. Classification of Matter

### a. Elements

**Elements** are substances that are composed of only one type of atom. Elements have chemical symbols (letters of their names) that are used for their representation in the periodic table. For example, the element Helium is displayed as He.

In nature, atoms of one element may be chemically bonded to other atoms of the same element. For example, hydrogen and oxygen are always diatomic, which means that they naturally exist as $H_2$ and $O_2$, respectively. Elemental sulfur exists as $S_8$. Many elements, like sodium, exist as single atoms in their elemental form.

### b. Compounds

A **compound** is a combination of two or more atoms of different elements in a precise proportion by mass. In a compound, atoms are held together by attractive forces called *chemical bonds*.

### c. Mixtures

A **mixture** is a combination of two or more compounds (or substances) that interact but are not bonded chemically with one another. Substances that make up a mixture can be separated by physical means.

## 7. Properties of Atoms

**Law of conservation of mass:** In a chemical reaction, matter cannot be created or destroyed—i.e., the mass of the reagents always equals the mass of the products. Likewise, the number of each type of atom will be equal on each side of the reaction.

**Law of constant (definite) proportion:** A chemical compound will always have the same proportion of elements by mass—e.g., water ($H_2O$) will always be 8/9 oxygen and 1/9 hydrogen by mass.

**Law of multiple proportions:** If two elements form more than one compound between them, then the ratios of the masses of the second element which combine with a fixed mass of the first element will be ratios of small whole numbers. For

example, 16 g of oxygen will react with 14 g of nitrogen to form NO and 28 g of nitrogen to form $N_2O$ (1:2 ratio).

# Questions

1. Which of the following statements about atoms is true?
   a. They have more protons than electrons.
   b. They have more electrons than protons.
   c. They are electrically neutral.
   d. They have as many neutrons as they have electrons.

2. What is the mass number of an atom with 60 protons, 60 electrons, and 75 neutrons?
   a. 120
   b. 135
   c. 75
   d. 195

3. What is the atomic number of an atom with 17 protons, 17 electrons, and 20 neutrons?
   a. 37
   b. 34
   c. 54
   d. 17

4. Two atoms, L and M, are isotopes. Which of the following properties would they NOT have in common?
   a. atomic number
   b. atomic mass
   c. chemical reactivity
   d. the number of protons in the nucleus

5. An atom with an atomic number of 58 and an atomic mass of 118 has
   a. 58 neutrons.
   b. 176 neutrons.
   c. 60 neutrons.
   d. 116 neutrons.

**6.** According to Dalton's theory, the only way a compound can consist of its elements in a definite ratio by mass is when it is made from the elements in

a. a definite ratio by volume.

b. a definite ratio by number of atoms.

c. multiple whole-number ratios by mass.

d. multiple whole-number ratios by volume.

**7.** Which of the following is a mixture?

a. sodium chloride

b. rice and beans

c. magnesium sulfate

d. water

**8.** The mass of an atom is almost entirely contributed by its

a. nucleus.

b. protons.

c. electrons and protons.

d. neutrons.

**9.** If an atom consists of 9 protons and 10 neutrons, its

a. atomic number is 10.

b. mass number is 10.

c. number of electrons is 9.

d. electrical charge is 9.

**10.** Which of the following is true of an atom?

a. It consists of protons, neutrons, and electrons.

b. It has a nucleus consisting of protons, neutrons, and electrons.

c. The protons are equal in number to the electrons, so the nucleus is electrically neutral.

d. All of the above are true.

# Answers

**1. c.** Atoms are electrically neutral; the number of electrons is equal to the number of protons.

**2. b.** Mass number is the number of protons plus the number of neutrons: $60 + 75 = 135$.

**3. d.** The atomic number is the number of protons—in this case, 17.

**4. b.** By definition, isotopes have different numbers of neutrons. Therefore, they differ in atomic weight.

**5. c.** The number of neutrons is equal to the atomic mass minus the atomic number (the number of protons): $118 - 58 = 60$.

**6. b.** This is part of Dalton's atomic theory.

**7. b.** Rice and beans are not chemically combined and can be separated into their constituent parts by physical means.

**8. a.** The protons and neutrons of an atom are found in the nucleus.

**9. c.** Atoms are electrically neutral. If there are 9 protons, each with a +1 charge, 9 electrons with a −1 charge are needed to balance the charge.

**10. a.** An atom consists of protons, neutrons, and electrons; the nucleus contains protons and neutrons. The protons are equal in number to the electrons, but the nucleus itself is not electrically neutral.

## B. Periodic Table (page 196)

### 1. Periodic Law

**Periodic law** is when the properties of the elements are a periodic function of their atomic number.

**Periodic table** is an arrangement of the elements according to similarity in their chemical properties and in order of increasing atomic number.

| IA | | | | | | | | | | | | | | | | VIIA | VIIIA |
|---|---|---|---|---|---|---|---|---|---|---|---|---|---|---|---|---|---|
| 1<br>**H**<br>1.00794 | IIA | | | | | | | | | | | IIIA | IVA | VA | VIA | 1<br>**H**<br>1.00794 | 2<br>**He**<br>4.002602 |
| 3<br>**Li**<br>6.941 | 4<br>**Be**<br>9.012182 | | | | | | | | | | | 5<br>**B**<br>10.811 | 6<br>**C**<br>12.0107 | 7<br>**N**<br>14.00674 | 8<br>**O**<br>15.9994 | 9<br>**F**<br>18.9984032 | 10<br>**Ne**<br>20.1797 |
| 11<br>**Na**<br>22.989770 | 12<br>**Mg**<br>24.3050 | IIIB | IVB | VB | VIB | VIIB | | VIIIB | | IB | IIB | 13<br>**Al**<br>26.981538 | 14<br>**Si**<br>28.0855 | 15<br>**P**<br>30.973761 | 16<br>**S**<br>32.066 | 17<br>**Cl**<br>35.4527 | 18<br>**Ar**<br>39.948 |
| 19<br>**K**<br>39.0983 | 20<br>**Ca**<br>40.078 | 21<br>**Sc**<br>44.955910 | 22<br>**Ti**<br>47.867 | 23<br>**V**<br>50.9415 | 24<br>**Cr**<br>51.9961 | 25<br>**Mn**<br>54.938049 | 26<br>**Fe**<br>55.845 | 27<br>**Co**<br>58.933200 | 28<br>**Ni**<br>58.6934 | 29<br>**Cu**<br>63.546 | 30<br>**Zn**<br>65.39 | 31<br>**Ga**<br>69.723 | 32<br>**Ge**<br>72.61 | 33<br>**As**<br>74.92160 | 34<br>**Se**<br>78.96 | 35<br>**Br**<br>79.904 | 36<br>**Kr**<br>83.80 |
| 37<br>**Rb**<br>85.4678 | 38<br>**Sr**<br>87.62 | 39<br>**Y**<br>88.90585 | 40<br>**Zr**<br>91.224 | 41<br>**Nb**<br>92.90638 | 42<br>**Mo**<br>95.94 | 43<br>**Tc**<br>(98) | 44<br>**Ru**<br>101.07 | 45<br>**Rh**<br>102.90550 | 46<br>**Pd**<br>106.42 | 47<br>**Ag**<br>107.8682 | 48<br>**Cd**<br>112.411 | 49<br>**In**<br>114.818 | 50<br>**Sn**<br>118.710 | 51<br>**Sb**<br>121.760 | 52<br>**Te**<br>127.60 | 53<br>**I**<br>126.90447 | 54<br>**Xe**<br>131.29 |
| 55<br>**Cs**<br>132.90545 | 56<br>**Ba**<br>137.327 | 57<br>**La***<br>138.9055 | 72<br>**Hf**<br>178.49 | 73<br>**Ta**<br>180.9479 | 74<br>**W**<br>183.84 | 75<br>**Re**<br>186.207 | 76<br>**Os**<br>190.23 | 77<br>**Ir**<br>192.217 | 78<br>**Pt**<br>195.078 | 79<br>**Au**<br>196.96655 | 80<br>**Hg**<br>200.59 | 81<br>**Tl**<br>204.3833 | 82<br>**Pb**<br>207.2 | 83<br>**Bi**<br>208.98038 | 84<br>**Po**<br>(209) | 85<br>**At**<br>(210) | 86<br>**Rn**<br>(222) |
| 87<br>**Fr**<br>(223) | 88<br>**Ra**<br>(226) | 89<br>**Ac****<br>(227) | 104<br>**Rf**<br>(261) | 105<br>**Db**<br>(262) | 106<br>**Sg**<br>(263) | 107<br>**Bh**<br>(262) | 108<br>**Hs**<br>(265) | 109<br>**Mt**<br>(266) | 110<br>**Ds**<br>(269) | 111<br>**Rg**<br>(281) | 112<br>**Cn**<br>(285) | 113<br>**Uut**<br>(286) | 114<br>**Uuq**<br>(289) | 115<br>**Uup**<br>(289) | 116<br>**Uuh**<br>(289) | 117<br>**Uus**<br>(294) | 118<br>**Uuo**<br>(293) |

| * Lanthanide series | 58<br>**Ce**<br>140.116 | 59<br>**Pr**<br>140.90765 | 60<br>**Nd**<br>144.24 | 61<br>**Pm**<br>(145) | 62<br>**Sm**<br>150.36 | 63<br>**Eu**<br>151.964 | 64<br>**Gd**<br>157.25 | 65<br>**Tb**<br>158.92534 | 66<br>**Dy**<br>162.50 | 67<br>**Ho**<br>164.93032 | 68<br>**Er**<br>167.26 | 69<br>**Tm**<br>168.93421 | 70<br>**Yb**<br>173.04 | 71<br>**Lu**<br>174.967 |
|---|---|---|---|---|---|---|---|---|---|---|---|---|---|---|
| ** Actinide series | 90<br>**Th**<br>232.0381 | 91<br>**Pa**<br>231.03588 | 92<br>**U**<br>238.0289 | 93<br>**Np**<br>(237) | 94<br>**Pu**<br>(244) | 95<br>**Am**<br>(243) | 96<br>**Cm**<br>(247) | 97<br>**Bk**<br>(247) | 98<br>**Cf**<br>(251) | 99<br>**Es**<br>(252) | 100<br>**Fm**<br>(257) | 101<br>**Md**<br>(258) | 102<br>**No**<br>(259) | 103<br>**Lr**<br>(262) |

## 2. Properties of the Periodic Table

### a. Periods

**Periods** are the horizontal rows of the periodic table of elements. Elements in the same period have the same number of electron shells (or levels).

### b. Groups

**Groups** are the vertical columns of elements with the same number of electrons in their outermost shell. The group number indicates the number of valence (or outermost) electrons. Elements in the same group share similar chemical properties.

### c. Metals

A **metal** is an element that is a good conductor of heat and electricity in addition to being shiny (reflecting light), malleable (easily bent), and ductile (made into wire). Metals are electropositive, having a greater tendency to lose their valence electrons. They are grouped in the left of the periodic table (groups I–III).

### d. Nonmetals

A **nonmetal** is an element with poor conducting properties. They are electronegative and accept electrons in their valence shell. They are found in the upper right-hand corner of the periodic table.

### e. Metalloids

A **metalloid** is an element with properties that are intermediate between those of metals and nonmetals, such as semiconductivity. They are also found between metals and nonmetals in the periodic table.

## 3. Electronic Structure of Atoms

### a. Bohr Atom

Niels Bohr's planetary model of the hydrogen atom, in which a nucleus is surrounded by orbits of electrons, resembles the solar system. Electrons could be excited by **quanta** of energy and move to an outer orbit (excited level). They could also emit radiation when falling to their original orbit (ground state).

### b. Orbitals

An **orbital** is the space where one or two paired electrons can be located. These are mathematical functions (or figures) with restricted zones, called **nodes**, and specific shapes—for example, *s* orbitals are spherical; *p* orbitals are dumbbell-shaped.

### c. Quantum Numbers

There are four quantum numbers that describe any electron in an atom. They are the principle quantum number (n), the orbital quantum number ($l$), the magnetic quantum number ($m_l$) and the spin quantum number ($m_s$).

- **Principle quantum number (n):** Determines the overall energy level of the electron. n is always a positive integer (n = 1, 2, 3, …). For a given principle quantum number (n), there are n − 1 possible orbital quantum numbers (0, 1, 2, … , n − 1). The principle quantum number defines the energy level of an electron. There are a maximum of $n^2$ orbitals and $2n^2$ electrons in an energy level.

- **Orbital quantum number ($l$):** Determines the shape of the orbital in which the electron resides (0 = s, 1 = p, 2 = d, 3 = f, etc.). For a given orbital quantum number ($l$), there are $2l + 1$ orbitals.

- **Magnetic quantum number ($m_l$):** Corresponds to a specific orbital in which the electron resides. For a given orbital quantum number, there are $2l + 1$ magnetic quantum numbers $(-l, -l + 1, -l + 2, …, 0, …, l - 2, l - 1, l)$.

- **Spin quantum number ($m_s$):** Describes the direction of electron spin, which may either be up $(+\frac{1}{2})$ or down $(-\frac{1}{2})$. Therefore, for two electrons to occupy the same orbital, they must be of opposite spins.

### d. Pauli Exclusion Principle

The **Pauli exclusion principle** states that no two electrons can possess the same four quantum numbers. As a consequence, each orbital holds a maximum of two electrons, and only if they are of opposite spin.

### e. Electron Configuration

**Electron Configuration** describes the exact arrangement of electrons (given in a superscript number) in successive shells (indicated by numbers 1, 2, 3, and so on) and orbitals (s, p, d, f) of an atom, starting with the innermost orbital.

For example, $1s^2\, 2s^2\, 2p^6$.

### f. Hund's Rule

**Hund's Rule** states that the most stable arrangement of electrons in the same energy level is the one in which electrons have parallel spins (same orientation).

### g. Outer Shell (or valence shell)

The **outer shell** is the last energy level in which loosely held electrons are contained. These are the electrons that engage in bonding and are therefore characteristic of the element.

## You Should Review

- periodic table: structure; specific names of the different groups (group I: alkali metal, group II: alkaline earth, group VII: halogens, etc.); the location of metals, nonmetals, and metalloids
- Bohr atom
- ground state
- quantization of energy
- quantum number
- Heisenberg uncertainty principle
- the maximum number of electrons that can be held in each energy level

## Questions

**11.** If the electron configuration of an element is written $1s^2\, 2s^2\, 2p_x^2\, 2p_y^2\, 2p_z^2\, 3s^1$, the element's atomic
   **a.** number is 11.
   **b.** number is 12.
   **c.** weight is 11.
   **d.** weight is 12.

**12.** Choose the proper group of symbols for the following elements: potassium, silver, mercury, lead, sodium, iron.
   **a.** Po, Ar, Hr, Pm, So, Fm
   **b.** Pb, Sl, Me, Le, Su, Io
   **c.** Pt, Sr, My, Pd, Sd, In
   **d.** K, Ag, Hg, Pb, Na, Fe

**13.** What is the maximum number of electrons that each p orbital can hold?
   **a.** 8
   **b.** 2
   **c.** 6
   **d.** 4

**14.** What is the maximum number of electrons that the second energy level can hold?
   **a.** 8
   **b.** 6
   **c.** 2
   **d.** 16

**15.** What is the name of the individual who proposed that the atom was similar to a solar system, with a dense nucleus and concentric circles around it?
   **a.** Hund
   **b.** Dalton
   **c.** Pauli
   **d.** Bohr

**16.** The horizontal rows of the periodic table are called
   **a.** families.
   **b.** groups.
   **c.** representative elements.
   **d.** periods.

**17.** Which of the following is an alkali metal (group IA)?
   **a.** calcium
   **b.** sodium
   **c.** aluminum
   **d.** alkanium

**18.** Who stated that an orbital can hold as many as two electrons if they have opposite spins, one clockwise and one counterclockwise?
   **a.** Hund
   **b.** Dalton
   **c.** Pauli
   **d.** Bohr

**19.** Which elements are strong conductors of electricity?
   **a.** metals
   **b.** nonmetals
   **c.** metalloids
   **d.** ions

**20.** If the electron configuration of an element is written: $1s^2\, 2s^2\, 2p^6\, 3s^2\, 3p^3$, the element's atomic
   **a.** number is 15.
   **b.** number is 5.
   **c.** weight is 15.
   **d.** weight is 5.

# Answers

**11. a.** Since there are 11 electrons in the element's electron configuration, the element has 11 protons and, therefore, an atomic number of 11.

**12. d.** See the periodic table.

**13. b.** Each p orbital holds two electrons. There are three p orbitals, holding a total of six electrons.

**14. a.** The second energy level has one s orbital and three p orbitals, holding a total of eight electrons.

**15. d.** Bohr proposed the model defined in the question.

**16. d.** By definition, the periods are the horizontal rows on the periodic table.

**17. b.** Sodium is an alkali metal.

**18. c.** The question defines the Pauli exclusion principle.

**19. a.** Metals, by definition, are strong conductors of electricity.

**20. a.** Since the element has 15 electrons, it also has 15 protons and an atomic number of 15.

## C. Chemical Bonds

### 1. Octet Rule

**Octet rule** states that atoms bond by surrounding themselves with eight (octet) outer electrons (two electrons for H). They tend to acquire the stability of their closest noble gases in the periodic table, either by losing (metals), gaining (nonmetals), or sharing electrons in their valence shell.

### 2. Ions
#### a. Anions

When an atom gains one or more electrons, it becomes a negatively charged entity called an **anion**. Most anions are nonmetallic. Their names are derived from the elemental name with an ending in the suffix, *-ide*. For example, a chlor*ide* ion ($Cl^-$) occurs when a chlorine atom (Cl) has gained one electron to achieve the octet structure of Argon, or Ar. An ox*ide* ion ($O^{2-}$) occurs when an oxygen atom (O) has acquired two electrons in its valence shell and has achieved the same stable electron configuration as Neon, or Ne.

#### b. Cations

A **cation** results when an atom loses one or more electrons, becoming positively charged. Most cations are metallic and have the same name as the metallic element. For example, lithium ion ($Li^+$) has one electron fewer than lithium atom (Li), having acquired the noble gas electron structure of Helium, or He.

### 3. Ionic Compounds

**Ionic compounds** are compounds formed by combining cations and anions. The attractive electrostatic force between a cation and an anion is called an **ionic bond**.

### 4. Molecular Compounds
#### a. Covalent Bonds

A **covalent bond** is a type of bond formed when two atoms share one or more pairs of electrons to achieve a complete octet of electrons.

#### b. Lewis Structures

**Lewis structures** are formulas for compounds in which each atom exhibits an octet of valence electrons. These are represented as dots, or as a line for a shared pair of electrons, thus leaving unshared pairs of electrons as pairs of dots.

unshared pairs of electrons

$H_2O$:

shared pairs of electrons

### c. Valence Shell Electron Pair Repulsion (VSEPR) Theory

The **VSEPR model** is based on electrostatic repulsion between electron pair orbitals. By pushing each other as far as possible, electron pairs dictate which geometry, or shape, a molecule will adopt. Molecules should be written as Lewis structures (see the preceding electron–dot notation).

### d. Electronegativity and Dipoles

**Electronegativity** is the ability of an atom in a bond to attract the electron density more than the other atom(s) in the bond. Electronegativity increases from left to right and from bottom to top in the periodic table. Thus, fluorine (F) is the most electronegative element of the periodic table, with the maximum value of 4.0 in the Pauling scale of electronegativity. The Pauling scale is a range of electronegativity values based on fluorine having the highest value at 4.0. These values have no units. Metals are electropositive, with a minimum electronegativity value of 0.8 on the Pauling scale for most alkali metals.

A **dipole** results in a covalent bond between two atoms of different electronegativity. Partial positive ($+\delta$) and negative ($-\delta$) charges develop at both ends of the bond, creating a dipole (i.e., two poles) oriented from the positive end to the negative end. For example: $H^{+\delta}-Cl^{-\delta}$

### 5. Hydrogen Bonds

**Hydrogen bonds** are weak bonds that form between dipoles of consecutive polar molecules (intermolecular) or polar groups of macromolecules (intramolecular), such as proteins and DNA, in which these bonds play an important structural role.

Electronegative atoms (such as F, N, or O) covalently bonded to H atoms are considered hydrogen bond donors. Electronegative atoms with free lone pairs of electrons in their Lewis structures act as hydrogen bond acceptors.

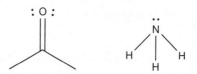

Acetone (($CH_3)_2CO$) is a hydrogen bond acceptor. Ammonia ($NH_3$) is a hydrogen bond donor and acceptor. Like ammonia, water is both a hydrogen bond donor and acceptor.

### 6. Polyatomic Ions

Polyatomic ions are groups of two or more covalently bonded atoms that possess a positive or negative charge. They form ionic compounds in the same way as single-atom ions. Polyatomic ions can be as simple as hydroxide ($OH^-$). Other common examples are ammonium ($NH_4^+$), phosphate ($PO_4^{3-}$), carbonate ($CO_3^{2-}$), nitrate ($NO_3^-$), and sulfate ($SO_4^{2-}$).

### You Should Review

- polyatomic ions
- molecular structures
- structures of water molecules and biological compounds

## Questions

**21.** The bond between oxygen and hydrogen atoms in a water molecule is a(n)
  **a.** hydrogen bond.
  **b.** polar covalent bond.
  **c.** nonpolar covalent bond.
  **d.** ionic bond.

**22.** Which of the following is a nonpolar covalent bond?
  **a.** the bond between two carbons
  **b.** the bond between sodium and chloride
  **c.** the bond between two water molecules
  **d.** the bond between nitrogen and hydrogen

**23.** The type of bond formed between two molecules of water is a
   **a.** polar covalent bond.
   **b.** hydrogen bond.
   **c.** nonpolar covalent bond.
   **d.** peptide bond.

**24.** Which of the following lists contains the formulas for these ions, in the order given: ammonium, silver, bicarbonate/hydrogen carbonate, nitrate, calcium, fluoride?
   **a.** $Am^-$, $Si^{++}$, $HCO_3^-$, $NA^+$, $CM^-$, $F^+$
   **b.** $AM^+$, $Ag^+$, $CO_3^{2-}$, $NO_3^-$, $Cal^+$, $Fl^-$
   **c.** $NH_4^-$, $Ag^+$, $HCO_3^-$, $NO_3^-$, $Cal^+$, $Fl^-$
   **d.** $NH_4^+$, $Ag^+$, $HCO_3^-$, $NO_3^-$, $Ca^{2+}$, $F^-$

**25.** If $X$ (atomic number 4) and $Y$ (atomic number 17) react, the formula of the compound formed will be
   **a.** $XY_2$.
   **b.** $YX_2$.
   **c.** $X_2Y_2$.
   **d.** $XY_4$.

**26.** To acquire an outer octet, an atom of element 19 has to
   **a.** lose one electron (and acquire a charge of +1).
   **b.** lose two electrons (and acquire a charge of +2).
   **c.** gain one electron (and acquire a charge of −1).
   **d.** gain two electrons (and acquire a charge of −2).

**27.** The most common ions of the elements of group VIIA have electrical charges of
   **a.** +7.
   **b.** −7.
   **c.** +1.
   **d.** −1.

**28.** Which of the following is true according to the octet rule?
   **a.** Ions of all Group IIA elements have electron configurations that conform to those of the noble gases and have charges of +1.
   **b.** The reactions of the active atoms of the representative elements of the periodic table generally lead to noble gas configurations.
   **c.** An ion of a metallic element that has lost electrons to achieve noble gas configuration is less active than an atom of the same element.
   **d.** The most reactive elements are generally those whose atoms are nearest, but not equal, to noble gas configurations.

**29.** Electron transfer is best described as a process
   **a.** by which ionic compounds are formed from atoms of their elements.
   **b.** in which a covalent bond is made.
   **c.** that occurs between two nonmetals.
   **d.** that occurs between two metals.

**30.** How many electrons do the following have in their outer levels: $S^{2-}$, $Na^+$, $Cl^-$, $Ar$, $Mg^{2+}$, and $Al^{3+}$?
   **a.** three
   **b.** five
   **c.** seven
   **d.** eight

## Answers

**21. b.** A covalent bond exists between H and O in the $H_2O$ molecule. Since the bond is formed between two elements with different electronegativities, it is polar.

**22. a.** The bond formed is covalent. Since it is between two identical elements, it is nonpolar.

**23. b.** Hydrogen bonds from the H of one water molecule to the O of another hold water molecules together.

**24. d.** The other choices give incorrect symbols for the elements or for the charge.

**25. a.** The electron configuration of $X$ is $1s^2 2s^2$, and the electron configuration of $Y$ is $1s^2 2s^2 2p^6 3s^2 3p^5$. $X$ needs to give away two electrons to achieve the stable noble gas configuration of He, which is $1s^2$. $Y$ needs to accept one electron to achieve the outer octet. Therefore, two $Y$ are needed to accept two electrons.

**26. a.** The electron configuration of element 19 is $1s^2 2s^2 2p^6 3s^2 3p^6 4s^1$. To achieve the outer octet, it must give away one electron, thus gaining a charge of +1.

**27. d.** Group VIIA elements need to accept one electron to achieve the outer octet, thus gaining a charge of −1.

**28. d.** The alkali metals (group I) and the halogens (group VIIA) are the most reactive and have atoms that are near but not equal to noble gas configurations.

**29. a.** Ionic compounds are formed between a metal and a nonmetal by electron transfer.

**30. d.** There are eight electrons in the outer shells of these ions.

## D. Chemical Equations and Stoichiometry

### 1. Molecular Weight

**Molecular weight** is the sum of the atomic weights of all the atoms in a molecular formula. It is the same as the molar mass (in grams) without the unit.

### 2. Moles

A **mole** of a particular substance is defined as the number of atoms in exactly 12 g of carbon-12. Experiments have established that number to be $6.02214199 \times 10^{23}$ particles per mole (**Avogadro's number**).

### 3. Chemical Equations
#### a. Balancing Equations
Chemical reactions can be balanced by a trial and error method.
- Write the correct formulas for all reactants and products.
- Compare the number of atoms on the reactant and product(s) sides.
- Rebalance and recheck if necessary.
- Always balance the heavier atoms before trying to balance lighter ones, such as H.
- Use fractions if necessary to reduce coefficients or use the smallest possible whole number.
- Verify (again!) that the number of atoms of each element is balanced.

#### b. Use of Moles in Chemical Equations
**Stoichiometry** establishes the quantities of reactants used and products obtained based on a balanced chemical equation.

$$\# \text{ moles} = \frac{\text{mass (in g)}}{\text{molar mass (in } \frac{\text{g}}{\text{mol}})}$$

### 4. Theoretical Yield
**Theoretical yield** is the amount of product expected in a chemical reaction based on the mass of the starting materials and the stoichiometry of the balanced chemical equation.

## 5. Percentage Yield

When a chemical reaction is run, oftentimes the amount of product recovered is less than what is predicted by stoichiometry. The **percentage yield** is the ratio of the experimental (actual) yield of the product divided by the theoretical yield.

$$\% \text{ yield} = \left(\frac{\text{actual yield}}{\text{theoretical yield}}\right) \times 100\%$$

## 6. Basic Types of Chemical Reactions

- Combination reactions:

  $A + B \rightarrow C$

  $2H_2 + O_2 \rightarrow 2H_2O$
- Decomposition reactions:

  $C \rightarrow A + B$

  $CaCO_3 \rightarrow CaO + CO_2$
- Single displacement reactions:

  $A + BC \rightarrow B + AC$

  $Zn + 2HCl \rightarrow H_2 + ZnCl_2$
- Double displacement reactions:

  $AB + CD \rightarrow AC + BD$

  $HCl + NaOH \rightarrow H_2O + NaCl$

### *You Should Review*

- balancing equations and using polyatomic ions in balancing equations

## Questions

**31.** The molecular weight (in amu) of aluminum carbonate, $Al_2(CO_3)_3$, is
   a. 55
   b. 114
   c. 234
   d. 201

**32.** The formula of carbon dioxide is $CO_2$. Its molecular weight is 44 amu. A sample of 11 grams of $CO_2$ contains
   a. 1.0 mole of carbon dioxide.
   b. 1.5 grams of carbon.
   c. 3.0 grams of carbon.
   d. 6.0 grams of oxygen.

**33.** How many grams are contained in 0.200 mol of calcium phosphate, $Ca_3(PO_4)_2$?
   a. 6.20
   b. 62.0
   c. 124
   d. 31.0

**34.** The symbol $5O_2$ signifies
   a. 5 atoms of oxygen.
   b. 80 grams of oxygen.
   c. 160 grams of oxygen.
   d. 5 grams of oxygen.

**35.** In the reaction
   $CaCl_2 + Na_2CO_3 \rightarrow CaCO_3 + 2NaCl$,
   if 0.5 mole of NaCl is to be formed,
   a. 1 mole of $Na_2CO_3$ is needed.
   b. 0.5 mole of $CaCO_3$ is also formed.
   c. 0.5 mole of $Na_2CO_3$ is needed.
   d. 0.25 mole of $CaCl_2$ is needed.

**36.** In the reaction $2Cu_2S + 3O_2 \rightarrow 2Cu_2O + 2SO_2$, if 24 moles of $Cu_2O$ are to be prepared, then how many moles of $O_2$ are needed?
   a. 24
   b. 36
   c. 16
   d. 27

**37.** Which of the following equations is balanced?
   a. $2H_2O_2 \rightarrow 2H_2O + O_2$
   b. $Ag + Cl_2 \rightarrow 2AgCl$
   c. $KClO_3 \rightarrow KCl + O_2$
   d. $Na + H_2O \rightarrow NaOH + H_2$

**38.** Butane ($C_4H_{10}$) burns with oxygen in the air according to the following equation:

$$2C_4H_{10} + 13O_2 \rightarrow 8CO_2 + 10H_2O$$

In one experiment, the supply of oxygen was limited to 98.0 g. How much butane can be burned by this much oxygen?

  **a.** 15.1 g $C_4H_{10}$
  **b.** 27.3 g $C_4H_{10}$
  **c.** 54.6 g $C_4H_{10}$
  **d.** 30.2 g $C_4H_{10}$

**39.** What type of chemical equation is $2NH_3 \rightarrow N_2 + 3H_2$?

  **a.** combination reaction
  **b.** decomposition reaction
  **c.** single displacement reaction
  **d.** double displacement reaction

**40.** Which of the following equations is balanced?

  **a.** $Mg + N_2 \rightarrow Mg_3N_2$
  **b.** $Fe + O_2 \rightarrow Fe_2O_3$
  **c.** $C_{12}H_{22}O_{11} \rightarrow 12C + 11H_2O$
  **d.** $Ca + H_2O \rightarrow Ca(OH)_2 + H_2$

## Answers

**31. c.** There are 2 atoms of Al, 3 atoms of C, and 9 atoms of O. Look at the atomic weights in the periodic table:

$2 \times Al = 2 \times 27 = 54$ amu

$3 \times C = 3 \times 12 = 36$ amu

$9 \times O = 9 \times 16 = 144$ amu

Then add them up to get the formula weight, which is 234 amu.

**32. c.** $11 \text{ g } CO_2 \times \frac{\text{mol C}}{44 \text{ g } CO_2} \times \frac{12 \text{ g}}{\text{mol C}} = 3.0 \text{ g}$

**33. b.** 1 mole of $Ca_3(PO_4)_2 = 310$ g;

$0.200 \text{ mol} \times \frac{310 \text{ g}}{\text{mol}} = 62 \text{ g}$

**34. c.** $5O_2 = 5 \text{ mol} \times \frac{32 \text{ g}}{\text{mol}} = 160 \text{ g}$

**35. d.** One mole of $CaCl_2$ would be needed to get 2 mol NaCl. Since 0.5 mol of NaCl, or 25% of 2 moles, is to be formed, 0.25 mol $CaCl_2$ (25% of 1 mole) is needed.

**36. b.** $24 \text{ mol } Cu_2O \times \frac{3 \text{ mol } O_2}{2 \text{ mol } Cu_2O} = 36 \text{ mol } O_2$

**37. a.** There are 4 H in the reactants and 4 H in the products, and 4 O in the reactants and 4 O in the products.

**38. b.** Normally, 2 moles of $C_4H_{10}$ react with 13 moles of $O_2$. The supply of oxygen is limited to 98 g, or 3.06 moles; $98.0 \text{ g } O_2 \times \frac{\text{mol } O_2}{32.0 \text{ g } O_2} \times \frac{2 \text{ mol } C_4H_{10}}{13 \text{ mol } O_2} \times \frac{58.0 \text{ g}}{\text{mol } C_4H_{10}} = 27.3 \text{ g}$

**39. b.** A decomposition reaction takes the form $C \rightarrow A + B$.

**40. c.** There are 12 C on both sides, 22 H on both sides, and 11 O on both sides.

### E. Energy and the States of Matter

#### 1. Solids

A **solid** is the state of matter characterized by a definite volume and shape. Solids are not compressible.

#### 2. Liquids

A **liquid** is a fluid state of matter characterized by a definite volume but no definite shape. Liquids are also slightly compressible.

## 3. Gases

All gases behave according to the following characteristics:

- They expand to assume the volume and shape of their container.
- Many gases mix evenly and completely when confined in the same container.
- Gas molecules collide with each other; they do not attract or repel each other.
- Gas molecules have a higher kinetic energy at higher temperatures.

## 4. Pressure

**Pressure** is force exerted over a unit area. The atmospheric pressure exerted by Earth's atmosphere is a function of the altitude and the weather conditions. It decreases with higher altitude. Some useful units of pressure are the atmosphere (atm): 1 atm = 760 mm Hg = 760 torr = 101,325 Pa (pascals).

## 5. Gas Laws

### a. Boyle's Law (at constant temperature)

The volume of a sample of gas decreases as its pressure increases. $(P \propto \frac{1}{V})$: $P_1 V_1 = P_2 V_2$

### b. Charles's Law (at constant pressure)

The volume of a sample of gas maintained at constant pressure increases with its temperature. $(V \propto T)$: $\frac{V_1}{T_1} = \frac{V_2}{T_2}$

### c. Gay-Lussac's Law (at constant volume)

The pressure of any sample of gas increases (maintained at constant volume) with the temperature. $(P \propto T)$: $\frac{P_1}{T_1} = \frac{P_2}{T_2}$

### d. Avogadro's Law (at constant T and P)

The volume of gas increases with the number of moles of gas present at constant temperature and pressure. $(V \propto n)$: $\frac{V_1}{n_1} = \frac{V_2}{n_2}$

Standard temperature and pressure (STP) condition is achieved at 273 K and 1 atm (760 torr) when one mole (or $6.023 \times 10^{23}$ particles) of any gas occupies a volume of 22.4 liters (molar volume at STP).

### e. Dalton's Law of Partial Pressure

In a mixture of gases, individual gases behave independently so that the total pressure is the sum of the partial pressures; $P_T = P_1 + P_2 + P_3 + \cdots$

### f. Graham's Law of Effusion

Graham's law of effusion states that:

$$\frac{\text{Effusion rate of A}}{\text{Effusion rate of B}} = \sqrt{\frac{\text{MW of B}}{\text{MW of A}}}$$

Graham's law states that the rate of effusion of two gases is inversely proportional to the square root of their molecular weights. For example, if hydrogen ($H_2$, MW = 2 g/mol) and oxygen ($O_2$, MW = 32 g/mol) are used to fill a balloon and a small pin hole is introduced, hydrogen will escape four times faster than oxygen.

$$\frac{k_{H_2}}{k_{O_2}} = \sqrt{\frac{32\frac{g}{mol}}{2\frac{g}{mol}}} = 4$$

### g. Ideal Gas Law

An ideal gas is a gas whose pressure, volume, and temperature obey the relation, $PV = nRT$ (a combination of Boyle's, Charles's, and Avogadro's laws), with $R$ being the gas constant. The same relation can also be expressed as: $\frac{P_1 V_1}{T_1} = \frac{P_2 V_2}{T_2}$

## You Should Review

- properties of gases, liquids, and solids
- kinetic theory of gases
- kinetic theory and chemical reactions

## Questions

**41.** A pressure of 740 mm Hg is the same as
a. 1 atm.
b. 0.974 atm.
c. 1.03 atm.
d. 0.740 atm.

**42.** What volume will 500 mL of gas initially at 25°C and 750 mm Hg occupy when conditions change to 25°C and 650 mm Hg?
a. 477 mL
b. 400 mL
c. 577 mL
d. 570 mL

**43.** Which law predicts that if the temperature (in Kelvin) doubles, the pressure will also double?
a. Boyle's law
b. Charles's law
c. Gay-Lussac's law
d. Dalton's law

**44.** Which of the following laws is related to this expression: $P_T = P_1 + P_2 + P_3$?
a. Boyle's law
b. Charles's law
c. Gay-Lussac's law
d. Dalton's law

**45.** Which of the following is NOT characteristic of gases?
a. They have a definite volume and shape.
b. They are low in density.
c. They are highly compressible.
d. They mix rapidly.

**46.** Gases that conform to the assumptions of kinetic theory are referred to as
a. kinetic gases.
b. natural gases.
c. ideal gases.
d. real gases.

**47.** What does the term *pressure* mean when applied to a gas?
a. weight
b. how heavy the gas is
c. mass divided by volume
d. force exerted per unit area

**48.** A sample of helium at 25°C occupies a volume of 725 ml at 730 mm Hg. What volume will it occupy at 25°C and 760 mm Hg?
a. 755 ml
b. 760 ml
c. 696 ml
d. 730 ml

**49.** A sample of nitrogen at 20°C in a volume of 875 ml has a pressure of 730 mm Hg. What will be its pressure at 20°C if the volume is changed to 955 ml?
a. 750 mm Hg
b. 658 mm Hg
c. 797 mm Hg
d. 669 mm Hg

**50.** A mixture consisting of 8.0 g of oxygen and 14 g of nitrogen is prepared in a container such that the total pressure is 750 mm Hg. The partial pressure of oxygen in the mixture is
a. 125 mm Hg.
b. 500 mm Hg.
c. 135 mm Hg.
d. 250 mm Hg.

## Answers

**41. b.** 760 mm Hg is equal to 1 atmosphere; $\frac{740 \text{ mm}}{760 \text{ mm}} = 0.974$.

**42. c.** Since temperature is constant, use Boyle's law: $P_1V_1 = P_2V_2$. In this case $P_1 = 750$ mmHg; $P_2 = 650$ mmHg; $V_1 = 500$ ml; $V_2 = x$.

$750 \times 500 = 650x$

$375,000 = 650x$

$\frac{375,000}{650} = x$

$577 \text{ ml} = x$

**43. c.** This is Gay-Lussac's law.

**44. d.** Dalton's law states that $P_T = P_1 + P_2 + P_3$.

**45. a.** Gases have low density, are highly compressible, and mix rapidly, but they do not have a definite volume and shape.

**46. c.** The assumptions of kinetic theory are applied to ideal gases.

**47. d.** Pressure refers to the force exerted per unit area.

**48. c.** Use Boyle's law: $P_1V_1 = P_2V_2$.

$730 \times 725 = 760V_2$

$529,250 = 760V_2$

$\frac{529,250}{760} = V_2$

$696 \text{ ml} = V_2$

**49. d.** Again, use Boyle's law: $P_1V_1 = P_2V_2$.

$730 \times 875 = P_2 \times 955$

$638,750 = 955 P_2$

$\frac{638,750}{955} = P_2$

$669 \text{ mm} = P_2$

**50. d.** $8.0 \text{ g O}_2 \times \frac{\text{mol O}_2}{32.0 \text{ g O}_2} = 0.25 \text{ mol O}_2$

$14 \text{ g N}_2 \times \frac{\text{mol N}_2}{28.0 \text{ g N}_2} = 0.50 \text{ mol N}_2$

$PO_2 = \frac{0.25}{0.25 + 0.50} \times 750 \text{ mmHg}$

$= 250 \text{ mmHg}$

## F. Solutions

### 1. Properties

**Solution** is a homogeneous mixture.
**Solute** is a substance dissolved in a solvent.
**Solvent** is a medium in which a solute is dissolved.

**Solvation** is the process of dissolving molecules of solute in a solvent.

## 2. Solubility

**Solubility** is the maximum amount of solute (in grams) that can be dissolved in a certain amount of solvent (in ml) at a particular temperature.

### a. Pressure

Solubility increases with pressure for a gas immersed in a liquid. Solubility of solids and liquids does not vary significantly with pressure.

### b. Temperature

Solubility of most solids and liquids increases with increasing temperature while decreasing for gases dissolved in liquids (gas molecules tend to escape).

## 3. Concentration of Solutions

**Percent concentration** expresses the concentration as a ratio of the weight (or the volume) of the solute over the weight (or the volume) of the solution. This ratio is then multiplied by 100.

$\frac{Weight}{volume}\% = \frac{\text{grams of solute}}{100 \text{ ml of solvent}}$

$\frac{Volume}{volume}\% = \frac{\text{volume of solute}}{100 \text{ ml volume of final solution}}$

$\frac{Weight}{weight}\% = \frac{\text{grams of solute}}{100 \text{ g of solution}}$

## 4. Molarity

**Molarity (M)** expresses the number of moles of solute per liter of solution. A 0.1 M NaOH aqueous (dissolved in water) solution has 0.1 mol of solute (NaOH) per 1 liter of water.

## 5. Dilution

$M_iV_i = M_fV_f$ ($i$ = initial; $f$ = final) established the equivalence between the initial and final concentrations. In dilution, equivalence must be achieved between the initial and final concentrations.

Since M (mol/L) × V (L) gives units of moles, this equation states that the amount of a substance must be constant before and after a dilution occurs, i.e., if 1 L of an aqueous solution containing 0.1 mol

(5.8 g) of NaCl is diluted by adding an additional liter of water, there will still be 0.1 mol (5.8 g) of NaCl in the solution.

## 6. Colloids

**Colloids** are stable mixtures in which particles of rather large sizes (ranging from 1 nm (nanometer) to 1 μm (micrometer)) are dispersed throughout another substance. Aerosols (liquid droplets or solid particles dispersed in a gas) such as fog can scatter a beam of light. This is called the **Tyndall effect**.

## 7. Water
### a. Properties

Water is the most abundant (and important, besides oxygen) substance on Earth. The O–H bonds are highly polar, and water forms networks of hydrogen bonds. It is found in large amounts in cells and blood. Water is an excellent solvent and has a high boiling point, high surface tension, high heat of vaporization, and low vapor pressure.

### b. High Heat Capacity and High Heat of Vaporization

**Heat capacity** is the amount of energy required to raise the temperature of a substance by 1° Celsius. The **specific heat capacity** is the energy required to raise the temperature of 1 g of a substance by 1°C. Water has a high heat capacity, absorbing and releasing large amounts of heat before changing its own temperature. It thus allows the body to maintain a steady temperature even when internal and/or external conditions would otherwise increase body temperature.

**Specific heat of vaporization** is the heat required to evaporate 1 gram of a liquid. Water's large heat of vaporization (540 calories/gram) requires large amounts of heat in order to vaporize it. During perspiration, water evaporates from the skin, and large amounts of heat are lost.

### c. Reactivity

Water is not reactive with most compounds, so it can serve to transport substances in the body. It takes part in most metabolic transformations (hydrolysis and dehydration reactions).

## You Should Review

- the characteristics of solutions and the properties of true solutions
- the types of solutions and how they compare
- saturated solutions
- supersaturated solutions
- dilute solutions
- concentrated solutions
- how water dissolves ionic compounds
- how water dissolves covalent compounds
- hydrates

## Questions

**51.** In a dilute solution of sodium chloride in water, the sodium chloride is the
  **a.** solvent.
  **b.** solute.
  **c.** precipitate.
  **d.** reactant.

**52.** To prepare 100 ml of 0.20 M NaCl solution from stock solution of 1.00 M NaCl, you should mix
  **a.** 20 ml of stock solution with 80 ml of water.
  **b.** 40 ml of stock solution with 60 ml of water.
  **c.** 20 ml of stock solution with 100 ml of water.
  **d.** 25 ml of stock solution with 75 ml of water.

**53.** How many grams of NaOH would be needed to make 250 ml of 0.200 M solution? (molecular weight of NaOH = 40.0 g/mol)

a. 8.00 g

b. 4.00 g

c. 2.00 g

d. 2.50 g

**54.** The number of moles of NaCl in 250 ml of a 0.300 M solution of NaCl is

a. 0.0750

b. 0.150

c. 0.250

d. 1.15

**55.** Which of the following properties of water is not dependent on the polar nature of water?

a. color

b. high boiling point

c. solvent power

d. high heat of vaporization

**56.** A substance has the formula $MgSO_4 \times 7H_2O$. How many grams of water are in 5.00 moles of this substance?

a. 7.00

b. 35.0

c. 126

d. 630

**57.** How many grams of sugar are needed to make 500 ml of a 5% (weight/volume) solution of sugar?

a. 20

b. 25

c. 50

d. 10

**58.** Which of the following types of bonds forms when a hydrogen atom binds to a highly electronegative atom and also partially binds to another atom?

a. coordinate covalent bond

b. hydrogen bond

c. ionic bond

d. covalent bond

**59.** Which of the following is NOT true of a solution?

a. Each component of a solution retains its original properties.

b. A solution is a heterogeneous mixture.

c. A solution is composed of a solute and solvent.

d. A solution involves two or more pure substances.

**60.** Which of the following is NOT a factor that affects solubility?

a. temperature

b. pressure

c. particle size

d. properties of the solvent

## Answers

**51. b.** The substance being dissolved is the solute, by definition.

**52. a.** You need 20 ml of stock solution; you would then fill the container with water to the 100 ml mark (80 ml $H_2O$).
$$M_i \times V_i = M_f \times V_f$$
$$1.0 \text{ M} \times V_i = 0.2 \text{ M} \times 100 \text{ ml}$$
$$1.0 \, V_i = 20$$
$$V_i = 20 \text{ ml}$$

**53. c.** $250 \text{ ml} \times \frac{0.2 \text{ mol NaOH}}{1,000 \text{ ml}} = 0.05 \text{ mol}$; $0.05 \text{ mol}$ $\times 40 \text{ g/mol} = 2.00 \text{ g}$

**54. a.** $250 \text{ ml} \times \frac{0.3 \text{ mol NaCl}}{1,000 \text{ ml}} = 0.0750 \text{ mol}$

**55. a.** The other properties listed are due to the polar nature of water.

**56. d.** There are 5 moles of $MgSO_4 \times 7H_2O$. There are 7 moles of water of $MgSO_4 \times 7H_2O$; $7 \times 5 = 35$ moles; $35 \text{ mol} \times 18 \text{ g/mol} = 630 \text{ g}$.

**57. b.** $5\% \frac{w}{v} = \frac{5 \text{ g solute}}{100 \text{ ml solution}}$

$$\frac{5 \text{ g}}{100 \text{ ml}} = \frac{x \text{ (solute needed)}}{500 \text{ ml (final volume)}}$$

$$\frac{5 \times 500}{100} = x$$
$$25 \text{ g} = x$$

**58. b.** Hydrogen atoms are capable of forming a partial bond between a highly electronegative atom and another atom.

**59. b.** A solution is a homogeneous mixture.

**60. c.** Temperature, pressure, and the properties of the solvent all affect solubility.

## G. Reaction Rates and Equilibrium

### 1. Equilibrium

**Equilibrium** is reached when two opposing reactions occur at the same rate. No change is observed in the system—e.g., for the reaction $A \leftrightarrow B$, the rate at which A is converted to B is the same rate that B is converted to A.

### 2. Equilibrium Constant

The **equilibrium constant**, $K$, for a reaction describes the concentrations of reactants and products for a chemical reaction at equilibrium. $K$ is often dependent on temperature. For a balanced chemical equation, $wA + xB \leftrightarrow yC + zD$, the equilibrium constant is written as:

$$K = \frac{[C]^y [D]^z}{[A]^w [B]^x}$$

where $[A]$, $[B]$, $[C]$, and $[D]$ are concentrations of reactants and products and $w$, $x$, $y$, and $z$ are the coefficients used to balance the chemical equation. If one of the reactants or products is a solid, it is not included in the equilibrium expression.

### 3. Activation Energy

**Activation energy** is the minimum amount of energy required for reactants to be transformed into products (i.e., to overcome the energy barrier between reactants and products). The higher the activation energy, the slower the reaction.

## 4. Endothermic versus Exothermic Reactions

**Endothermic reactions** are reactions that consume energy in order to take place. Anabolic reactions are endothermic.

**Exothermic reactions** are energy-releasing reactions. Most catabolic and oxidative reactions are exothermic.

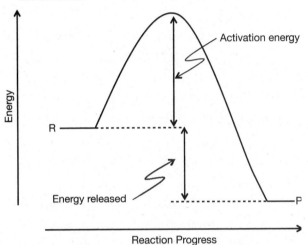

Reaction diagram for an exothermic reaction

## 5. Factors Affecting the Rate of Reaction

### a. Temperature

Rates of reactions increase with temperature, as more collisions between particles occur at higher temperatures.

### b. Particle Size

Smaller particles react faster, as they collide often at any given temperature and concentration.

### c. Concentration

A high concentration of reacting particles increases the rate of chemical reactions between them.

### d. Catalysis

**Catalysts** speed the reaction rate by lowering the activation energy of the reaction. They are not consumed in the reaction.

## 6. Reversible Reactions

A double arrow (⇆) designates reversible (two-way) chemical reactions. If arrows differ in length, the longer arrow indicates the major (faster) direction in which the reaction proceeds.

## 7. Le Chatelier's Principle

**Le Chatelier's Principle** states that when a system at equilibrium experiences a change (e.g., in concentration, temperature, or partial pressure), it will respond to counteract this change and establish a new equilibrium. For example, increasing the concentration of compounds on the right side of a chemical equation will shift the equilibrium to the left.

### *You Should Review*

- Le Chatelier's principle and the different stresses that can be placed on chemical processes
- equilibrium constants
- energy diagrams

# Questions

**61.** Which of the following is NOT true of reversible chemical reactions?
  **a.** A chemical reaction is never complete.
  **b.** The products of the reaction also react to reform the original reactants.
  **c.** When the reaction is finished, both reactants and products are present in equal amounts.
  **d.** The reaction can result in an equilibrium.

**62.** Which is an example of an exothermic change?
  **a.** sublimation
  **b.** condensation
  **c.** melting
  **d.** evaporation

**63.** Which is NOT an example of an endothermic change?
   **a.** melting
   **b.** sublimation
   **c.** freezing
   **d.** evaporation

**64.** The following reaction is exothermic: $AgNO_3 + NaCl \rightleftharpoons AgCl + NaNO_3$. How will the equilibrium be changed if the temperature is increased?
   **a.** Equilibrium will shift to the right.
   **b.** Equilibrium will shift to the left.
   **c.** The reaction will not proceed.
   **d.** Equilibrium will not change.

## Answers

**61. c.** The fact that a reaction is complete does not mean that both reactants and products are present in equal amounts.
**62. b.** Condensation is an example of a reaction in which energy is given off.
**63. c.** Freezing does not absorb energy.
**64. b.** When the temperature is increased, the equilibrium shifts to the left.

### H. Acids and Bases

#### 1. Definitions

**Acids** are proton donors (according to the Brønsted Theory) or electron acceptors (according to the Lewis Theory). Acids release protons ($H^+$) and form anionic conjugate bases (negatively charged ions). Strong acids completely dissociate in water. Acids have a sour taste.

| COMMON STRONG ACIDS |
| --- |
| Hydrochloric (HCl) |
| Hydrobromic (HBr) |
| Hydroiodic (HI) |
| Perchloric ($HClO_4$) |
| Sulfuric ($H_2SO_4$) |

**Bases** are proton acceptors (Brønsted) or electron donors (Lewis). When dissolved in water, strong bases such as NaOH dissociate to release hydroxide ions and sodium cations. Bases have a bitter taste and feel slippery like soap.

#### 2. Reactions of Acids

Common reactions include:

- metal + acid → salt + hydrogen
  $Zn + 2HCl \rightarrow ZnCl_2 + H_2$
- base + acid → salt + water
  $NaOH + HNO_3 \rightarrow NaNO_3 + H_2O$

- metal oxide + acid → salt + water
  $CaO + 2HNO_3 \rightarrow Ca(NO_3)_2 + H_2O$
- metal carbonate + acid → salt + carbonic acid (unstable)
  $NaHCO_3 + HCl \rightarrow NaCl + H_2CO_3$
  $(H_2CO_3 \rightarrow H_2O + CO_2)$

## 3. Autoionization of Water

In pure water, $2H_2O \underset{\rightarrow}{\leftarrow} H_3O^+ + OH^-$.
$[H_3O^+] = [OH^-]$.
The ion product of water is Kw:
$Kw = [H_3O^+] \times [OH^-] = 1 \times 10^{-14}$. Thus, in pure water: $[H_3O^+] = [OH^-] = 1 \times 10^{-7}$ moles/liter.

## 4. pH

**$pH = -\log[H^+]$.** The **pH** measures the negative logarithm (for presentation of very small numbers in a large scale) of the hydrogen ion concentration (in moles/liter). The pH scale runs from 0 to 14, with acids in the lower end of the scale (smaller than pH 7) and bases at the higher end (greater than pH 7).

## 5. Buffers

**Buffer** is a solution of a weak base and its conjugate acid (weak also) that prevents drastic changes in pH. The weak base reacts with any $H^+$ ions that could increase acidity, and the weak conjugate acid reacts with $OH^-$ ions that may increase the basicity of the solution.

### a. Carbonic Acid/Bicarbonate Buffer

Blood pH must be maintained at pH 7.40 by a buffer system consisting of the couple $H_2CO_3$ (carbonic acid) and $HCO_3^-$ (bicarbonate).

Neutralization of acid:
$HCO_3^- + H^+ \rightarrow H_2CO_3$

Neutralization of base:
$H_2CO_3 + NaOH \rightarrow NaHCO_3 + H_2O$

### b. Phosphate Buffer

The principal buffer system inside cells in blood consists of the couple $H_2PO_4^-$ and $HPO_4^{-2}$.

Neutralization of acid:
$HPO_4^{-2} + H^+ \rightarrow H_2PO_4^-$

Neutralization of base:
$H_2PO_4^- + OH^- \rightarrow HPO_4^{-2} + H_2O$

## 6. Titration

**Titration** is a technique used to determine the unknown concentration of an analyte of interest by reaching it with a known quantity of a reagent. In an acid–base titration, an acid or base of unknown concentration is reacted with a known amount of base or acid.

### a. Equivalence Point

In an acid–base titration, the **equivalence point** is reached when the amount of titrant (acid or base of known concentration) is equal to the amount of analyte (base or acid of unknown concentration) and the solution is of neutral pH.

### b. Normality (N)

**Normality** is the number of equivalents of the solute per liter of solution. 1 N solution of acid (or base) contains 1 equivalent of an acid (or base) per liter of solution.

## You Should Review

- monoprotic, diprotic, and triprotic acids
- organic and inorganic acids
- Arrhenius acids and bases
- Brønsted-Lowry acids and bases
- reactions of acids
- activity series of metals
- solubilities of salts
- ionic equations
- buffer systems in the body
- metabolic acidosis and alkalosis
- respiratory acidosis and alkalosis

## Questions

**65.** What is the formula of sulfuric acid?
   a. $HNO_3$
   b. $H_2SO_4$
   c. HCl
   d. $H_2CO_3$

**66.** What is the formula of the hydronium ion?
   a. $H^+$
   b. $NH_4^+$
   c. $H_3O^+$
   d. $H_2O^+$

**67.** The pH of a blood sample is 7.40 at room temperature. The pOH is therefore
   a. 6.60
   b. 7.40
   c. $6 \times 10^{-6}$
   d. $4 \times 10^{-7}$

**68.** As the concentration of hydrogen ions in a solution decreases,
   a. the pH numerically decreases.
   b. the pH numerically increases.
   c. the product of the concentrations $[H^+] \times [OH^-]$ comes closer to $1 \times 10^{-14}$.
   d. the solution becomes more acidic.

**69.** The pH of an alkaline solution is
   a. 14.
   b. less than 7.
   c. more than 14.
   d. more than 7.

**70.** A base is a substance that dissociates in water into one or more _____ ions and one or more _____.
   a. hydrogen . . . anions
   b. hydrogen . . . cations
   c. hydroxide . . . anions
   d. hydroxide . . . cations

**71.** An acid is a substance that dissociates in water into one or more _____ ions and one or more _____.
   a. hydrogen . . . anions
   b. hydrogen . . . cations
   c. hydroxide . . . anions
   d. hydroxide . . . cations

**72.** A pH of 4 denotes _____ times fewer _____ than a pH of 3.
   a. 10 . . . hydrogen ions
   b. 4 . . . hydrogen ions
   c. 10 . . . water molecules
   d. 20 . . . hydroxide ions

**73.** Which of the following is considered to be neutral on the pH scale?
   a. pure water
   b. pure saliva
   c. pure blood
   d. pure urine

**74.** A substance that functions to prevent rapid, drastic changes in the pH of a body fluid by changing strong acids and bases into weak acids and bases is called a(n)
   a. salt.
   b. buffer.
   c. enzyme.
   d. coenzyme.

**75.** Complete the following equation:
$NaHCO_3 + HCl \rightarrow NaCl^+$
   a. $HCO_3$
   b. $H_2CO_3$
   c. HCl
   d. $H_2PO_4$

## Answers

**65. b.** The formula is $H_2SO_4$.

**66. c.** The formula is $H_3O^+$.

**67. a.** The ion product constant of $H_2O$ is $1 \times 10^{-14}$;
$[H^+] [OH^-] = \frac{1 \times 10^{-14}}{1 \times 10^{-7.40}} = 1 \times 10^{-6.60}$;
pOH = 6.60
or
pH + pOH = 14.00
pOH = 14.00 − 7.40 = 6.60

**68. b.** As the concentration of hydrogen ions decreases, the pH becomes more basic and increases.

**69. d.** On the pH scale, 1–7 is acidic, 7 is neutral, and 7–14 is alkaline.

**70. d.** By definition, when a base dissociates in water, it produces one or more $OH^-$ and one or more cations.

**71. a.** By definition, when an acid dissociates in water, it produces one or more $H^+$ and one or more anions.

**72. a.** An increase of one pH unit is a tenfold decrease in hydrogen ions.

**73. a.** The pH of pure $H_2O$ is 7. $[H^+] = [OH^-]$

**74. b.** This is the definition of a buffer.

**75. b.** Metal bicarbonate + an acid → salt + carbonic acid.

## I. Oxidation-Reduction

### 1. Oxidation State

**Oxidation state** (or **oxidation number**) is the number of charges carried by an ion in an atom, or the number of charges that an atom would have in a [neutral] molecule if electrons were transferred completely. Oxidation numbers enable the identification of oxidized (increase in oxidation number) and reduced (reduction in oxidation number) elements.

The sum of the oxidation numbers of all atoms in the formula of a neutral compound is zero (or equal to the charge on the ion for a polyatomic ion).

### 2. Oxidation-Reduction (Redox) Reactions

**Oxidation** corresponds to a loss of electrons.

**Reduction** corresponds to a gain of electrons.

**Redox (reduction-oxidation) reaction** involves an electron transfer between the oxidizing (oxidizes another by accepting its electrons) and the reducing (reduces another by donating electrons) agents.

**Example:**  $2Na + Cl_2 \rightarrow 2NaCl$
$Na \rightarrow Na^+ + e^-$
Oxidation Number:  0  +1  −1
(Na is oxidized to $Na^+$)

**Example:**
$Cl + e^- \rightarrow Cl^-$
Oxidation Number:  0  −1  −1
(Cl is reduced to $Cl^-$)
Sum: $Na + Cl \rightarrow Na^+ + Cl^-$

### You Should Review

- redox reactions: cellular respiration, combustion, rusting
- oxidizing agents
- reducing agents

## Questions

**76.** The number of electrons lost during oxidation must always equal the
  **a.** charge of the ion.
  **b.** total change in oxidation number.
  **c.** number of electrons gained in the reduction.
  **d.** number of electrons gained by the reducing agent.

**77.** What is the oxidation number for nitrogen in $HNO_3$?
  **a.** −2
  **b.** +5
  **c.** −1
  **d.** −5

# Answers

**76. c.** The number of electrons lost during oxidation must always equal the number of electrons gained in the reduction.

**77. b.** $H = +1$; $O_3 = 3 \times -2 = -6$

$+1 + N - 6 = 0$

$N = +5$

## J. Nuclear Chemistry

### 1. Characteristics of Radioactivity

**Radioactivity** is the process by which unstable nuclei break-down spontaneously, emitting particles and/or electromagnetic radiation (i.e., energy) also called **nuclear radiation.**

Heavy elements (atomic numbers 83 to 92) are naturally radioactive, and many more (the transuranium elements: atomic numbers 93 to 118) are generated in laboratories.

### 2. Alpha Emission

An **alpha particle** (symbol: $^4_2He$ or $\alpha$) corresponds to the nucleus of a helium atom (having two protons and two neutrons) that is spontaneously emitted by a nuclear breakdown or decay.

$\alpha$-particles are of low energy and therefore low penetrating (a lab coat is sufficient to block their penetration), but they can be dangerous if inhaled or ingested.

### 3. Beta Emission

A **beta particle** (symbol: $^0_{-1}e$ or $\beta^-$) is an electron released with high speed by a radioactive nucleus in which neutrons are converted into protons and electrons ($\beta$-particles). $\beta$-particles are medium-penetrating radiation requiring dense material and several layers of clothing to block their penetration. They are dangerous if inhaled or ingested.

### 4. Gamma Emission

**Gamma rays** (symbol: $\gamma$) are a massless and chargeless form of radiation (pure energy). They are the most-penetrating form of radiation, similar to X-rays, and can only be stopped by barriers of heavy materials such as concrete or lead. They are extremely dangerous and can cause damage to the human body.

### 5. Transmutation

Nuclear **transmutation** is the conversion of one element or isotope into another. This process may be spontaneous (through $\alpha$- or $\beta$-decay) and result in lighter elements, or it may occur when nuclei are bombarded by other particles (protons or neutrons) or nuclei, resulting in heavier elements.

During nuclear reaction, there is:

1. conservation of mass number
2. conservation of atomic number

For example, U-238 undergoes $\alpha$-decay to form Th-234

$$^{238}_{92}U \rightarrow {}^{234}_{90}Th + {}^4_2He$$

### 6. Half-Life

**Half-life** (symbol: $t_{\frac{1}{2}}$) is the time required for the concentration of the nuclei in a given sample to decrease to half of its initial concentration. Half-life is specific to a radioactive element and varies widely (from a fraction of a second for Tc-43 to millions of years for U-238).

### 7. Nuclear Fusion

**Nuclear fusion** is the process by which small nuclei are combined (fused) into larger, more stable ones with the release of a large amount of energy. Fusion reactions take place at very high temperatures. They are also known as thermonuclear reactions. Examples are our Sun and H-bombs.

### 8. Nuclear Fission

**Nuclear fission** is the process by which a heavier, usually less stable, nucleus splits into smaller nuclei and neutrons. The process releases a large amount of energy and neutrons that can set up a **chain reaction**

(or self-sustaining nuclear fission reaction) with a more and more uncontrollable release of energy (a highly exothermic reaction) and neutrons.

## 9. Radioactive Isotopes

A **radioactive isotope (radioisotope)** is an unstable isotope of an element that decays into a more stable isotope of a different element. They are of great use in medicine as tracers in the body to help monitor particular atoms in chemical and biological reactions. In this way, they aid with diagnosis and treatment. Doctors use Iodine (-131 and -123) and Technetium-99 because of their short half-lives. A short half-life means a radioisotope decays into a stable (nonradioactive) substance in a relatively short time.

### You Should Review

- nuclear reactions
- writing balanced nuclear equations
- radiocarbon dating
- the principles of nuclear power
- the use of radioisotopes and their detection in nuclear medicine
- the dangers of ionizing radiation
- radiation sickness/biological effects of radiation
- units of radiation measurement

## Questions

**78.** The time required for $\frac{1}{2}$ of the atoms in a sample of a radioactive element to decay is known as the element's
   **a.** decay period.
   **b.** life time.
   **c.** radioactive period.
   **d.** half-life.

**79.** The least penetrating radiation given off by a radioactive substance consists of
   **a.** alpha particles.
   **b.** beta particles.
   **c.** gamma rays.
   **d.** X-rays.

**80.** The half-life of a given element is 70 years. How long will it take 5.0 g of this element to be reduced to 1.25 g?
   **a.** 70 years
   **b.** 140 years
   **c.** 210 years
   **d.** 35 years

**81.** If element $^{210}_{83}A$ gives off an alpha particle, what is the atomic number and mass of the resulting element B?
   **a.** $^{210}_{81}B$
   **b.** $^{206}_{81}B$
   **c.** $^{206}_{83}B$
   **d.** $^{204}_{81}B$

**82.** If element $^{238}_{92}B$ gives off a beta particle and gamma rays, what is the resulting element?
   **a.** $^{238}_{93}B$
   **b.** $^{234}_{90}B$
   **c.** $^{239}_{92}B$
   **d.** $^{239}_{91}B$

**83.** What is the missing product?
   $^{42}_{17}X \rightarrow ^{42}_{18}Y + ?$
   **a.** $^{4}_{2}He$
   **b.** $\gamma$
   **c.** $^{0}_{1}e$
   **d.** $^{0}_{-1}\beta$

**84.** What is the missing product?
   $^{60}_{24}A \rightarrow ^{60}_{24}B + ?$
   **a.** $^{4}_{2}He$
   **b.** $\gamma$
   **c.** $^{0}_{-1}e$
   **d.** $^{0}_{1}\beta$

# Answers

**78. d.** The question gives the definition of half-life.

**79. a.** Alpha particles give off the least penetrating radiation.

**80. b.** In 70 years, there will be $\frac{1}{2} \times 5.0 = 2.5$ g. In 70 more years (140 total), there will be $\frac{1}{2} \times 2.5 = 1.25$ g.

**81. b.** Giving off an alpha particle is equivalent to giving off a helium nucleus.
$$_{83}^{210}A - {}_2^4He = {}_{81}^{206}B$$

**82. a.** When a beta particle is given off, the nucleus has the same mass number, but the atomic number is greater by one since a neutron is converted to a proton and an electron.

**83. d.** A beta particle allows the mass to remain the same and increases the atomic number by 1.

**84. b.** Gamma rays are not particles and therefore do not change the atomic number or atomic mass.

## K. Organic Compounds

### 1. Definition

**Organic compounds** are compounds made predominantly of carbon, hydrogen, and heteroatoms such as oxygen, nitrogen, the halogens, phosphorus, sulfur, and others.

### 2. Stereoisomers

**Stereoisomers** are two molecules that have the same molecular formula and structure but different spatial orientation with respect to the median axis or plane of the molecule. Their three-dimensional shapes are, therefore, different.

### 3. Carbohydrates
#### a. Function

Carbohydrates (or sugars) serve as the main source of energy for living organisms. They are made of one, two, or more rings of carbon, hydrogen, and oxygen. The names of carbohydrates end with the suffix, *-ose* (for example, *glucose* and *fructose*).

#### b. Monosaccharides

**Monosaccharides** are the simplest carbohydrate structures made of one ring that can contain five C atoms, called a **pentose**, or six C atoms, called a **hexose**. An example of a pentose is ribose, which is a constituent of RNA. One example of a hexose is galactose, which is derived from milk-sugar lactose.

#### c. Disaccharides

**Disaccharides** are dimeric sugars made of two monosaccharides joined together in a reaction that releases a molecule of water (dehydration). The bond between the two sugar molecules is called a glycosidic linkage and can have either an axial ($\beta$-glycoside) or an equatorial ($\alpha$-glycoside) orientation with respect to the ring conformation.

> Examples:
> **Maltose** is two glucose molecules joined together, found in starch.
> **Lactose** is one galactose joined to one glucose, found in milk.
> **Sucrose** is one fructose joined to one glucose, found in table sugar.

#### d. Polysaccharides

**Polysaccharides** are polymers, or a long chain of repeating monosaccharide units.

- **Starch** is a mixture of two kinds of polymers of $\alpha$ glucose (linear amylose and amylopectin). Amylose contains glucose molecules joined together by $\alpha$-glycosidic linkages, while amylopectin has an addition of branching at C-6. They are the storage form of polysaccharides in plants.
- **Glycogen** consists of glucose molecules linked by $\alpha$-glycosidic linkage (C-1 and C-4) and branched (C-6) by $\alpha$-glycosidic linkage. Glycogen is the storage form of glucose in animals (in liver and skeletal muscle).

- **Cellulose** consists of glucose molecules joined together by β-glycosidic linkage. Cellulose is found in plants and cannot be digested by humans because they lack the necessary enzyme.

### e. Condensation and Hydrolysis

**Condensation** is the process of bonding separate monosaccharide subunits together into a disaccharide and/or a polysaccharide. It is also called **dehydration synthesis**, as one molecule of water is lost in the process. It is carried out by specific enzymes.

**Hydrolysis** is the reverse process of condensation as a water molecule and specific enzymes, called hydrolases, break the glycosidic linkages in disaccharides and polysaccharides into their constituting monosaccharides.

## 4. Lipids

### a. Function

**Lipids** are a diverse group of compounds that are insoluble in water and polar solvents but soluble in nonpolar solvents. Lipids are stored in the body as a source of energy and contain twice the energy provided by equal amounts of carbohydrates.

### b. Triglycerides

**Triglycerides** are lipids formed by condensation of glycerol (one molecule) with fatty acids (three molecules). They can be saturated (all fatty acids containing only C–C single bonds) or unsaturated (presence of one or more C=C double bonds). Triglycerides are found in the adipose cells of the body (neutral fat) and are metabolized by the enzyme lipase during hydrolysis, producing fatty acids and glycerol.

### c. Ketone Bodies

There are three **ketone bodies** formed during the breakdown (metabolism) of fats: acetoacetate, β-hydroxybutyrate, and acetone. They are produced to meet the energy requirements of other tissues. Fatty acids—produced by the hydrolysis of triglycerides—are converted to ketone bodies in the liver. They are removed by the kidneys (**ketosuria**), but if they are found in excess in the blood (**ketonemia**), ketone bodies can cause a decrease of the blood pH, and **ketoacidosis** may result. In **ketouria**, acetone is exhaled via the lungs. The whole process is called **ketosis**. Ketosuria and ketonemia are common in patients with diabetes mellitus and in cases of prolonged starvation.

### d. Phospholipids

**Phospholipids** are lipids containing a phosphate group. They are the main constituents of cellular membranes.

### e. Steroids

**Steroids** are organic compounds characterized by a core structure known as **gonane** (three cyclohexane—six carbon rings and one cyclopentane—or five C rings fused together). Steroids differ by the functional groups attached to the gonane core. Cholesterol is an example of a steroid and is a precursor for the steroid hormones such as the sex hormones (androgens and estrogens) and the corticosteroids (hormones of the adrenal cortex).

## 5. Proteins

### a. Functions

Every organism contains thousands of different proteins with a variety of functions: structure (collagen, histones), transport (hemoglobin, serum albumin), defense (antibodies, fibrinogen for blood coagulation), control and regulation (insulin), catalysis (enzymes), and storage.

### b. Structure

Proteins (also called polypeptides) are long chains of amino acids joined together by covalent bonds of the same type (peptide or amide bonds). There are 20 naturally occurring amino acids, each characterized by an amino group at one end and a carboxylic acid group at the other end. Different proteins have different numbers and types of additional functional groups.

The sequence of amino acids in the long chain defines the **primary structure** of a protein.

A **secondary structure** is determined when several residues, linked by hydrogen bonds, conform to a given combination (for example, the α-helix or β-sheet).

**Tertiary structure** refers to the three-dimensionally folded conformation of a protein. This is the biologically active conformation.

A **quaternary structure** can result when two or more individual proteins assemble into two or more polypeptide chains.

**Conjugated proteins** are complexes of proteins with other biomolecules (for example, glycoproteins, also called sugar proteins).

### c. Enzymes

**Enzymes** are biological catalysts whose role is to increase the rate of chemical (metabolic) reactions without being consumed in the reaction. They do so by lowering the activation energy of a reaction by binding specifically into the active site of their substrates in a "lock and key" or "induced-fit" mechanism. They do not change the nature of the reaction (in fact, any change is associated with a malfunctioning enzyme, the onset of a disease) or its outcome.

Enzyme activity is influenced by:

- temperature: proteins can be destroyed at high temperatures, and their action is slowed at low temperatures.
- pH: enzymes are active in a certain range of pH.
- concentration of cofactors and coenzymes (vitamins)
- concentration of enzymes and substrates
- feedback reactions

Enzyme names are derived from their substrate names with the addition of the suffix -*ase*. An example is *sucrase* (substrate is sucrose). There are categories of enzymes according to the reactions they catalyze (for example, the kinases for phosphorylation).

Enzymes are often found in multienzyme systems that operate by simple negative feedback.

$$
\begin{array}{llll}
\text{enzyme 1} & \text{enzyme 2} & \text{enzyme 3} & \text{enzyme 4} \\
A \underset{\rightarrow}{\overset{\leftarrow}{\phantom{x}}} B & B \underset{\rightarrow}{\overset{\leftarrow}{\phantom{x}}} C & C \underset{\rightarrow}{\overset{\leftarrow}{\phantom{x}}} D & D \underset{\rightarrow}{\overset{\leftarrow}{\phantom{x}}} E_1 \\
 & & & \rightarrow E_2 \\
 & & & \text{enzyme 5}
\end{array}
$$

### d. Protein Denaturation

**Protein denaturation** occurs when a protein's configuration is changed by the destruction of the secondary and tertiary structures (reduced to the primary structure). Common denaturing agents are alcohol, heat, and heavy metal salts.

## You Should Review

- stereoisomers
- the structure of monosaccharides and hemiacetals
- the structure of disaccharides and acetals, glycosides
- reducing sugars
- stereoisomers and enzymes in carbohydrate metabolism
- digestion and synthesis of carbohydrates
- ketoacidosis, ketonemia, acetone breath, chemical structures of ketone bodies, gluconeogenesis
- functions of proteins
- protein synthesis and amino acid structures
- organic functional groups in proteins
- enzyme-catalyzed reactions
- vitamins, metal ion activators
- enzyme nomenclature
- multienzyme systems, simple negative feedback

$$
\begin{array}{ccccccccc}
E & + & S & \rightarrow & ES & \rightarrow & E & + & P \\
\textit{enzyme} & & \textit{substrate} & & \textit{enzyme-substrate} & & \textit{enzyme} & & \textit{product} \\
 & & & & \textit{complex} & & & &
\end{array}
$$

# Questions

**85.** The elements found in carbohydrates are
  **a.** oxygen, carbon, and hydrogen.
  **b.** zinc, hydrogen, and iron.
  **c.** carbon, iron, and oxygen.
  **d.** hydrogen, iron, and carbon.

**86.** Steroids are classified as
  **a.** carbohydrates.
  **b.** nucleic acids.
  **c.** lipids.
  **d.** proteins.

**87.** The primary function of food carbohydrates in the body is to
  **a.** provide for the storage of glycogen in cells.
  **b.** maintain the constancy of the blood sugar.
  **c.** maintain energy production within the cells.
  **d.** contribute to the structure of the cells.

**88.** A high level of ketone bodies in urine indicates marked increase in the metabolism of
  **a.** carbohydrates.
  **b.** fats.
  **c.** proteins.
  **d.** nucleic acids.

**89.** Which polysaccharide is a branched polymer of α-glucose found in the liver and muscle cells?
  **a.** amylase
  **b.** cellulose
  **c.** glycogen
  **d.** amylopectin

**90.** An enzyme that catalyzes the hydrolysis of a triglyceride (fat) is
  **a.** a catalose.
  **b.** an esterase.
  **c.** an amidose.
  **d.** lactose.

**91.** The site on an enzyme molecule that does the catalytic work is called the
  **a.** binding site.
  **b.** allosteric site.
  **c.** lock.
  **d.** active site.

**92.** In the multienzyme sequence shown here, molecules of E are able to fit to the enzyme $E_1$ and prevent the conversion of A to B. What is this action of E called?

$$E_1 \qquad E_2 \qquad E_3 \qquad E_4$$
$$A \rightarrow B \rightarrow C \rightarrow D \rightarrow E$$

  **a.** effector inhibition
  **b.** allosteric inhibition
  **c.** feedback inhibition
  **d.** competitive inhibition by nonproduct

**93.** The carbohydrate sucrose is broken down by the enzyme sucrase into
  **a.** glucose and fructose.
  **b.** galactose and glucose.
  **c.** two glucose molecules.
  **d.** glucose and zylose.

**94.** The bonds between amino acids in a polypeptide are
  **a.** glycosidic bonds.
  **b.** ester bonds.
  **c.** peptide bonds.
  **d.** hydrogen bonds.

## Answers

**85. a.** By definition, carbohydrates are made of oxygen, carbon, and hydrogen.

**86. c.** Steroids are a subcategory of lipids.

**87. c.** Glucose, a monosaccharide, is the primary energy source in the body.

**88. b.** Ketone bodies are formed from free fatty acids.

**89. c.** Glycogen is a branched polymer of $\alpha$-glucose, which is found stored in limited amounts in the liver and muscle cells.

**90. b.** A fat is formed from one molecule of glycerol and three fatty acids, which are combined by three ester bonds. To break these bonds, an esterase is needed.

**91. d.** The active site is where the substrate is broken down.

**92. c.** E stops $E_1$ from converting A to B.

**93. a.** The disaccharide sucrose is broken down into glucose and fructose by sucrase.

**94. c.** Peptide bonds are formed between adjacent amino acids in a polypeptide chain.

## III. Other Concepts You Should Be Familiar With

### A. The Scientific Method

#### 1. General

The scientific method is based upon **observations** that lead to the formulation of a **hypothesis** in an attempt to make a comprehensive guess. Only reproducible **experiments** will confirm the hypothesis and eventually develop into a **theory** supported by all the facts.

#### 2. The Science of Chemistry

**Chemistry** is the study of the structures, properties, and transformations of atoms and molecules.

### B. Metric System

**Metric system** is the standard system for recording measurements. It is a decimal system, with the basic unit and its subunits separated by increasing and decreasing powers of ten. Some of the basic units of measurement are:

- Length: meter (m)
- Volume: liter (l)
- Mass: kilogram (kg)
- Time: the second (s)
- Temperature: Centigrade (°C)
- Amount of substance: mole (mol)

### C. Unit Conversion: The Factor Label Method

A **conversion factor** establishes a relationship of equivalence in measurement between two different units. It is expressed as a fraction. For instance, for 1 kg = 2.2 lbs., the conversion factor is $\frac{1 \text{ kg}}{2.2 \text{ lbs.}}$, or $\frac{2.2 \text{ lbs.}}{1 \text{ kg}}$.

**Example:**

Convert 50 cm to m:

Since 100 cm = 1 m, the conversion factor is

$\frac{1 \text{ m}}{100 \text{ cm}}$ or $\frac{100 \text{ cm}}{1 \text{ m}}$

So, 50 cm $\times (\frac{1 \text{m}}{100 \text{ cm}}) = 0.50$ m

**Example:**

How many grams are in 0.45 lbs.? (1 lb. = 453.6 g)
Conversion factor: $\frac{1 \text{ lb.}}{453.6 \text{ g}}$ or $\frac{453.6 \text{ g}}{1 \text{ lb.}}$
Since we need an answer in grams, we will use the conversion factor that has the grams in the numerator.
So, 0.45 lb. $\times (\frac{453.6 \text{ g}}{1 \text{ lb.}}) = 204.1$ g.

## D. Significant Figures

The number of significant figures in any physical quantity or measurement is the number of digits known precisely to be accurate. The rules for counting significant figures are the following:

- Zeros sandwiched between nonzero digits are significant. For example, both 400.005 and 400,005 have six significant figures.
- Zeros that locate the decimal place (place holder) on the left are not significant. For example, 0.045 ml, 0.0045 ml, and 0.00045 ml each have two significant figures.
- Trailing zeros to the right of the decimal point are significant if the number is greater than 1. For example, 4.56000 has six significant figures.
- For numbers smaller than 1, only zeros to the right of the first significant digit are significant. For example, 0.020 has two significant figures.
- Trailing zeros are not significant in a non-decimal number. For example, 5,500 has two significant figures.

## E. Error, Accuracy, Precision, and Uncertainty

**Error** is the difference between a value obtained experimentally and the standard value accepted by the scientific community.

**Accuracy** establishes how close in agreement a measurement is with the accepted value.

**Precision** of a measurement is the degree to which successive measurements agree with each other (average deviation is minimized).

**Uncertainty** expresses the doubt associated with the accuracy of any single measurement.

## F. Functional Groups in Organic Chemistry

### 1. Alkene

### 2. Alcohol

### 3. Aldehyde

### 4. Ketone

### 5. Carboxylic Acid

### 6. Amine

### 7. Amide

**8. Ester**

**9. Aromatic**

**10. Alkyne**

$$-C\equiv C-$$

**11. Ether**

$$-O-$$

**12. Disulfide**

$$-S-S-$$

# IV. Suggested Sources for Further Study

## Study Guides

Klein, David R. *Organic Chemistry as a Second Language* (New York: John Wiley & Sons, 2004).

Klein, David R. *Organic Chemistry as a Second Language: First Semester Topics, 3rd Edition.* (New York: John Wiley & Sons, 2011).

Varma-Nelson, Pratibha and Mark S. Cracolice. *Peer-Led Team Learning General, Organic, and Biological Chemistry* (New York: Prentice Hall, 2001).

## Textbooks

Chang, Raymond. *General Chemistry: The Essential Concepts, 3rd Edition* (New York: McGraw-Hill, 2003).

Chang, Raymond and Overby, Jason. *General Chemistry: The Essential Concepts, 6th Edition.* (New York: McGraw-Hill, 2011).

Kotz, John C., and Paul M. Treichel. *Chemistry and Chemical Reactivity, 5th Edition* (Pacific Grove, CA: Brooks/Cole, 2003).

Kotz, John C., et al. *Chemistry & Chemical Reactivity, 8th Edition.* (Pacific Grove, CA: Brooks/Cole, 2011).

Timberlake, Karen C. *General, Organic, and Biological Chemistry: Structures of Life, Platinum Edition* (Redwood City, CA: Benjamin-Cummings, 2004).

Timberlake, Karen C. *General, Organic, and Biological Chemistry: Structures of Life, 4th Edition.* (New York: Prentice Hall, 2012).

Wade, Leroy G. Jr. *Organic Chemistry, Fifth Edition* (New York: Prentice Hall, 2003).

Wade, Leroy G. Jr. *Organic Chemistry, 8th Edition.* (New York: Prentice Hall, 2012).

C H A P T E R

# GENERAL SCIENCE REVIEW

## *CHAPTER SUMMARY*

This chapter highlights the core concepts you need to know for the general science section of most nursing school entrance exams—essential topics such as the scientific method, formation of the universe, evolution, and biodiversity. Use this chapter as a study aid to review important concepts and test yourself with sample questions.

## General Science Review: Important Concepts

## I. General Introduction

### A. Description of How Nursing School Entrance Exams Test General Science

Nursing school entrance exams do not all measure scientific knowledge in the same way. The natural sciences section (which is comprised of chemistry, biology, and health) of the Registered Nursing School Aptitude Exam (RNSAE) and the Aptitude for Practical Nursing Exam (APNE) is made up of approximately 90 multiple-choice questions. The Nurse Entrance Test (NET) has reading comprehension questions that focus on the sciences.

The following subject areas are important for you to know for your exam: history and methods of science, the cosmos, basics of matter, evolution and life, earth works, biodiversity, ecology, and global environmental challenges.

## B. How to Use This Chapter

This chapter covers all the subject areas just listed. Use the information about core topics and the practice questions in this chapter to guide you as you prepare for your exam, but remember that this chapter should not be your only resource. Review scientific concepts more comprehensively in the suggested materials listed at the end of this chapter or in your own textbooks.

After you read each subject heading in this chapter, answer the practice questions that follow. These questions are designed to reflect the type of questions you will find on your nursing school entrance exam. Once you have answered the sample questions, you can target the content areas where you need the most review.

Plan your study time effectively so that you have enough preparation for the test. Familiarizing yourself with real test questions and brushing up on important natural science topics in a good college-level textbook will build your confidence and lessen your test anxiety.

# II. Main Topics

## A. History and Methods of Science

Everywhere you look in our present world, science is evident, from the technology of medicine to our understanding of how stars are made. Here you have an overview of what science is and how it works.

### 1. Giants of Science

How did science begin? Who were the early discoverers of this way of exploring nature? It is important to look back and review some of these giants of science.

### a. Ancient Greeks

(Some dates are approximate.)

*Thales (624–546 BCE)*, called the "father of philosophy," said the universe was ultimately made of water (one of the four ancient Greek elements of water, fire, earth, and air).

*Pythagorus (560–480 BCE)* discovered the mathematics of musical harmony and the properties of right triangles (triangles with one 90° angle in them).

*Hippocrates (460–370 BCE)* was called the "father of medicine."

*Plato (427–347 BCE)* was a major philosopher who wrote the dialogues of Socrates and was influential in championing logical thinking.

*Aristotle (384–322 BCE)* was a student of Plato and tutor of Alexander the Great. He wrote volumes on the knowledge of everything, from plants to the heavens and politics.

*Euclid (325–270 BCE)* accomplished major work in geometry.

*Archimedes (287–212 BCE)* discovered the law of buoyancy and density, legend has it, during a bath, which allowed a king to verify the amount of gold in a crown. He accomplished major work in geometry and was first to calculate the surface area and volume of a sphere.

### b. Originators of Modern Science

*Nicholas Copernicus (1473–1543)*, Polish. His book showed that the motions of the sun, moon, and planets in the sky could be explained by assuming that the planets go around the sun and that Earth is a planet as well. The book had so much influence that we still talk about the "Copernican Revolution."

*Francis Bacon (1561–1626)*, English. He wrote early books on how to do science, emphasizing experiments and inductive reasoning to make generalizations.

*Galileo Galilei (1564–1642)*, Italian. Galileo studied the swing of a pendulum, found that bodies of different masses fall at the same rate, and distinguished acceleration from velocity. He first saw the moons of Jupiter and craters on Earth's moon.

*Johannes Kepler (1571–1630)*, German. Kepler described the laws of planetary motion and declared that the paths of planets around the sun are ellipses, not circles.

*René Descartes (1596–1650)*, French. This father of modern philosophy invented coordinate geometry (the *x–y* axis) and said "I think, therefore I am."

*Robert Hooke (1635–1703)*, English. Hooke published the book *Micrographia*, with detailed drawings of life under a microscope. He named the little units he saw in cork "cells," which became the general word used in biology.

*Anton von Leeuwenhoek (1632–1723)*, Dutch. He perfected the microscope and made many discoveries, such as human sperm cells.

*Sir Isaac Newton (1643–1727)*, English. Newton discovered the law of gravity, discovered how a prism splits light into colors, invented a new form of math called calculus, and set forth the laws of motion (such as "every action has an equal and opposite reaction").

*Pierre-Simon Laplace (1749–1827)*, French. Laplace applied math to the solar system in a new level of detail and correctly surmised that the solar system was formed by condensation from a gas nebula.

### c. Science Goes Full Tilt

*James Hutton (1726–1797)*, Scottish. This "father of geology" realized the antiquity of Earth.

*John Dalton (1766–1844)*, English. Dalton was a chemist whose theory of atoms explained why elements combined into molecules in constant proportions.

*Sir Charles Lyell (1797–1875)*, Scottish. This geologist championed "uniformitarianism," the idea that small constant changes over time created Earth today.

*Baron Alexander von Humboldt (1769–1850)*, German. Baron von Humboldt was a geologist and world traveler. The "Humbolt Current" off the west coast of South America is named after him.

*Matthias Jakob Schleiden (1804–1881)*, German. Schleiden contributed the cell theory for plants, which says that all plants are made of cells.

*Charles Darwin (1809–1882)*, English. Darwin's book, *The Origin of Species by Means of Natural Selection*, started a new field of science, evolutionary biology. He traveled extensively in South America and discovered many new species both modern and extinct.

*Theodor Schwann (1810–1882)*, German. Schwann contributed the cell theory for animals, which says that all animals are made of cells, and coined the term "metabolism."

*Gregor Mendel (1822–1884)*, Austrian. Mendel studied the heredity of pea plants, which led to the modern science of genetics.

*Louis Pasteur (1822–1895)*, French. Pasteur invented biochemistry, discovered right-handed and left-handed crystals, worked with yeast to prove that life only came from other life, and developed the germ theory of disease.

*Thomas Henry Huxley (1825–1895)*, English. Huxley championed the theory of evolution for technical and popular audiences and became known as "Darwin's Bulldog."

*Lord Kelvin (1824–1907)*, Scottish. Kelvin made new calculations on heat and analyzed the history of Earth.

*James Clerk Maxwell (1831–1870)*, Scottish. Maxwell developed mathematical laws of electromagnetism, now known as "Maxwell's equations."

*Dmitri Mendeleyev (1834–1907),* Russian. Mendeleyev discovered the arrangement of elements in repeating sequences of properties, and thereby created the first periodic table of chemistry. He predicted new elements, which were, in fact, found.

*Ernst Mach (1838–1916),* Austrian. Mach was a physicist who is honored by our use of the name "Mach 1" for the speed of sound, "Mach 2" for twice the speed of sound, and so forth.

*Sigmund Freud (1856–1939),* Austrian. Freud developed a theory of dreams and the unconscious.

### d. The Last 100 Years

*Albert Einstein (1879–1955),* German-Swiss. Einstein computed the size of atoms. He developed the special and general theories of relativity for light and gravity, respectively. He also described the concept of four-dimensional space-time and made famous the equation $E = mc^2$, which describes the relationship between energy (E) and mass (m).

*Alfred Lothar Wegener (1880–1930),* German. Wegener proposed that all continents were once a single large one and had drifted apart in a "continental drift."

*Niels Bohr (1885–1962),* Danish. He described the Bohr model of the atom, in which electrons orbit around a nucleus like planets around the sun.

*Werner Karl Heisenberg (1901–1976),* German. Heisenberg developed the uncertainty principle of quantum physics.

*Erwin Schrödinger (1887–1961),* Austrian. Schrödinger developed wave mechanics to explain the structure of atoms.

*Francis Crick (1916–2004),* English. Crick was a codiscoverer of the double helix structure of DNA.

*James Watson (1928– ),* American. Watson was also a codiscoverer of the double helix structure of DNA and is a leader in the Human Genome Project.

## 2. Methods

What makes science special among ways of knowing are its specific methods that uncover the truths of nature in ways that can be repeated by anyone. For example, after Galileo saw the moons of Jupiter, anyone could look at Jupiter through a telescope and see them. Science does not accept any revelations said to be available only to visionary individuals.

### a. Scientific Method

The scientific method is used in all branches of science to study the natural world. The method outlines a series of five principal steps that scientists must undertake in order to test and verify their ideas.

**Formulate the problem:** Develop a question, the solution to which explains an order or process in nature.

**Collect data:** Research background information and make observations that are related to the problem.

**Form a hypothesis:** Develop an educated guess based on your observations and background research that will answer the question. The hypothesis must be logical and testable—experiments must be possible that can disprove the hypothesis.

**Do experiments:** Conduct experiments to test the hypothesis. A hypothesis can be disproved, but never absolutely proved—it may change with new evidence! Experiments must be repeatable, free of bias, and adequately controlled.

**Analyze the data:** Look at the results of your experiments and determine if they are consistent with your hypothesis. If not, develop a new hypothesis that is consistent with all available data. Begin the scientific method again with this new hypothesis!

Successful hypotheses lead scientists to make predictions about the natural world that allow the hypothesis to be tested further.

### b. Conducting Good Experiments

Experiments are tests designed to evaluate a hypothesis. In a good experiment, only one variable is changed at a time and all other variables are kept constant—this is to ensure that any change is a result of only that variable. Often in an experiment, two systems are compared where in one system nothing is changed (the **control**), and in the other, the aspect to be tested is altered (the formal **experiment**). The results of the two systems are then compared.

**Example:** Louis Pasteur took two flasks of sterilized meat broth and configured their long necks so that air could go into both. But for one (the experiment), dust normally in the air was blocked. In the other (the control), the dust along with the air could get in (as would usually be the situation, note that the baseline is the control).

In Pasteur's experiment, he observed that the meat broth spoiled in the control flask open to both air and dust but not in the other experiment flask where dust was excluded. Experiments consist of independent variables, which are usually consciously varied by the experimenter (in Pasteur's case, the presence or absence of dust). Experiments also have dependent variables, which, in our example, is state of the broth, which is affected by (and therefore is dependent upon) the independent variables. Often, experiments are not a simple two-part system, but also include some variable that is shifted across a range of values, to be compared to the control.

If you were Pasteur, you might predict that using a different kind of meat broth would give the same results, thus confirming the original experiment. More remarkably, you might predict the existence of small, invisible organisms in the dust of air as the cause of the spoiling of the meat broth (microbes in air were in fact discovered).

**Hypothesis and theory:** In everyday language, the word *theory* is often used to imply that something is only believed, but not yet proven. However, to scientists, a theory is a set of well-substantiated observations and explanations for something. A scientific theory is accepted as fact and is based on scientific observations.

The process of experiment is cyclic. That is, the experiment leads to new ideas for further experiments. The cycle of the scientific method is repeated.

### c. How Truth Is Forged

The ancient Greeks never formalized the process of experimentation in the way that happened in Europe after Galileo's time.

*Laws versus rules.* When phenomena eventually become explained, they become laws of science. This term is most appropriate in physics and chemistry. Biology, in contrast, includes so many creatures and types of ecosystems that there are often exceptions to the norm. Biologists refer to rules instead of laws.

*What determines scientific truth?* The famous philosopher of science, Karl Popper, said that experiments never prove; they only fail to disprove. He therefore said one should design experiments with the aim to falsify. Popper's concept has been influential. So how is truth known? As more and more experiments fail to falsify a specific hypothesis, the hypothesis comes to be known as true.

**Paradigm shift** is a term coined by the philosopher of the process of science, Thomas Kuhn, that refers to what happens when new scientific discoveries overturn an entire body of knowledge. Einstein's theories of relativity were a paradigm shift.

**Reductionism** occurs when smaller entities interacting as a system explain a phenomenon. **Holism** is sometimes contrasted to reductionism—it looks to the context, the larger system surrounding the phenomenon being studied, as key to the explanation.

*Truth changes as science progresses.* Does that mean that anything goes, or that anything is possible? All scientific truth is tentative, but not arbitrary. Truth is won by many practitioners, checking each other's results and trying new ideas for experiments, over and over.

### d. Graphs, Calculations, and Models

Detailed data from experiments are often plotted as points or lines on **graphs** with *x*- and *y*-axes.

> *x*-**axis:** the horizontal axis that, by convention, varies along the numerical range of the independent variable (either time or some other property being changed by the experimenter, such as temperature).
> *y*-**axis:** the vertical axis that contains the result being measured, which is called the dependent variable.

**Three-dimensional graphs** are graphs that use two horizontal axes for two independent variables (*x,y*) and a vertical axis called the *z*-axis for the dependent variable.

**Calculations** are crucial to science. Important tools are measurements, which then might be analyzed by algebra (to relate variables), calculus (to look at changes in time and changes in rates of processes in time), and statistics (to look at large amounts of data that have inherent variability).

**Models** are conceptual or mathematical systems that serve as explanations for phenomena. Models can be simple, such as Copernicus's model of the solar system. But usually the term *model* refers to conceptual systems that are more complex, such as today's computer models of the weather that include hundreds of equations.

### 3. Measurements

Measurements are so important to science that a practitioner once said, "the only things that count are things that can be counted." This may seem like a stretch, but it captures the importance of measure-ment. For example, the Egyptians knew how to lay out right triangles to measure areas of land and to site the pyramids. The word *geometry* comes from ancient Greek, meaning "Earth-measurement."

### a. Units Are Crucial

Two types of units are used in the world: the metric system and the English system (used only in the United States). The units in the English system include pounds, quarts, feet, inches, miles, and degrees Fahrenheit. The metric system, used by most of the world and by scientists, is the universal language of science. Here are some units in the metric system, which uses factors of ten smaller or larger to develop the names.

> *Length:* meter (m)
>> micrometer (μm), also called a micron (.000001 m)
>> millimeter (mm) (.001 m)
>> centimeter (cm) (.01 m)
>> kilometer (km) (1,000 m)
> *Time:* second (s). Time in the metric system does not use factors (or powers) of ten, except for units under a second (hundredths of a second, milliseconds, microseconds, and so forth).
>> minute (min.)
>> hour (h. or hr.)
>> day (d.)
>> year (y. or yr.)

Note that there is another "second" in use as well. Consider: For degrees latitude and longitude, the 360° of the circle is divided into smaller units called "minutes" (60 to each degree, note this is not a minute of time) and "seconds" (60 seconds to a minute of degree).

> *Mass:* gram (g)
>> micrograms (μg) (.000001 g)
>> milligrams (mg) (.001 g)
>> gram (g)
>> kilograms (kg) (1,000 g)

metric tons (t; 1,000 kilograms to a
metric ton)

*Volume:* liter (L)

milliliters (mL) (.001 L)

the cubic meter (1,000 L = 1 m$^3$)

*Temperature:* The degree Centigrade (°C, sometimes also called degree Celsius). An interval
of one degree C is $\frac{9}{5}$ times larger than the
interval of one degree F. To convert the
numerical scale of °F into the numerical scale
of °C, use the equation $x\,°C = \frac{5}{9}(y\,°F - 32)$.
The freezing point of water is 0 °C or 32 °F.

*Energy:* The joule (J), or calorie (cal); 1 cal =
4.184 J. Note that 1 calorie of energy in food
(Cal) is actually a kilocalorie of energy in the
metric system. Therefore, 1 Cal = 1,000 cal =
1 kcal. Also, power is energy summed over
time. Therefore, another term for energy is
the kilowatt-hour (kW-h) [or joule second
(J.S.)].

*Power:* watt (W)

milliwatts (mW)

kilowatts (kW)

## b. Powers of Ten and Constants

Powers of ten with prefix names in the metric system:

$10^{-12}$ pico (p), one-trillionth
$10^{-9}$ nano (n), one-billionth
$10^{-6}$ micro (μ), one-millionth
$10^{-3}$ milli (m), one-thousandth
$10^{-2}$ centi (c), one-hundredth
$10^3$ kilo (k), thousand
$10^6$ mega (M), million
$10^9$ giga (G), billion
$10^{12}$ tera (T), trillion
$10^{15}$ peta (P), quadrillion

**Constants:** Relating properties in the calculations of science has resulted in universal constants
for major laws. These constants are units that work
out to multiply the other properties in a way that
makes the total units equal on both sides of scientific equations. You do not have to memorize the
numbers, but you should be familiar with the existence and use of these constants.

**Avogadro's number (Na or n):** In one mole of
any element, there is an Avogadro's number of constituent particles (usually atoms or molecules). This
number can also be used for the number of molecules of a substance in a chemical mix.

$N_A = 6.022 \times 10^{23}$ mole$^{-1}$

**Speed of light in a vacuum (*c*):** $3.0 \times 10^8 \frac{m}{s}$.

**Universal gas constant (*R*):** used to relate pressure, temperature, and volume of a gas in the gas law.

$R = 8.314 \frac{J}{mol \times K}$ or $0.08206 \frac{L \times atm}{mol \times K}$

**Stefan-Boltzman constant (σ):** used to relate the
energy of radiation of a material body (say, the sun)
to its surface temperature.

$\sigma = 5.67 \times 10^{-8} \frac{J}{s \times m^2 \times K^{-4}}$

## You Should Review

- major scientists
- major experiments and findings
- units of metric system
- powers of ten

# Questions

1. Who wrote *The Origin of Species by Means of Natural Selection*, which established the theory of evolution?
   a. Charles Darwin
   b. William Gilbert
   c. Aristotle
   d. René Descartes

2. If you are measuring how water chemistry changes in a river in the days after a flood, the time measurement is the
   a. independent variable.
   b. independent constant.
   c. dependent variable.
   d. dependent constant.

3. The prefix *tera-* refers to which unit in the metric system?
   a. thousand
   b. trillion
   c. ten thousand
   d. three

4. This codiscoverer published one of the giant papers in the history of science in 1953 on the double helix structure of DNA.
   a. Albert Einstein
   b. Francis Crick
   c. Ernst Mach
   d. Niels Bohr

5. Mathematics provides science with analytical tools. The branch of mathematics that deals with changes in the rates of changes of variables over time is
   a. algebra.
   b. calculus.
   c. statistics.
   d. tensor analysis.

6. To compute the number of molecules in 2 moles of oxygen gas, you would use
   a. Avogadro's number.
   b. Einstein's speed of light.
   c. the Stefan-Boltzman constant.
   d. Planck's constant.

7. Who discovered the circulation of the blood?
   a. Galileo
   b. Archimedes
   c. Schleiden
   d. Harvey

8. Which sequence best described the sequence of the classical scientific method?
   a. experiment, prediction, idea, hypothesis
   b. idea, experiment, hypothesis, prediction
   c. prediction, idea, hypothesis, experiment
   d. hypothesis, prediction, idea, experiment

9. How many milliwatts are in 10 watts?
   a. 10,000
   b. 1,000
   c. 100
   d. 10

10. What famous equation did Einstein write?
    a. $F = ma$
    b. $E = mc^2$
    c. $PV = nRT$
    d. $A = \pi r^2$

# Answers

**1. a.** Darwin's world-shaking book on evolution was published in England in 1859. William Gilbert (1544–1603), also English, theorized correctly that Earth was a giant magnet, thereby explaining why compass needles work as they do. See pages 226–227 for the others.

**2. a.** The independent variable in this case is time, because that is what is changing by itself. On the other hand, the river chemistry is the dependent variable, because it is changing as a function of time. Choices **b** and **d** are made up.

**3. b.** The prefix *tera-* refers to trillion. For example, a teragram is a trillion grams.

**4. b.** Francis Crick not only discovered the double helix structure of DNA, but also went on to figure out the genetic code that coded for amino acids that are assembled into proteins. He died in 2004. See page 228 for the others.

**5. b.** Calculus can take derivatives of variables, which gives rates of changes in the variables.

**6. a.** Avogadro's number is a unit of the specific number of atoms or molecules found in one mole of a substance.

**7. d.** William Harvey (1578–1657) was an English physician who discovered that blood makes a closed circuit around the body. See pages 226–227 for the others.

**8. b.** First, you have an idea. Then, you create an experiment, derive an hypothesis of why the experiment worked (or did not work), and, finally, make predictions, which then lead to other experiments. Language can be tricky, because "idea" and "hypothesis" can have similar meanings. However, the sequences in the other answer choices do not make sense.

**9. a.** Because there are 1,000 milliwatts in one watt, in 10 watts there are 10,000 milliwatts.

**10. b.** $E = mc^2$ computes the energy ($E$) inherent in mass ($m$) itself, which is multiplied by one of the important constants of physics, the speed of light ($c$), which is squared in this case. The equation in choice **a** was written by Newton. The equation in choice **c** is the universal gas law. The equation in choice **d** is for the area of a circle.

## B. The Cosmos

### 1. First Billion Years of the Universe

It is believed that our universe began with an event called the Big Bang, which was followed by the formation of galaxies about a billion years later.

The Big Bang theory is a set of explanations for how the universe began. It states that the universe was once very small and densely compacted. The theory goes on to explain that about fourteen billion years ago, the universe began expanding outward, and it continues to expand outward today.

#### a. Evidence for the Expanding Universe

In the 1920s, American astronomer Edwin Hubble measured the distances to a number of galaxies and their spectra of light, which provided crucial evidence that the universe is expanding.

**Spectra:** All elements, if above 0 K (absolute zero on the Kelvin scale of temperature, which is approximately −273°C), glow at particular wavelengths. These are along different wavelengths of the electromagnetic (EM) spectrum, which spans from the very long wavelengths of radio waves to the ultra short wavelengths of X-rays. The wavelengths that our eyes see are called visible light. Visible red has a longer wavelength than blue. The particular wavelengths for each element form patterns, which are characteristic of that element, and which might be called *photon-prints*, after the patterns of the EM photons. As the numerous EM emissions from a star pass through gases that contain particular elements, elements also absorb wavelengths in their characteristic patterns. Thus, both emission spectra and absorption spectra can provide astronomers with information about the elements in outer space.

**Hubble's Observations:** By examining spectra, Hubble found that compared to the photon-prints of elements on Earth, those elements found in the galaxies of deep space are shifted toward the red; in other words, the wavelengths are longer. This could only occur if the galaxies were moving away from Earth. (If the galaxies were moving toward us, the shift in the wavelengths of the patterns would have been toward the blue, which was not observed.)

Hubble had discovered the expanding universe. By extrapolating the expansion back in time, astronomers concluded that the expansion started with a single explosive event known as the Big Bang.

If all galaxies are moving away from us, does that imply that we are at the center? No, because inhabitants of any galaxy would also observe that they appear to be at the center. It is like raisins in an expanding raisin cake. To each raisin, all the others are moving away.

We can look back in time as we look out into space, because the light reaching us was emitted long ago. Because the speed of light is finite (fast but finite), the light from stars in our own galaxy hundred of thousands of years ago or stars in other galaxies billions of years ago is just now reaching us.

## b. The Big Bang

The Big Bang occurred about 13.7 billion years ago (with an uncertainty of a few hundred million years).

*At one microsecond (following the Big Bang):* The universe as a whole had a temperature of about a trillion degrees K. Matter as we know it, as stable atoms, does not exist at this temperature.

*Between the first microsecond and one second:* Matter and antimatter nearly annihilated each other.

**Antimatter** is a form of matter that is the mirror opposite of matter in all aspects. For a positively charged particle, for example, the antiparticle is negatively charged. Particles and their antiparticles have

the same masses. The key point is that when particles and antiparticles meet, they explode into pure energy, in an amount dictated by Einstein's famous equation $E = mc^2$. We know that antiparticles exist because they can be made in high-energy physics experiments.

In the early universe, there was an imbalance between matter and antimatter, to the extent of about one part in 200 million. Therefore, in the matter-antimatter annihilation, only one part in 200 million remained as matter, and the rest became energy.

*At one second:* The universe was about a billion degrees K. This was "cool" enough for protons, neutrons, and electrons to exist as stable particles, which physicists call "subatomic" particles because they are basic constituents of atoms.

Note that the proton by itself is the nucleus of a hydrogen atom.

## c. Formation of First Atoms

At around 300,000 years after the Big Bang, the temperature of the universe had dropped to about 3,000 K (close to the temperature of our sun's surface). This was cool enough for electrons to remain bound to nuclei (of protons and neutrons), thus creating atoms. (In contrast, at hotter temperatures, electrons are stripped off nuclei, and atoms cannot exist.)

Astronomers talk about this event by saying that "the universe became transparent." Before this point, freely moving electrons (in the state of matter known as **plasma**, a kind of matter-energy "fog") blocked the propagation of electromagnetic radiation such as light. This crucial event separated matter and energy. Except for small amounts absorbed over time by interactions with matter, this ongoing energy has been traveling throughout the universe ever since, stretching and cooling with the ongoing expansion.

In 1965, this radiation was detected. It is called the **cosmic background radiation.** Its temperature, which represents the average temperature of the current state of the universe, is 2.7 K, very close to absolute zero. (Locally, places like Earth and the sun, of course, are much hotter.)

At this point of formation of atoms, both theoretical calculations and actual measurements have shown that matter consisted of 76 percent hydrogen and 24 percent helium, with a trace of lithium. No other elements existed.

### d. Formation of Stars and Galaxies

Stars and galaxies formed between 1 million and a billion years after the Big Bang. Stars are created when gas clouds in space are pulled together by gravity and condense. During the condensation, the gas becomes hotter and hotter. If the density and temperature are high enough, the protostar ignites and is sustained as a glowing star by nuclear fusion.

Stars exist within large, gravitationally bound groupings called **galaxies**. Our Milky Way galaxy has about 100 billion stars, which go through births and lifetimes. In special cases, extremely large masses can contract so much that light itself cannot escape; they are called **black holes**. Many galaxies are believed to have black holes in their centers. Our galaxy has a central black hole.

The contraction of the matter of the universe into galaxies could only have occurred from some initial lumpiness in the universe, which was predicted to be still present in the cosmic background radiation. Satellites such as the Cosmic Background Explorer did indeed find such **inhomogeneities**, which indicate differences in the distribution of energy in space from the time the universe became transparent. These differences are small, only + or −27 microdegrees warmer and cooler than the average 2.7 K, but they are a crucial confirmation for the Big Bang theory. Our universe now contains about 100 billion galaxies.

### 2. Birth of Chemical Elements in Stars

All elements heavier than the primordial triplet of elements, primarily hydrogen and helium with a trace of lithium, are created in stars.

### a. Nuclear Fusion

Stars are hot and are able to emit radiation into space because of fusion reactions deep within their cores. Nuclear fusion is a type of nuclear reaction in which the nuclei of relatively light atoms combine to form a heavier atom. In the process, tremendous amounts of energy are given off. For atoms from hydrogen up to the atomic weight of iron, energy is released when atoms are fused to make larger atoms. This is because the protons and neutrons inside the nuclei of the larger atoms (again, up to iron) contain less mass per subatomic particle and therefore less energy according to Einstein's equation. The excess energy of fusion is released as heat and radiation.

### b. Sequence of Births of Elements

Inside stars, the first element to be fused is hydrogen, the most abundant primordial element. Under intense temperature and pressure, two hydrogen atoms are fused into one atom of helium, releasing energy and making stars hot, thus sustaining further fusion reactions. When the hydrogen is used up, helium is fused into carbon, and then the carbon and some helium are fused into oxygen. All the elements up to iron can be made in this way. Note the sequence of how elements are made: Hydrogen (H) → Helium (He) → Carbon (C) → Oxygen (O). All these fusion reactions release energy.

### c. Supernovas and the Dispersal of Elements

Stars can run out of matter to fuel fusion; they can "die." Some stars die by throwing off gases, then wither into small, smoldering white dwarfs.

Very massive stars, on the order of ten times the mass of our sun, can create supernova explosions at their deaths. One supernova, for example, occurred in our galaxy in A.D. 1066 and created what is now known as the Crab Nebula. Ancient people observed this bright new star in the sky before it faded.

Supernovas are important parts of how our universe works because they do two special things. First, all elements heavier than iron (such as gold and uranium) are made in the intense heat and pressure of the supernova. Second, the supernovas disperse all the elements inside the former star out into space. We can see these elements in the emission and absorption spectra in the regions surrounding former sites of supernovas. In the dispersal of elements by supernovas, there are elements made earlier in fusion reactions during the long, ordinary lifetime of the star, as well as the new elements made only in the supernova itself.

The elements dispersed into space can eventually gather into gas clouds and might contract, after mixing with remnants of other supernovas, into totally new stars and planets.

## 3. Formation of Earth
### a. Age of Sun and Earth
About five billion years ago, a gas cloud condensed into the star that is now our sun, which has been burning since that birth.

Around the sun, the gas cloud condensed into smaller bodies (picture small whirlpools of contraction around a large, central one). What started as dust grains coalesced into rocks, then boulders, then objects the size of mountains. By collisions and gravitational attraction, which held the bodies together, the objects grew. Sometimes, the collisions created smaller bodies but, on the whole, growth in size ruled. Earth formed about 4.5 billion years ago.

### b. Methods of Dating
To date the formation of stars and planets, scientists use radioactive clocks. Very large atoms, such as those of uranium, can have unstable nuclei. These unstable nuclei restructure into nuclei that are slightly smaller by giving off radioactive particles (there is also a kind of radioactive decay that only gives off energy). The new atom might also be radioactive, and thus, the process continues until it

reaches an atom that is perfectly stable. Lead-206, for example, is the stable daughter-product of what started as Uranium-238 (the numbers refer to the atomic weights, or the number of protons and neutrons in the atom's nucleus). When molten or gaseous, the lead-206 is driven off; the radioactive clock is thereby "reset." We can use the clock to date when rocks formed. The oldest Earth rocks are 3.9 billion years old, the oldest moon rocks 4.1 billion years old, and most meteorites about 4.6 billion years old. Because Earth and the moon would have been molten even after they formed (see the following paragraph), the date of the meteorites is taken to be the time that Earth condensed (4.6 billion years ago, or, rounded to the nearest half billion, about four and a half billion years ago).

### c. Formation of the Moon
Though it was once thought that the moon might have condensed separately around the Earth, the following scenario is now known to be true (from multiple lines of evidence). A few hundred million years after the formation of Earth, a rogue body about the size of Mars, which had an odd orbit around the Sun, smashed into Earth. Material from both the colliding body and Earth flew off and condensed around Earth to form the moon. The moon was much closer then and has been slowly moving away from Earth ever since.

## 4. Exploration of the Solar System
From the dawn of time, humans have looked up at the stars. Only in the past half century have we been able to look back on Earth itself with satellite cameras and even human eyes.

### a. From Satellites to Humans in Space
**Sputnik**, which means "fellow traveler" in Russian, was launched by the U.S.S.R. in 1957. It was the first artificial satellite in orbit.

**Vanguard** was the first U.S. satellite, launched in 1958.

In the manned U.S. space program, the *Mercury* program put solo humans in orbit, the *Gemini* program put teams of two into orbit, and the *Apollo* program, with teams of three, aimed for the moon. The first manned moon landing came in 1969. The Russians had the first space station, called Mir (for "peace"), but eventually it could not be maintained and fell to Earth. The International Space Station, led by the efforts of the United States, is currently in orbit, and every half year or so, there are changes of crew. Russia has supplied the rockets for these changes in recent years, following the grounding of the U.S. Space Shuttles after the second total loss of a space shuttle crew in 2003, during the Space Shuttle *Columbia*'s disastrous reentry into Earth's atmosphere.

### b. Discoveries from Venus

Astronomers cannot see surface features of the planet Venus because of its thick clouds. Several U.S. and Russian probes have measured properties of the Venusian atmosphere and even mapped the surface from orbit, using various wavelengths that can penetrate the clouds. Despite its similar size to Earth, Venus is very different. It is extremely hot, partly because it is closer to the Sun, but mostly because the atmosphere is about 600 times more massive than that of Earth and consists mostly of carbon dioxide. This amount of $CO_2$ produces an intense greenhouse effect, keeping the planet hot. There is no water vapor or oxygen in the atmosphere.

### c. Discoveries from Mars

In the mid-1970s, the Viking probe successfully landed on Mars and measured properties of the soil, seeking signs of life. None was found, but scientists now believe that there is a possibility for life in cracks in rocks, well beneath the surface. Unusual bacteria are found in similar sites deep under the surface of Earth.

In 2004, the United States successfully deployed two more rovers on the surface of Mars. They have analyzed minerals and concluded, through multiple lines of evidence, that Mars was once wet. Rivers flowed, and there was possibly a shallow ocean. Again, compared to Earth, the atmosphere of Mars is very foreign. The thin atmosphere (about 7% that of Earth) is, like that of Venus, mostly made up of carbon dioxide. There is only a faint trace of oxygen and little nitrogen (the two most abundant gases in Earth's atmosphere).

## 5. Mysteries of the Cosmos

### a. Dark Matter

When astronomers use the law of gravity to compute what the spin of galaxies (such as ours) should be, given the presence of a known amount of matter, they find that there must be a significant amount of matter that is "dark," or unseen and unknown.

The dark matter is about six times the mass of the known, ordinary matter of stars and gas clouds.

### b. Dark Energy

Certain kinds of supernovas explode with a fixed real brilliance. Astronomers have mapped these "standard candles," and, knowing their real brilliance, their apparent brilliance to us on Earth, and their red shifts, can calculate their distances and ages. A startling fact has emerged, which has been borne out by other lines of evidence as well: The expansion of the universe has been accelerating since the Big Bang.

What is causing the expansion? It is some kind of energy that we cannot currently see. It is therefore known as **dark energy**.

Using Einstein's equation $E = mc^2$, any amount of energy can be computed as an equivalent mass. Therefore, scientists can ask about the amounts of dark energy, dark matter, and the universe's third constituent of known, ordinary matter and energy. Here are the results:

Dark energy: 73% (most of the substance of the universe)

Dark matter: 23%

Ordinary matter and energy: 4%

### c. Life and Intelligence Elsewhere

Are we alone? The research program called *SETI (the Search for Extraterrestrial Intelligence)* seeks answers to this question. It assumes that other intelligent civilizations might send out signals to space. So far, no definite signals have been found.

By measuring wobbles in stars, which are caused by planets circling the stars and perturbing the stars with their gravity, astronomers do know that many stars have planets around them. To date, this technique locates only very large planets, assumed to be similar to the gas giants of our solar system, Jupiter and Saturn. More than 600 planets around other stars are currently known. The first stars of the universe could not have had planets of heavy elements, such as iron. Early planets could not have had carbon, a crucial element for life as we know it. This is because iron and carbon are made in the fusion reactions inside stars. Therefore, the density of carbon increases over time, as stars go through lifetimes and more stars form. Is there a critical density of carbon needed for life? Perhaps we are alone (or nearly so) because just around the time of formation of Earth the density of carbon reached a value high enough to form life. This is a possible explanation for our apparent aloneness, but more work on the history and composition of the cosmos needs to be done.

### You Should Review

- Big Bang theory
- formation of stars and galaxies
- dating methods
- supernovas
- formation of Earth and moon
- characteristics of planets in the solar system
- discoveries from space exploration
- dark matter and dark energy

## Questions

**11.** What feature of our universe is demonstrated by the "red shift"?
- **a.** an increase in supernovas
- **b.** the contraction of black holes
- **c.** the expansion of the universe
- **d.** the decrease in gravity

**12.** What of the following did not occur at about 300,000 years after the Big Bang?
- **a.** Matter was left over from matter-antimatter annihilation.
- **b.** The universe became transparent.
- **c.** The first atoms formed.
- **d.** Electrons started orbits around atomic nuclei.

**13.** What is the current temperature of the universe, as indicated by the cosmic background radiation?
- **a.** 2.7°C
- **b.** −2.7 K
- **c.** −2.7°C
- **d.** 2.7 K

**14.** In the stages of nuclear fusion inside stars, which element in the list is the ultimate building block for all the others?
- **a.** hydrogen
- **b.** helium
- **c.** carbon
- **d.** oxygen

**15.** A supernova is observed in a star that is a distance of 500 light years from Earth. That means we now see the star
- **a.** as it was 500 years in the past.
- **b.** as it was 500 years after the Big Bang.
- **c.** as it will be 500 years in the future.
- **d.** as it is today.

**16.** We can date very old rocks because of what fact?
   **a.** Uranium turns into platinum.
   **b.** Uranium turns into lead.
   **c.** Lead turns into uranium.
   **d.** Gold turns into uranium.

**17.** How did the moon form?
   **a.** A large body crashed into Earth soon after its own formation.
   **b.** A gas cloud condensed around Earth at the same time Earth itself condensed.
   **c.** Early Earth was unstable and split into the moon and what became Earth.
   **d.** The moon was captured by Earth early on.

**18.** Which planet is about the same size as Earth, has a blanket of thick clouds, and has a surface temperature that could melt lead?
   **a.** Mercury
   **b.** Jupiter
   **c.** Titan
   **d.** Venus

**19.** Which country was the first to launch a satellite?
   **a.** Union of Soviet Socialist Republics (U.S.S.R.)
   **b.** United States
   **c.** China
   **d.** European Union

**20.** What is the main piece of evidence for dark energy?
   **a.** black holes found in the centers of most galaxies
   **b.** discovery of cosmic background radiation
   **c.** rotations of galaxies not explained by our known, ordinary matter and energy
   **d.** acceleration of the expansion of the universe

## Answers

**11. c.** All galaxies have red shifts in the signatures of elements in their spectra of light, which shows that the galaxies are all moving away from each other, and therefore that the universe is expanding.

**12. a.** This event (matter left over from matter-antimatter annihilation) occurred less than a second after the Big Bang. Choices **c** and **d** are two ways of describing the same event, which happened at about 300,000 years following the Big Bang. Choice **b** describes what happened during atom formation, which also occurred during this time period.

**13. d.** K for Kelvin refers to the temperature scale that uses absolute zero as the "zero" point. Note that it is written as just "K" not "°K." You can figure this out if you know that 0 K refers to absolute zero and that the average temperature of the universe is very close to absolute zero. Negative K makes no sense. The choices **a** and **c** are too warm, given that 0°C is about 273 K.

**14. a.** Hydrogen is the building block for other elements inside stars. It is the simplest element, with one proton and one electron.

**15. a.** We see the star as it was 500 years in the past because light can only travel at a finite speed (fast but finite, the *c* in Einstein's famous equation). A light year is the distance that light travels in a year. When we look out into space, we also are looking back in time.

**16. b.** Uranium, a radioactive element, decays and turns into lead, which is stable. The amount of a particular isotope of lead present gives the amount of time that has passed since the rock formed, and any lead that was present prior to rock formation would have been purged while in a gaseous or molten state during formation.

**17. a.** A large body crashed into Earth soon after its own formation. From this collision, material went into space and recondensed to form the moon, in addition to restructuring the surface of Earth. This was after Earth had already condensed.

**18. d.** Venus has a super-thick atmosphere of carbon dioxide that creates high surface temperatures. Choice **c** is not a planet but a moon of Saturn.

**19. a.** The Union of Soviet Socialist Republics first launched a satellite into Earth's orbit. (This country has since broken up into a number of countries, but the largest part of the former U.S.S.R. is Russia.) Choice **d**, the European Union, did not exist at the time of the first satellite's launch.

**20. d.** The existence of dark energy is evidenced by the accelerating expansion of the universe. We know this by measuring the distances to certain types of supernovas in distant galaxies, which serve as standard candles of known brightness.

## C. Basics of Matter

### 1. Physics

**Physics** is the study of the constituents and forces that govern matter at its most elementary level.

#### a. Atoms

The word **atom** comes from the ancient Greek *atomos*, meaning "indivisible." Atoms are the most finely divided parts of matter that possess the characteristics of a particular element, such as copper, gold, carbon, or hydrogen.

Atoms are not actually indivisible. Atoms not in molecules or ions are electrically neutral and contain equal amounts of positive and negative electrical charges. The positive charge is concentrated in a tiny central massive region called the **nucleus**. The negative charge is in one or more tiny electrons, which orbit the nucleus, bound to it by electrical attraction.

The nucleus also has parts: **protons** and **neutrons**. Protons are positively charged, and neutrons are neutral. Their masses are nearly (but not exactly) the same. The mass of a proton or neutron is about 2,000 times the mass of an electron.

**Quantum theory** made the picture of the atom more complete though more difficult to visualize. According to quantum mechanics, the electrons do not orbit the nucleus like planets around a star but exist in spaces that are more like clouds of probability. An electron can exist anywhere in its cloud (its range of possible places), popping in and out of existence in different sites within its cloud, which fades out with distance from the nucleus.

The atoms of a particular element all have the same number of protons in their nuclei (which determines the charge of the nucleus, thus the number of electrons around the nucleus, and thus the chemistry of the element). But atoms of elements can vary in the number of neutrons in their nuclei; therefore atoms of an element can vary in their masses. Atoms of the same element that possess different numbers of neutrons are called **isotopes**.

**Example:**

Most atoms of the element carbon contain 6 protons and 6 neutrons in their nuclei. This is carbon-12 (atomic number 6, atomic weight 12). About 1 in 100 atoms of carbon have 6 protons and 7 neutrons in their nuclei. This is carbon-13 (atomic number 6, atomic weight 13). An even smaller fraction of carbon is carbon-14. It has 6 protons and 8 neutrons in the nucleus. Also, it is radioactive, which means it is inherently unstable and will decay in the following manner: One neutron converts to a proton plus an electron that is shot out at great energy from the nucleus (note that the electron was created by the conversion—it was not "in" the nucleus.) This is **beta decay**, which is governed by the weak nuclear force. After beta decay, the atom is no longer carbon; it is nitrogen, with 7 protons and 7 neutrons, and is now perfectly stable. Other radioactive isotopes, such as those of uranium, can decay in another manner called **alpha decay**, when a bound particle of 2 protons and 2 neutrons (a He nucleus) is ejected.

### b. Quarks and Charges

From the discoveries of quantum mechanics, protons and neutrons were found to be made of **quarks**. There are six flavors (types) of quarks according to the Standard Model (the current framework used to describe elementary particles): up, down, top, bottom, charm, and strange. Combinations of quarks make up some subatomic particles. For example, the proton is made of two "up" quarks and one "down" quark. The neutron is made of one "up" quark and two "down" quarks. Other combinations of quarks create other kinds of particles in a quantum mechanical "zoo," such as **mesons**. This zoo also contains chargeless particles called **neutrinos** with a mass much less than that of electrons.

### c. Essential Concepts

**Velocity** (*v*) is distance (*d*) covered per unit time (*t*): $v = \frac{d}{t}$.

**Acceleration** (*a*) is the change in velocity over an interval of time. It can be written as $a = \frac{\Delta v}{\Delta t}$ ($\Delta$ = difference, or, in the terms of calculus, **derivative**). If velocity is a change in position, then acceleration is the change in velocity.

**Newtonian concept of force** (*F*): $F = m \times a$. It takes force to accelerate a mass (*m*). Honoring Newton, the metric unit of force is called a Newton (*N*). Its units are $\frac{\text{kg} \times \text{m}}{\text{s}^2}$ (the force it takes to accelerate one kilogram by one meter by second over the course of one second).

**Momentum** is mass times velocity. A car traveling at 60 mph has twice the momentum of a car with the same mass traveling at 30 mph.

Objects traveling not in straight lines but in curved paths have angular properties—**angular velocity**, **angular acceleration**, and **angular momentum**. In the governing equations one must also account for the change in the angle. Earth has a huge angular momentum because of its huge mass.

Forces can be **static** as well as **dynamic**. **Pressure** (for example, the pressure that exists inside a balloon blown up with air) is expressed as $\frac{N}{m^2}$, a force per area on the inner surface of the balloon. But once it is blown up, the balloon does not keep expanding. This is because there is an equal and opposite force exerted by the stretched skin of the balloon and the outside air pressure. The balloon remains at the same size (except for slowly leaking) because the two forces, from air and skin, exactly balance each other.

**Electricity** is an entire special topic in physics.

**Voltage** is the difference in electrical force that can drive electrons from one place to another; the unit is the volt.

**Amperage** is the actual amount of flow of electricity, or electrons; the unit is the ampere or amp.

**Resistance** is the resistance to the flow of electricity, which varies among materials; the unit is the ohm. The watt (*W*) is the rate at which work is done when 1 amp flows through an electrical force of 1 volt.

Another important topic in physics is waves. **Waves** are characterized by **frequency** (cycles per unit of time) and by **wavelength** (distance traveled by one cycle). Amplitude (strength) is another characteristic. For example, sound consists of traveling waves of compression and expansion in air (or water). Light waves (standing waves) are electromagnetic, which can travel in a vacuum.

### d. Basic Forces

Physicists recognize four forces that are ultimately fundamental.

1. **Gravity** attracts two masses toward each other. Newton wrote the main equation of gravity, and Einstein's general theory of relativity more completely explained gravity as a warping by matter of space-time. The force of gravity obeys an inverse-square law: the strength of the force decreases as the square of the distance from the source increases.

2. **Electromagnetism** (*EM*) is the force that exists between charged particles. It is attractive when the charges are opposite (positive and negative) and repulsive when the charges are the same (both positive or both negative). Electromagnetism holds atoms together—the EM force in various forms is the secret to the chemical bond. The EM force, like gravity, obeys an inverse square law. Its main theoretical formulation is in Maxwell's equations.

3. **Weak nuclear force**, which has a very short range and is responsible for certain kinds of interactions within the atom, governs a particular kind of radioactive decay called **beta decay**, in which a neutron converts to a proton plus an electron and antineutrino.

4. **Strong nuclear force** is the major stabilizer of the atomic nucleus and governs interactions among the quarks that make up the protons and neutrons. Unlike forces such as gravity and EM that diminish with distance, strong nuclear force strengthens with distance. The more that quarks are separated, the more strongly they are bound to each other. This is why free quarks have never been observed.

## 2. Chemistry

Chemistry studies the interactions of atoms, how they form molecules, and the interactions of those molecules, which range from simple ions to complex organic molecules.

### a. Atoms and the Periodic Table

The naturally occurring elements contain from 1 proton (hydrogen) to 92 protons (uranium) in the nuclei of their atoms. Elements with more protons have been made artificially in experiments of high-energy physics.

The electrons around each nucleus fill, in sequence, what are called **shells**. These shells, and the number of electrons in them, determine the chemical properties of the elements, such as crystal geometry, electrical conductivity, and, most importantly, their bonding properties with other atoms to form molecules.

The first shell can hold two electrons. The second shell can hold eight electrons (in two subshells of *s* with two and one *p* with six). The third shell can hold 18 electrons (in three subshells of *s* with two, three *p* with six, one *d* with 10, and so on). Things become more complicated as the elements move into higher **atomic numbers**, with, for example, phenomena such as a lower subshell filling after a more outer shell contains electrons. But basically, for most of the chemistry we need to consider, the outermost shell will have eight electrons when it is full. (Note that the first shell only holds two electrons.)

These shells of electrons, and the fact that shells can be full or less than full, create **cycles** in the properties of elements. For example, elements with full shells include helium, neon, and argon. These elements are in the family of elements called **noble gases**, which almost never combine with other elements (they don't need the other elements to create a full shell of electrons because they are already full).

There is a tendency, driven by energy considerations, for atoms to achieve complete shells of electrons. They may do this by either losing or gaining electrons, depending on which direction makes creating the full shell "easier."

For example, elements with one electron in an outer shell will tend to give up that electron in a chemical bond with a different atom. Elements with seven electrons in the outer shell will tend to grab an electron in a chemical bond with another atom. An example is table salt, NaCl. By themselves, atoms of sodium (Na) have one outer electron, whereas those of chlorine (Cl) have seven outer electrons. In chemical contact, sodium gives up an electron to chlorine, thereby both achieving full shells. They bond into a solid crystal (salt) of an alternating, three-dimensional lattice of Na ions and Cl ions.

The outer shell that is chemically active by virtue of this tendency to give up or gain electrons is called the **valence shell** of atoms.

Depending on the strength of the tendency to gain or lose electrons and the "needs" of chemical partners, **chemical bonds** exist in different types. **Ionic bonds** occur when one element completely gives up electrons and the other element gains. An example is table salt, where the sodium atoms, having lost electrons, become ions with a positive charge (+1), and the chlorine atoms, having gained electrons, become ions with a negative charge (−1). In another kind of bond, called a **covalent bond**, electrons are shared in pairs. In a covalent bond, the resulting atoms in the bond do not become ions, but they still can have a slight charge polarization. The complexities of forces between atoms in chemical bonds and between molecules with charged surfaces create other types of bonds, like hydrogen bonds and the bonds from van der Waal forces.

## b. Chemical Reactions

**Chemical reactions** occur when chemical reactants change into products. Reactions can be as simple as salt dissolving its ions into water, or as complex as two organic molecules brought together into a larger one in the presence of an enzyme. In a chemical reaction, substances called *reactants* undergo a chemical change so that new chemical substances are formed. The new substances are called *products*.

Chemical reactions can be expressed with chemical equations, in which the reactants are on the right side of the equation and products are on the left side. By convention, chemical equations are written with an arrow taking the reactants into the state of products.

Chemical reactions must be balanced according to the **law of conservation of matter**: Matter can be neither created nor destroyed. (Changes in the nucleus, for example, from nuclear fusion, nuclear fission, or radioactive decay, are not chemical reactions, which involve only the electrons of atoms, not their nuclei.) For instance, the number of atoms of oxygen in the reactants has to equal the number of atoms of oxygen in the products.

Reactions can give off energy (**exothermic**). These tend to occur spontaneously (but not instantaneously). Some reactions require energy supplied from the environment—these are called **endothermic**.

Many important chemical reactions are known as **oxidation-reduction reactions**. One element gains electrons (is reduced). A different element loses electrons (is oxidized). The word **reduced** refers to the fact that the gain in electrons reduces the oxidation state of the atom in the chemical compound.

**Acids** are substances whose dissolution in water creates hydrogen ions (H+). **Bases** are substances whose dissolution accepts hydrogen ions in water. The **pH scale** is the measure of acidity or basicity that ranges from 0 to 14, with 7 being neutral, values below 7 being acidic, and those above 7 being basic.

## c. States of Matter

**Solid:** the state of matter in which atoms or molecules are bound tightly and move together as a unit. Some solids are mathematically regular in their atomic structure (such as crystals). Other solids can be more amorphous (such as coal).

**Liquid:** the state of matter in which atoms or molecules can glide past each other and are loosely bound but not attached to specific neighbors. However, in liquids, the molecules still have some degree of coherence to each other.

**Gas:** the state of matter in which atoms or molecules are totally free of each other. In air, for example, the molecules of nitrogen and oxygen travel as independent units, only bumping into other molecules (this bumping creates the gas pressure).

The different states of matter contain different amounts of energy. The energy required to change a substance from solid to liquid is called the **heat of fusion** (fusion here means melting). The energy required to change a substance from liquid to gas is called the **heat of vaporization**. The heats of fusion and vaporization occur at constant temperatures, depending on the substance. It requires energy to heat water to the boiling point, but then more energy is needed—at that constant boiling point temperature—to turn the water into steam. Only after the water has become steam can more energy raise the temperature of the steam itself. These heats of fusion and vaporization are unique for all substances, as are the freezing and boiling temperatures. Water, for example, has a heat of vaporization of 549 calories per gram.

When temperatures are extreme (as in the center of the sun), electrons are stripped from their nuclei. The resulting state of matter is called a **plasma** (often, plasma is called a fourth state of matter).

### d. Organic and Inorganic Molecules

Organic molecules contain a reduced form of carbon, or carbon with a slightly negative charge from the stronger attraction (electron affinity) of electrons in sharing with other atoms, notably hydrogen. Carbon has four electrons in its outer energy level, thus requiring four more to complete the shell of eight. Carbon can bond with itself in chains, a virtually unique feature of its atomic structure (silicon also has this special characteristic). Pure forms of carbon include diamonds, graphite, and the recently discovered form of carbon in a hollow sphere of 60 atoms called buckminster-fullerene, or "buckyball."

Organic molecules are the stuff of life. Therefore, organic chemistry is the chemistry of life itself. There are important classes of organic molecules in living things.

**Proteins** are organic molecules made from smaller organic components called **amino acids**. Amino acids contain the element nitrogen. **Enzymes** and many structural parts of cells are all types of proteins. **Hemoglobin** in our blood is a protein.

**Carbohydrates** are organic molecules of carbon in chains that are fairly short, with side groups that branch off the chains and consist of hydrogen and hydrogen-oxygen (hydroxy) groups. The chemical formulae for carbohydrates often look like they consist of carbon plus multiples of water (for example, $C_6H_{12}O_6$)—thus, the name carbo-hydrates. Examples are sugars such as sucrose and lactose, and starch. The important structural molecule of plants—cellulose—is also a carbohydrate.

**Lipids** are very long chains of carbon atoms, with side groups that are primarily single hydrogen atoms. Other side groups also occur. Examples of lipids are the molecules in various kinds of oils (saturated versus unsaturated). Lipids are crucial components of the membranes of cells, which all consist of complex lipids called **phospholipids** because they have a phosphate group at one end. Most lipids are insoluble in water.

**Nucleic acids**, such as DNA and RNA, form important coding molecules inside cells for the genetics of living things.

**Inorganic chemistry** deals with the chemistry of everything that is not organic. This includes, for example, the chemical reactions between simple charged ions dissolved in water, and the structures of crystals, with their different planes of cleavage. Inorganic chemistry includes many kinds of reactions among molecules in Earth's atmosphere.

## 3. Energy

### a. First Law of Thermodynamics

**Work** is force times distance and has the same units as energy. The metric unit of energy is the joule (J, therefore $1 J = 1 N \cdot m$). The unit is named after James Prescott Joule (1818–1889), one of the founders of the concept of the conservation of energy.

In the first law of thermodynamics, energy can neither be created nor destroyed, but only transformed.

One of the amazing discoveries in the history of science was the gradual realization that types of energy can be equivalent in value, which is the manifestation of the first law. How can the warmth of our body or the strength of our arms come from the food we eat? Joule discovered the mechanical equivalent to heat—that, indeed, mechanical motion and heat could be put into equivalent terms as forms of energy. In heat, the unit is the calorie. In the mechanical equivalent of heat, $4.18 J = 1$ calorie. One feature shared by all forms of energy is that they can be converted into heat, or work.

### b. Second Law of Thermodynamics

All forms of energy can be converted to heat, but heat cannot be converted to all other forms of energy with equal efficiency. In a sense, heat is the most degraded form of energy because it is least convertible. This fact—that not all forms of energy are equal in "quality"—led to what is known today as the second law of thermodynamics.

The key property of this law is **entropy**. This is often taken to mean "disorder." Indeed, there is a relationship between the order of matter and its entropy content. Thus, a gas has higher entropy than a solid because compared to the molecular chaos of a gas, the solid has atoms and molecules in relatively neat arrangements.

Physicist Ludwig Boltzmann (1844–1906) worked out the relationship between entropy and the number of states possibly occupied by a state of matter. He had the equation for entropy put on his gravestone.

In general, entropy will increase over time. Disorder increases. A hot cup of tea placed in an ordinary room will cool off. Its energy went into the room's air. Thus, the tea cooled off by many degrees as the room warmed up a tiny amount of temperature (because it has a bigger mass). Because the heat, as energy, went from a more concentrated state (in the tea) to a more diffuse state (in the room's air), there was an increase in entropy of the tea-and-room considered as a system. A concentrated amount of heat at a high temperature is not as degraded as a diffuse amount of heat at a lower temperature. In fact, the unit of entropy is the heat per unit degree Celsius, in other words, the $\frac{calorie}{°C}$. (Note from this definition that one calorie of heat at a lower temperature has a higher entropy than one calorie at a higher temperature.) A state of higher entropy is a more disorderly and more degraded state of energy. These considerations are essential for the industrial world—for example, in the design and operation of electrical power plants.

Entropy can sometimes decrease. Energy can become more useful (less degraded). For example, in plant photosynthesis, carbon dioxide and water are transformed into carbohydrates, which are food energy that we can eat. The carbon dioxide and water have a higher entropy than do the same atoms arranged into the carbohydrate molecules. In this case, entropy decreased, which is an apparent violation of the second law. But photosynthesis uses the solar energy of sunlight, which itself is a very low form of entropy. One can compute the efficiency of photosynthesis, which is the efficiency of the conversion of solar energy into chemical energy of food. The wasted light (this waste is an unavoidable part of the process) goes off as heat from the plant. This heat is an increase in entropy. When we combine the entropies for the two processes (1. some part of the sunlight, along with carbon dioxide and water, goes into carbohydrates in an entropy decrease; and 2. the other part of sunlight goes into heat in an entropy increase), it turns out that the increase dominates.

Local decreases in entropy have always been found to co-occur with increases in entropy on a larger scale, when more factors are included. Therefore, some prefer to state the second law as the fact that in any process that transforms energy, the net entropy of the universe always increases.

### c. Types of Energy

**Heat** (also called **thermal energy**), on a molecular scale, whether for a solid, liquid, or gas, is the motion of molecules. In a solid, the atoms or molecules do not go anywhere; they vibrate in place. In a gas, higher temperatures mean faster velocities for the molecules. As a cup of hot tea cools, the fast molecules of the tea hit the molecules of the tea cup, which causes them to vibrate faster; these, in turn, come in contact with the molecules of air around the cup, causing the air molecules to move faster. The air molecules that are faster collide into the slower ones, causing them to move. Thus, the heat moves outward into the air as the cup cools. In addition to this **conduction** of heat, heat can also move by **convection**, as when waves of air waft upward from a hot highway during midday in summer. Heat can also move by **radiation**, which is why your hands held even to the sides of a campfire perimeter are warmed.

**Mechanical energy** is the energy of motion (for example, water in a waterfall that can turn a turbine). As a very high quality (low entropy) form of energy, mechanical motion can be easily converted into other high quality forms, such as electricity.

**Light** is an electromagnetic wave that travels in a vacuum at the universal constant velocity, the speed of light. The energy of an individual quantum packet of light in this wave (a photon) is higher for shorter wavelengths. Thus, a blue photon has higher energy than a red photon, and an ultraviolet photon has even higher energy. A very high energy photon would be the X-ray. A low energy photon is the microwave.

**Electricity** is moving electrons. In direct current (DC, as from a battery), electrons actually move from the negative pole to the positive pole. Eventually, the battery becomes dead when the electrons that can move have all done so. In alternating current (AC, 60 cycles per second here in the United States), electrons are vibrated back and forth, first toward one direction in the wire, then toward the other direction. They do not actually travel. We use AC for most power needs because it is safer at the high voltages needed for long distance transmission from power plants to individual homes.

**Nuclear energy** is the energy inherent in the nuclei of certain atoms. For example, nuclear power plants use the nuclear energy of a uranium isotope (U-235), which can be split in a controlled chain reaction of nuclear fission. This source of energy turns water to steam to spin a turbine, and thereby generates electricity. In the sun, the form of nuclear energy is nuclear fusion, in which hydrogen is fused to helium with the release of energy.

**Work** is formally defined as force times distance ($w = F \times d$). For example, to lift a heavy box from the ground is to do work. You exert a force, counter to that of gravity, to lift the mass through a distance. Work has the same units as energy because work requires the expenditure of energy. Where has the energy gone? Some went into body heat as your muscles were used. Some went into lifting the box, now above the ground, and now a form of potential energy.

**Gravitational and mechanical potential energy:** There are many forms of potential energy, which usually means that energy is being held in a static arrangement of matter in some form, with the potential to be released and turned into some other form of energy, such as kinetic or electrical or heat (thermal). An object lifted above the ground has potential energy due to gravity. Potential energy also resides in the mechanical tension of a pressed or stretched spring.

**Chemical potential energy** exists when two or more substances are capable of undergoing a chemical reaction that could potentially release energy in an exothermic reaction. One example is food and the oxygen in the air. That pair has the chemical potential to "burn" together and release energy. We do this when consuming the food. Our cells convert the energy into other molecules that can store energy. This stored energy can then be used to construct the other molecules we need to live.

**Kinetic energy** is similar to mechanical energy and is called the energy of motion. It is proportional to the square of the velocity of an object.

$$KE = \frac{1}{2}mv^2 \ (m = \text{mass of the object}, v = \text{velocity})$$

## You Should Review

- laws of motion, gravitation, momentum
- light and magnetism
- electricity
- structure of the atom
- periodic table
- chemical bonds
- forms of energy
- first and second laws of energy thermodynamics

# Questions

**21.** Which variant of the most common type of atom of an element has a different number of neutrons in the nucleus?
  a. epitope
  b. isotope
  c. moletope
  d. entrope

**22.** Which of the following is a true statement?
  a. Velocity is the rate of change of time.
  b. Acceleration is the rate of change of velocity.
  c. Velocity is the rate of change of acceleration.
  d. Acceleration is the rate of change of time.

**23.** A bicycle tire has air pressure inside it. Which concept in physics is the pressure most closely related to?
  a. energy
  b. momentum
  c. wave
  d. force

**24.** Which force gets stronger as the distance increases?
  a. strong nuclear force
  b. gravity
  c. weak nuclear force
  d. electromagnetism

**25.** When a sodium atom gives up an electron to enter into an ionic bond with chorine in table salt, it does so because
  a. it requires a electrical charge of +1.
  b. it requires an electrical charge of −1.
  c. it creates a negative potential energy.
  d. it achieves a full electron shell.

**26.** Dissolving $H_2SO_4$ in water creates an acid by increasing the
  a. sulfate ions.
  b. water ions.
  c. hydrogen ions.
  d. oxygen ions.

**27.** Which organic molecule contains nitrogen?
  **a.** carbohydrate
  **b.** lipid
  **c.** cellulose
  **d.** protein

**28.** What is the first law of thermodynamics?
  **a.** Matter can be neither created nor destroyed, but only transformed.
  **b.** Energy moves from higher forms to lower forms.
  **c.** Energy can be neither created nor destroyed, but only transformed.
  **d.** Matter moves from higher forms to lower forms.

**29.** It is a fact that heat leaving a teacup never goes back in. Some have called this the "arrow of time." This concept is most closely related to
  **a.** energy.
  **b.** entropy.
  **c.** reactions.
  **d.** expanding universe.

**30.** Moving electrons are best described as
  **a.** electricity.
  **b.** heat.
  **c.** kinetic energy.
  **d.** light.

## Answers

**21. b.** Epitope refers to cell biology; the others are nonsense words.

**22. b.** Velocity is a change in distance; acceleration is a change in velocity.

**23. d.** Pressure is, in fact, a force, usually expressed as force per unit of area (force per square inch or force per square centimeter, in the case of the tire).

**24. a.** The strong nuclear force exhibits this counterintuitive behavior.

**25. d.** The sodium atom has 1 electron in its outermost shell; by losing 1 electron, it achieves a full shell (the next innermost one was already full). The sodium atom achieves an electrical charge of +1, which is the result of, not the reason for, giving up an electron.

**26. c.** Hydrogen ions come directly from putting $H_2SO_4$ into solution.

**27. d.** The amino acids that make up proteins all have nitrogen atoms in them. Cellulose is a form of carbohydrate.

**28. c.** Thermodynamics covers the properties of energy, and the first law is about the conservation of energy.

**29. b.** In the teacup example, even though it involves the transfer of energy, the governing rule is the law of the increase in entropy.

**30. a.** Electricity is electrons in motion.

## D. Evolution and Life

### 1. Origin of Life

Life on Earth has persisted for nearly four billion years. How did it begin?

#### a. Formation of Organic Molecules

In 1953, a Nobel Prize–winning experiment by Harold Urey and Stanley Miller created organic molecules by passing a spark through a mixture of gases, such as methane and ammonia, which are presumed constituents of an early Earth atmosphere. Zapping inorganic molecules with energy—a possible analogy to lightning in ancient Earth's atmosphere—could create certain constituents for life.

Other possible sources of organic molecules are space, because organic molecules do occur in certain types of meteorites, and deep sea vents, where raw chemicals from inner Earth provide a source of materials and chemical energy.

### b. Concentration of Organic Molecules

To form life, organic molecules need to be concentrated. Darwin had the concept of a warm, little pond as a site for the origin of life. Lagoons that periodically flooded and then dried up might have concentrated organic molecules during the dry stages.

Scientists are not sure of the temperature of early Earth at the time of the formation of life. Some say that early Earth was cold enough for ice to at least occasionally form, and the freezing of water, which excludes any organic molecules present, could have concentrated organic molecules at the surfaces of ice.

Clay minerals are complex, and some scientists have suggested clay as a template for the concentration, and even organization, of organic molecules into more complex networks on the way to life.

As a possible source of organic molecules, deep sea vents are also candidates, due to their necessary concentration. In fact, in recent years, various lab experiments have increased the odds that the vents—with hot water rich in minerals and abundant complex minerals—were sites of key steps in the origin of life.

### c. Membranes

All cells today have membranes that separate inside from outside and regulate the exchange of matter and energy.

Organic molecules (lipids) from certain kinds of meteorites, when added in water, spontaneously form spherical vesicles (liposomes). According to some, these gifts from space could have created the molecular vesicles that became protocells, within which ran self-perpetuating chemical reactions, a step on the way to real life.

The details of how the origin of life went from simple organic molecules, perhaps enclosed in membranes, to real cells with the genetic machinery of proteins and DNA are still unknown. Many scientists claim that RNA served as the first genetic material and was only later supplanted by DNA, at which time RNA then took on the role of helper molecule in that machinery.

### d. Evidence in the Rocks

Evidence for early life is of two types.

An isotope of carbon, carbon-13, is set in a special ratio to ordinary carbon-12 when carbon passes through living metabolisms. Some evidence of this isotopic signature of early life has been found in rocks as old as 3.9 billion years old.

Scientists (micropaleontologists) find ancient rocks, slice them, and look through a microscope to seek direct visual evidence of cells. There are indications of cells in rocks from 3.5 billion years ago.

To gain clues to the origin of life, scientists seek organisms generally known as **extremophiles** across Earth. These are bacteria or archaea adapted to (and requiring) extreme conditions of acid or temperature to live (acidophiles, thermophiles, and others).

## 2. Recipe for Evolution

### a. Inheritance, Variation, and Selection

**Inheritance** is when organisms in each generation share many of the same features as their predecessors because the DNA is copied from parent to offspring.

**Variation:** Often, offspring are not exactly like the parents. Variation is key because this serves as the raw material that can be molded by evolution into new structures and types of creatures.

**Selection (natural selection)** is defined as survival of the fittest. Not all offspring live long enough for themselves to put forth the next generation.

Those that can withstand drought, or seek out food most efficiently, or run the swiftest, survive. The filtering process of death upon life selects certain types of creatures to carry on.

In summary, evolution is modification by natural selection. The process repeats: inheritance, variation, selection. It operates over and over as generations roll along, and it has been doing so for nearly four billion years.

### b. DNA and Mutations

The molecule **DNA (deoxyribonucleic acid)** is key to inheritance and variation. It is the famous double helix, with double strands of alternating sugar and phosphate units, between which are set rungs of the genetic code. The code is made of four bases: adenine (A), cytosine (C), thymine (T), and guanine (G). Base A always pairs with base T, and base C always pairs with base G. The double helix allows a way for DNA to make copies. In the copying process, DNA unravels, and because of the rule of pairing (A-T, C-G), the code on both individual strands can be completed and each made double again, as the complementary bases are added rung by rung. This copying creates faithful inheritance.

Mistakes, or mutations, in copying sometimes occur randomly. Most mutations are detrimental to the offspring. But some can be beneficial (for example, a mutation might create a more effective pore in the cell membrane for the transport of nutrients into the cell).

The simplest type is **base substitution**, in which one type of base nucleotide is removed and a base of another type is incorrectly substituted. In another kind of mutation, entire genes can be duplicated and put somewhere else into the DNA. If the original gene continues with its function, the duplicated gene has the potential to mutate into what possibly could be a new and beneficial structure or function.

There can be insertions and deletions from sections of the code.

All the types of mutations potentially serve as variation in the process of evolution.

How is the genetic code translated? Triplets of bases are read off and code for single amino acids (there are 20 of these). Amino acids are assembled in chains that then fold into complex, bulbous shapes of proteins. Many proteins are active enzymes, while others are structural. Enzymes facilitate the assembly of other types of molecules through chemical reactions inside cells.

### c. "Blind Watchmaker" of Natural Selection

Before evolution was accepted, a story about a watch found on a beach was used as a parable to suggest the presence of a creator for all life forms. A watch, being so complex, obviously had a watchmaker. The scientist and master writer of evolution, Richard Dawkins, coined the phrase the "blind watchmaker." Evolution creates wondrous organisms, even though there is no maker, and because the process is "blind," it doesn't know where it is going.

## 3. Types of Cells

### a. Prokaryotes

**Prokaryotic cells** were the earliest type of cell. They are small and simple. The word *prokaryote* means "before" (*pro*) and "kernel" (*karyote*), signifying that the prokaryotes are single cells with no central "kernel," or nucleus. Prokaryotes have their DNA floating in the cytyplasm and do not contain membrane-bound organelles. Today, there are two types of prokaryotic organisms: **archaea** and **bacteria**. Prokaryotes reproduce asexually, primarily by binary fission when the cell copies itself and splits into two identical daughter cells. Bacteria also have ways to exchange parts of their genomes with different bacteria of the same species, or even other species.

### b. Eukaryotes

Eukaryotes are larger cells that make up animal and plant matter and fungi. Some types of single-celled creatures, such as amoebas and paramecia, are also eukaryotes. The word *eukaryote* means "good" (*eu*) and "kernel" (*karyote*), signifying that eukaryotic cells have a central, membrane-bound nucleus, which houses the DNA for these complex cells. Eukaryotic cells also have other membrane-bound organelles inside them, which support special functions for the cells. All eukaryotic cells have **mitochondria**, which are powerplant organelles that take food nutrients and create high-energy molecules used elsewhere in the cell for various metabolic tasks. Plant cells have another organelle, called the **chloroplast**, which contains the photosynthetic machinery for the plant cell. Eukaryotic cells have internal structures, like wires and tent posts, called, respectively, **microfilaments** and **microtubules**. These allow the big cells to take on complex shapes (and even creep along as the amoeba does).

Eukaryotic cells can reproduce by mitosis (for example, paramecia or our skin cells). In addition, multicellular eukaryotes (animals, plants, fungi) have sexual reproduction for the entire organism, which uses **meiosis** to generate sex cells with half the genetic components (sperm and egg).

### c. Cell Evolution by Symbiosis

The eukaryotic cell evolved about two billion years ago, at about the same time that Earth's atmosphere shifted from anaerobic (with virtually no oxygen) to a level of oxygen about ten percent of the current amount. The eukaryotic cell evolved from a symbiotic merger between a large prokaryote and a smaller prokaryote, which eventually became the mitochondrion of the new, eukaryotic type of cell. **Symbiosis** means working together, and the two cells that merged had specific ways to help the other (probably by sharing metabolic products). Eventually, this merger became permanent. Genes were transferred from the small, embedded cell into the genome of the larger host. One strong piece of evidence in support of this ancient merger is the fact that today's mitochondria still have a remnant of useful DNA inside them. Also, mitochondria are about the same size as typical bacteria.

The chloroplast also came about from a symbiotic merger between something like today's **cyanobacteria** (a type of photosynthesizing, chlorophyll-containing bacterium). As in the case of the mitochondrion, most of the DNA from the symbiotic cyanobacteria migrated into the genome of the larger host cell, but there still exists a remnant DNA for a few proteins in the modern cell's chloroplast. Again, the size of the chloroplast is also about right for the theory.

Because all eukaryotic cells have mitochondria but only some have chloroplasts, the symbiotic event that created the mitochondria came first. Scientists do not know how the nucleus itself evolved.

### d. The Universal Tree of Life

All life possesses DNA and much of the same genetic machinery. This is strong evidence that all current life shares a universal ancestry. In addition, all organisms manufacture proteins at cell sites called **ribosomes**, where amino acids are linked into chains on the way to forming proteins. The ribosome contains some structural RNA as a permanent subunit. All organisms thus contain rRNA (ribosomal RNA). This rRNA varies from organism to organism because rRNA mutated over time. The closer in structure the rRNA is between two organisms, the more closely related they are.

Scientists can construct a tree of all life, using the degree of similarity of rRNA as the metric to distinguish and group organisms. The rRNA tree of life reveals three major lobes: the eukaryotes, the archaea (a type of prokaryote), and the bacteria (another type of prokaryote). Eukaryotes most likely gained some of their genetic material from the archaea and some from the bacteria.

The universal tree of life constructed from the patterns of rRNA shows that most of the organisms near the trunk (prokaryotes living today that presumably are similar to those that lived long ago, when the tree was near its trunk stage in evolutionary time) are **hyperthermophilic** (they require high temperatures). These creatures might indicate a very high temperature origin for life. Such temperatures would have occurred at the deep sea vents, or possibly over the entire Earth.

## 4. Multicellular Life

The eukaryotic cells gave rise in evolution to true multicellular life forms: fungi, plants, and animals.

### a. Earliest Evidence

Evidence of the first multicelled creatures is obscure because their soft bodies meant they were rarely preserved as fossils. Scientists use fossil and genetic evidence from the universal tree of life to estimate the date of the origin of multicellularity at about one billion years ago. That means that for nearly three-fourths of the history of life, all creatures were single-celled.

**Ediacaran fauna** was an early type of multicellular life that lived about 600 MYA (million years ago). Scientists named these strange, flat creatures found in many shapes and sizes after the Ediacara Hills of Australia, where their fossils were first found. Some scientists believe that the Ediacarans went extinct when predators evolved.

### b. Cambrian Explosion

The **Cambrian explosion** was the geological time period of ten million years that began around 540 million years ago, in which suddenly all kinds of animals with hard parts (which is why they were preserved) "exploded" into the fossil record. The hard parts—shells of various types—used calcium from ocean water. Except for the absence of vertebrates, the Cambrian explosion formed most of the basic body plans of animals. The action was all underwater, with **arthropods** (such as **crustaceans** called **trilobites**) and bizarre creatures crawling on the sea floor while others swam and sported formidable jaws. Scientists have not yet determined the trigger for this blossoming of life.

### c. Evolution of Trees and Fungi

The **Devonian period** was a period roughly between 300 and 400 million years ago in which new types of creatures emerged. Important adaptations made this evolution possible. For land plants, these developments included: (1) molecules such as **cellulose** and **lignin** that could give structure to stems and trunks and lift plants up into the air, and (2) **vascular tissues** in the stems, trunks, and roots that could transport water and mineral ions up from the roots to the photosynthetic parts (via tubes called the **xylem**) and transport manufactured food downward from the photosynthetic parts to the roots (via tubes called the **phloem**).

The fossil record shows that plants evolved from tiny, moss-sized beings into tall trees over a period of about 20 million years. No flowering plants (**angiosperms**) existed yet. Fossil evidence shows that fungal cells (visible as microscopic fossils) occurred inside the roots of ancient plants. Apparently, these fungi lived in a symbiotic partnership with plants like some kinds of fungus do today. These fungi live as microscopic underground threads, called **hyphae**.

### d. Animals

What makes an animal an animal? One defining characteristic is a **blastula stage** (a hollow ball of cells) during early embryonic development.

**Vertebrates** evolved in the ocean as fish.

Animal life came ashore during the Devonian period as fishlike creatures with four legs (tetrapods). Besides the legs, lungs were another key development for what became **amphibians**.

To become fully terrestrial, vertebrates had to solve the problem of living in the desiccating air. **Reptiles** became terrestrial with adaptations like a water-retaining amnion (sac) in their embryo stages, a waterproof egg, and a watertight skin of scales.

**Mammals** evolved around 200 million years ago from mammal-like reptiles, which had split off as a branch of reptiles about 260 million years ago. Adaptations of mammals include hair and nursing the young with mammary glands.

## 5. Mass Extinctions

In just the last 20 years, we have discovered what caused the extinction of the dinosaurs. The answer has given scientists new understanding into what factors contributed to the story of life.

### a. Origin of the Dinosaurs

Dinosaurs are a diverse group of animals that diverged from early reptiles 220 million years ago. An important adaptation in dinosaurs was a new kind of hip joint that allowed many early (and late) dinosaurs to run bipedally. Species of dinosaurs came and went over the course of more than one hundred and fifty million years, until their sudden extinction 65 million years ago.

### b. Evidence for Impacts from Space

Objects from space occasionally strike Earth—evidence includes the meteor crater in northern Arizona and the Sudbury crater in Canada. The longer the time period between impacts, the greater the chance of a devastating impact. (Small objects enter Earth's atmosphere every night, and burn up, i.e., shooting stars.) On the moon and Mars, where little or no geological change occurs, scientists see evidence of large impacts (craters). On Earth, as wind and water shift sediments, and continents rise and fall, most craters are buried or erased.

### c. End of Cretaceous and End of Dinosaurs

In the 1980s, an unusually large amount of a rare element called iridium (Ir) was discovered in a centimeter-thick clay layer in rocks in Italy, dating from the time of the dinosaur extinction. This anomaly of iridium was subsequently found all over the world.

Iridium only occurs at such large concentrations in meteorites. This discovery pointed to a large impactor (comet or asteroid) as the source of the iridium and the cause of the mass extinction 65 MYA. Such an object would have smashed into Earth at a speed of 20 km/sec and is estimated to have been about the size of Manhattan (10 km, or 6 miles, in diameter).

A few years later, evidence from gravity patterns revealed a crater buried under sediments in the Yucatan Peninsula of Mexico. About 200 km in diameter (about the estimated size of the crater made by a 10 km object), it dates to exactly 65 million years ago, the end of what geologists call the **Cretaceous** (K) and the beginning of the **Tertiary** (T). A wealth of other types of evidence for the **K-T impact** has been found, including material ejected close to the impact and shocked minerals, as well as chemical evidence for worldwide fires and other environmental disruptions.

At the K-T boundary, 65 million years ago, many other types of life also went extinct on all scales, all the way down to the plankton. One group of creatures survived that had been alive at the time of the K-T extinction and were directly descended from the dinosaurs: birds. And, fortunately for us, mammals also survived, probably because the mammals back then were only the size of rats and could weather the catastrophe in underground burrows.

### d. End of Permian

Another large extinction occurred 250 million years ago at the end of the **Permian era** that marked the beginning of the **Triassic** (the P-T boundary). It came just before either dinosaurs or mammals existed, during an age of giant amphibians and early reptiles. Some paleontologists have called this the "Great Dying." What caused it is not yet known.

### e. Other Mass Extinctions

Species are always going extinct. But once in a while comes a mass extinction, which we know from the fossil record. In some cases, scientists name climate change or large impacts as the cause.

Though the stories of individual mass extinctions are still being assembled from field data, the discovery of the K-T impact and the mass extinction of the dinosaurs has given us new insight into how precarious life on Earth has been and how evolution has been subjected to random shocks from space. What if the impact had been larger? And what if it had not taken place? Before the dinosaurs went extinct, mammals had remained small for over a hundred million years. In the millions of years following the demise of the dinosaurs, mammals evolved into a huge variety of species, some of them as big as hippopotamuses and elephants. In terms of evolutionary biology, the mammals radiated. Without the K-T extinction, this radiation would not have occurred.

## 6. Human Evolution

### a. Gorillas, Chimps, and the Hominid Tree of Life

The molecular clock, the rate at which certain proteins mutate over time, has been used to date the divergences of evolutionary lineages of humans from the great apes: orangutans, gorillas, and chimpanzees.

> At about 12–15 MYA, the lineage leading to orangutans diverges.
> At about 8–10 MYA, the lineage leading to modern gorillas diverges.
> At about 5–7 MYA, humans and chimps share a common ancestor. Many lines of evidence—from morphology to genetics—show that chimpanzees are our closest living animal relative.

### b. Many Species of Hominids

*Australopithecus* is the genus that evolved in Africa after the hominids' divergence with chimps.

*Australopithecus afarensis* is the species thought to be a human ancestor; the fossil named "Lucy" represents this species and lived about 3.2 million years ago. It had a brain size equivalent to the modern chimp's (humans' famed evolutionary brain growth had not yet begun), but the species stood upright, and its legs, feet, spine, pelvis, and skull were adapted to upright living. Some paleontologists suggest that living upright freed the hands to carry objects (although there were no real stone tools yet), which then caused selective pressure for more braininess.

*Homo* is the genus of the modern human, which evolved 2.3 to 2.4 million years ago. An early important species in the genus *Homo* is *Homo erectus*, which evolved in Africa but spread over wide parts of the world, as far as China and other parts of Asia. Most paleontologists think a closely related species, *Homo ergaster*, is more likely our direct ancestor. Compared to *Australopithecus*, the brains and bodies of *H. erectus* and *H. ergaster* are larger. Scientists have found evidence that these early hominids used some of the first stone tools—crudely chipped rocks—which were likely made for cutting meat, scraping, and pounding.

There were other species of genus *Homo* in the time between 500,000 to 200,000 years ago. Paleontologists are still sorting out (and discovering) evidence. Some of these species reached Europe and evolved, by 150,000 years ago, into *Homo neanderthalensis*, the Neanderthals. They were large and powerfully muscular, with brow ridges above their eyes and slightly bigger brains than humans have today. Though the word Neanderthal is sometimes used to mean "dumb," these creatures are considered intelligent. Why did they go extinct? Was it from competition with our species? Was it climate change? They did survive in Europe and Russia during a deep ice age. Scientists do not know for sure.

*Homo sapiens*, the species of modern humans, originated in Africa about 200,000 years ago. *Homo sapiens* migrated from Africa into the Middle East and even shared land with Neanderthals in some cases. Over this span of human evolution, from *Australopithecus afarensis* to *Homo sapiens*, brain size increased about threefold. Human brains (relative to body size) are much larger than the mammalian average and enormous even for the brains of primates.

### c. The Creative Explosion

A creative explosion occurred between about 60,000 to 30,000 years ago and included complex tool making (using animal bones for needles, harpoons, and other craft items), clothing, and elaborate burial practices. An early sculpture from Germany shows what seems to be a standing man with a lion's head. Was this a shaman? Does this signal the birth of myths? (Some scholars claim we will find evidence for art even earlier, when the time period of 100,000 years ago is examined more carefully in Africa.) By 30,000 years ago, we have evidence of elaborate color paintings of animals deep within caves, usually featuring the animals that were hunted. Were these the sites for rituals? For initiation ceremonies?

A find in the Ukraine, dated at about 15,000 years ago, shows that the people constructed dome homes out of mammoth bones and probably covered them with mammoth hides. Thus, they had architecture.

What was their language? Scholars tend to agree that by the time of cave art and elaborate bone tools and carvings, language was used to educate the young and to organize complex social dynamics. But did language come even earlier? Was the creative explosion due to a final genetic advance, or was it all cultural? Scientists do not yet have the answers.

### d. Evolutionary Psychology

**Evolutionary psychology** is the study of the evolution of human behavior, and is considered controversial by some because scientists are limited in studying the minds and emotions of ancestral humans. No other mammal species wages war—although male chimps have been observed in similar behavior, forming a band to kill a solitary individual in a competing band. Humans also cooperate to an unprecedented degree. In a central African jungle lives another kind of ape called the bonobo. Unlike the male-dominated chimp, the bonobo has a female-bonded society and uses sex as a social lubricant. Chimps and bonobos diverged genetically 2 to 3 million years ago, after their shared lineage diverged from the lineage that led to humans. Evolutionary psychologists study chimps and bonobos to investigate how the behavior of humans may have evolved.

The human brain contains an organ, called the **amygdala**, that senses danger and creates the emotion of fear. Humans share this organ with other mammals and most vertebrates. But humans can also project into the future more than any other creature. We know we are going to die. Evolutionary psychologists investigate whether this knowledge is linked with the origin of religion.

## You Should Review

- cell evolution
- prokaryotic and eukaryotic cells
- major events of evolution
- major adaptations leading to new kinds of organisms
- steps in human evolution
- mass extinctions

## Questions

**31.** The four bases of DNA are
   **a.** ACEG.
   **b.** CMEP.
   **c.** TAGC.
   **d.** MGPA.

**32.** Considering the question of the origin of life on Earth, which is NOT a possible source of organic molecules?
a. dissolution of rocks
b. lightning in the atmosphere
c. deep sea vents
d. meteorites from space

**33.** Which cell type has a nucleus?
a. bikaryotic
b. prokaryotic
c. eukaryotic
d. postkaryotic

**34.** For what fraction of the span of life's existence on Earth was life only microbial?
a. $\frac{1}{1}$
b. $\frac{3}{4}$
c. $\frac{1}{2}$
d. $\frac{1}{5}$

**35.** A lichen is a symbiosis between which two organisms?
a. animal-plant
b. algae-fungi
c. plant-fungi
d. animal-algae

**36.** What was the mass extinction that ended the reign of the dinosaurs?
a. Cretaceous-Tertiary
b. Permian-Triassic
c. Triassic-Jurassic
d. Carboniferous-Permian

**37.** The most direct ancestor of the mammals was a
a. mammal-like amphibian.
b. mammal-like reptile.
c. mammal-like fish.
d. mammal-like crocodile.

**38.** Which animal today is the direct descendant of the dinosaurs?
a. ostrich
b. white shark
c. African lion
d. humpback whale

**39.** About how many times larger are the brains of humans today, compared to our Australopithecine ancestors about three million years ago?
a. 2 times
b. 5 times
c. 8 times
d. 3 times

**40.** Which is the second oldest, relatively, in terms of evolution?
a. *Homo erectus*
b. *Homo sapiens*
c. *Homo neanderthalensis*
d. *Australopithecus*

## Answers

**31. c.** The four DNA bases are thymine, adenine, guanine, and cytosine.

**32. a.** Dissolution of rocks creates ions in water, but this has nothing to do with actually forming organic molecules. All the other choices are definite possibilities.

**33. c.** Eukaryotic cells have a nucleus. The word means "good (or true) kernel."

**34. b.** Life became single celled nearly four billion years ago, but multicellular life did not evolve until about one billion years ago. Therefore, the time period over which life was only microbial was $\frac{3}{4}$ of the total span of life.

**35. b.** A lichen on a rock is a working partnership (a symbiosis) between a green algae and a nutrient-gathering fungi.

**36. a.** The Cretaceous-Tertiary event caused the extinction of the dinosaurs about 65 million years ago. (This is also called the K-T boundary—K for Cretaceous, in geologist's terminology.)

**37. b.** Because fish evolved into amphibians, which evolved into reptiles, the ancestor of mammals was a mammal-like reptile. Crocodiles came much later.

**38. a.** The ostrich, like all birds, is a descendent of the dinosaurs.

**39. d.** Human brains are 3 times larger than those of our Australopithecine ancestors.

**40. a.** *Homo erectus* came after *Australopithecus* but well before *Homo neanderthalensis* and *Homo sapiens*.

## E. Earth Works

### 1. Continental Drift and Plate Tectonics

#### a. History

In 1912, German scientist Alfred Wegener proposed that continents could move around, or "drift." One of Wegener's clues to the drift was the fact that the east coast of South America could fit into the lower half of the west coast of Africa, almost like two puzzle pieces. Wegener also pointed to evidence in South America, Africa, India, and Australia for ice sheets at about the same time (300 million years ago), which made no sense with the continents in their present positions because some of these sites are at today's equator.

Modern geologists have evidence that continents have shifted positions radically throughout Earth's history. For example, if molten rock (**magma**) is slightly magnetic when it cools to become solid rock, it takes on the magnetic field of Earth, which depends on latitude. Rocks near the poles have signatures of ancient latitudes near the equator and vice versa.

#### b. Seafloor Spreading

In the 1960s, new lines of evidence supported the idea of shifting continents, but the focus changed to the spreading ocean floor. Ships drilled and brought to the surface cores from the ocean's rocky floor and analyzed them for periodic reversals in Earth's magnetic fields in the lava that came to the surface.

On both sides of the Atlantic Ocean's mid-ocean ridge, stripes showed times when Earth's magnetic field was normal and reversed. The ocean's floor had been growing over time, and the Atlantic Ocean is slowly increasing in size. This ocean floor was like a tape recorder of the history of seafloor spreading. The Atlantic Ocean spreads at a rate of 1–2 inches per year (consider that rate over tens of millions of years). They also analyzed the seafloor to find out its age at various points outward from the mid-ocean ridge. They saw that the seafloor is very young close to the ridge and gets progressively older moving outward from the ridge in both directions. This implies that new seafloor is being created at the ridge and is spreading outward from the ridge.

Finally, scientists had a mechanism for continental drift. It wasn't that the continents drifted, but that they were moved by changes in the ocean's floor. Seafloor spreading replaced continents drifting.

### c. Subduction Zones and Plate Tectonics

If the Atlantic Ocean is growing, what about the other oceans? Because Earth is a constant size, the other oceans cannot also be growing. However, there is a north-south underwater volcanic ridge in the Eastern Pacific that is spreading even several times faster than the Mid-Atlantic Ridge. Eventually, the solution was found in the discovery of what are called **subduction zones**. These are regions where ocean crust disappears by diving down into the depths of Earth, or subducting. The loss of ocean floor in subduction zones balances the creation of new ocean floor in mid-ocean ridges.

The modern theory of **plate tectonics** was thus born. Earth's geological activities have always been called **tectonism**. What about the term **plate**? Think of an egg shell with patterns of cracks in it, creating zones of the shell, and that's the crust of Earth. Earth's surface is divided into a number of major plates. Sometimes, continents ride within the areas of the plates; sometimes edges of continents coincide with edges of other plates. From some of the edges of the plates emerge new ocean crust from mid-ocean ridges and seafloor spreading. Into other cracks, ocean crust subducts (the western coast of South America and the ocean trench regions of the western Pacific are examples). Plates grow and shrink in size with the geological ages. Thus, continents shift positions.

South America, Africa, and Antarctica were all joined as recently as 200 million years ago.

Plate tectonics is an overarching theory that solves many separate mysteries about geology. What made mountain ranges? Why do earthquakes and volcanoes occur where they do? Why is there a "Ring of Fire" around the outer edge of the Pacific Ocean, a ring with huge numbers of earthquakes and volcanoes? It turns out that earthquakes and volcanoes tend to occur at the boundaries between two plates because that is where geological activity happens.

The Pacific Ring of Fire occurs because the Pacific Ocean is ringed by many plate edges. The famous San Andreas Fault in California, which is the origin of California's earthquakes, is a plate boundary where the two plates are sliding past each other, neither subducting nor spreading apart. The towering Andes mountain chain along the western coast of South America has been lifted up by a plate plunging under South America from the west, putting pressure from below to lift the mountains up.

### d. Earth Over Time and the Geologic Time Scale

Earth coalesced from planetary materials brought together by gravity about 4.6 billion years ago (BYA). Geologic time is divided into segments of various length, with eons lasting half a billion years or more and eras lasting several hundred million years.

The **Hadean** Eon (4.6–3.8 billion years ago) was the earliest eon and means "time of hell." Earth still experienced many bombardments from space throughout this eon.

The **Archean** Eon (3.8–2.5 BYA) was when single-celled life originated.

The **Proterozoic** Eon (about 2.5 BYA–545 MYA) was the time of the first great rise in oxygen and evolution of eukaryotic cell about 2 BYA. Near the end of the eon, multicelled life evolved. There is also evidence for massive ice ages, which came close to covering the entire Earth in ice sheets.

The **Phanerozoic** is the current eon, which can be further divided into eras. The **Paleozoic** Era (545–250 MYA) started with the Cambrian explosion of life and by its end, plants had evolved into tall trees. Giant amphibians and early reptiles were the dominant life on land.

The **Mesozoic** Era (250–65 MYA) is subdivided into three main periods called the Triassic, Jurassic, and Cretaceous. The Jurassic was the reign of dinosaurs. The mass extinction at 65 MYA ended the dinosaurs' existence and the Mesozoic period.

The **Cenozoic** period (from 65 MYA to today) is the age of mammals. The **Pleistocene** epoch (a subdivision of the Cenozoic period) lasting from 2.5 MYA to 12,000 years ago, was the time of the growth and then retreat of giant ice sheets in cycles of about 100,000 years each. During the height of the last ice age, for example, ice sheets a mile thick covered all of Canada and extended as far south as New York City. Sea level was 100 meters lower, and the ocean was therefore far offshore of its present location. At the final deglaciation, about 10,000 years ago, geologists end the Pleistocene and start a new epoch, called the **Holocene** (for "wholly recent"). Because humans are perturbing so much of the planet, there has been the suggestion that we have inaugurated what should be called a new epoch, perhaps the "anthropocene," the "human-made recent."

## 2. Earth's Layers

### a. Core and Mantle

When Earth formed 4.6 billion years ago, the heat generated from all the impacts that formed it, and heat emitted from the large amounts of radioactive rock, put Earth into a molten state. Being molten, elements and minerals could separate according to their densities. The heavier materials sunk toward Earth's center. The lighter materials floated nearer to the surface.

Earth's metallic core is solid near the center and liquid farther out. It is about 1,200 kilometers thick and mostly made of iron, with smaller amounts of nickel and other elements.

Circulation of the liquid iron in the core generates Earth's magnetic field. This field is related to Earth's spin, but the north and south magnetic poles are not in the same locations as the north and south poles of Earth's spin axis.

Outside the core is the layer called the **mantle**. With a thickness of about 2,800 km, the mantle reaches to 10 to 50 km below the surface. The upper layer of the mantle belongs to the lithosphere (see the following section). Then, below the lithosphere and

about 250 km thick, is a layer of the mantle called the **aesthenosphere**. This is crucial because although it is made of rock, the aesthenosphere can move like putty over long time periods. The circulation of the aesthenosphere is one main factor in plate tectonics.

When Earth's crust enters subduction zones, the material sinks back down into the aesthenosphere, melting and joining with the deep Earth material of the mantle.

### b. Lithosphere

Lithosphere (literally "rock-sphere"), the uppermost and lightest layer of the Earth, consists of the outermost crust and a thin upper part of mantle. Below the lithosphere, the rock is malleable (the putty of the aesthenosphere). The lithosphere itself, being cooler, is brittle. The border between lithosphere and aesthenosphere is defined by this change in behavior of the rock, from brittle to malleable.

The crust under the ocean's water is thin, about 10 km deep.

The crust under the continents is thick, about 50 km deep.

### c. Oceans

The average depth of the ocean is about 4 km. Around the continents, the ocean is shallow, about 100 to 300 meters deep. This so-called continental shelf is really part of the continental mass. Heading seaward from the continental shelf, the bottom of the ocean drops downward in a steep slope. This region is called the **continental slope**.

At its deepest, much of the ocean is between 3 and 5 km deep. Exceptions are the very deep trenches, which are formed where slabs of ocean floor are subducting downward into the mantle at plate boundaries. Other exceptions are the mid-ocean ridges, which are mountain ranges underwater where new crust is forming, as described above.

In certain regions of the Earth, plumes of magma in semi-permanent tubes from the mantle rise into the lithosphere. These are **hotspots**. The

Hawaiian islands have been formed by a hotspot. As the Pacific plate moves westward (its motion created by plate tectonics), the plate moves over the hotspot (which remains approximately stationary). The Hawaiian islands have been formed, one by one, sequentially, as the Pacific plate has moved over the hotspot over tens of millions of years. Therefore, the oldest Hawaiian island is the one furthest to the west, Kauai. The most recent Hawaiian island, with active volcanoes, is the "big island," called Hawaii itself. Because new ocean floor (crust) is continually being formed and then subducted, the average age of the oldest ocean floor is about 100 million years.

### d. Continents

The continents are also part of the crust, but are much thicker than the ocean-floor crust. Continents that are elevated because of mountain ranges also have deep roots below. The continental masses, in a sense, float on the heavier aesthenosphere.

Continents form when relatively light magma bursts from below to the surface, solidifying as rock. Plate movements that rub bits of crust together can cause continents to grow as the lightest material ends up staying on the surface.

Geologists believe that early Earth had almost no continents or, at most, very small ones. Continents have generally been growing throughout time because once the light rock reaches the surface, it tends to stay there.

A distinctive feature of continents is mountain ranges, which rise and then are eroded away over tens of millions of years or more. Rocks on continents can be very old. Some of the oldest, more than three billion years old, are found in Canada and Australia.

## 3. Rocks and Minerals

### a. Igneous

**Igneous** rock, which was once very hot and molten, makes up most of Earth's crust. Molten magma from under Earth's surface becomes igneous rock when it cools and solidifies. Volcanoes create *extrusive* igneous rock. Molten intrusions under the surface create *intrusive* igneous rock. The base of the ocean's floor is igneous rock that emerged at mid-ocean ridges. Types of igneous rock include granite, rhyolite, gabbro, and basalt.

Igneous rocks have crystals of minerals that form when the magma cools and becomes rock. The slower the cooling, the larger the crystals. Therefore, crystals are larger in intrusive igneous rocks.

### b. Sedimentary

**Sedimentary** rock is formed by the processes of weathering, erosion, and sedimentation. Over time, little pieces of rock and soil are broken down into even smaller pieces by the forces of wind, water, and living organisms. These pieces are called sediments. The sediments pile up and eventually become so numerous that the weight of the sediments on top compacts those below into solid rock. Sedimentary rock may also be formed by the precipitation of chemicals from seawater. This type of rock makes up most of Earth's surface. Fossil evidence for the origin of life comes from sedimentary rocks (3.5–3.9 BYA).

Some types of sedimentary rock are made from physical particles cemented together: conglomerate (from sedimented gravel), sandstone (from sedimented sand), siltstone (from sedimented silt), and shale (from sedimented mud). Note that this sequence progresses from coarse to fine particles.

Some types of sedimentary rock are made primarily from chemical precipitation: limestone (from the mineral calcite) and dolostone (from the mineral dolomite). Calcite and dolomite are calcium carbonate and calcium-magnesium carbonate, respectively. These precipitates are biogenic, created by organisms that precipitate shells. The shells were later fused into rock. Examples of limestone are the white cliffs of Dover in England and much of Indiana, Illinois, and Florida. Other types of sedimentary rock are created from precipitation during the evaporation of seawater: halite (salt) and gypsum (calcium sulfate).

### c. Metamorphic

**Metamorphic** rock is created when either igneous, sedimentary, or another metamorphic rock is subjected to great heat and pressure. Rock already at Earth's surface can be buried deep, creating heat and pressure, or trapped in a mountain-building event, which squeezes the rock and twists the sediments. The mineral structure is changed although the rock is not melted (which would turn it back into igneous rock). Some types of metamorphic rock include slate (from shale), marble (from limestone), and quartzite (from sandstone).

### d. Element Abundances

Rocks are made of specific minerals with definite chemical compositions and crystal structures. The minerals can be classed by hardness. Diamond, of course, is the hardest—a number ten on Mohs Scale of Hardness. Talc is the softest, at number one on the scale. Other examples include calcite (hardness of 3) and quartz (hardness of 7).

What elements make up the crust of the continents? Here are the main elements and their abundance percentages, rounded off to whole numbers: oxygen (45%), silicon (27%), aluminum (8%), iron (6%), calcium (5%), magnesium (3%), sodium (2%), potassium (2%), and titanium (1%). Hydrogen, manganese, phosphorus, and all the others make up the rest.

The large amount of oxygen and silicon in the crust means that many of its constituent minerals are silicon oxides, or silicates. Other elements join in to create different kinds of silicates, such as magnesium-iron silicates, magnesium-aluminum silicates, and so forth.

Elements are shifted from rock to the ocean by two processes. In physical weathering, bits of rock are sloughed off and transported by rivers to the ocean. In chemical weathering, minerals are actually dissolved in water and then transported to the ocean. In this way, one kind of rock contributes to the chemistry of future kinds of rock. Rocks are thereby recycled and reformed.

## 4. Structure of the Biosphere

The biosphere is the thin, dynamic upper layer of our planet that includes air, water, soil, and life.

### a. Atmosphere

The atmosphere contains a mixture of gases: nitrogen ($N_2$, 78.08%), oxygen ($O_2$, 20.95%), and argon (Ar, 0.93%). These three gases make up most of dry air; all the other gases are only 0.04% of the total. Of these, the most abundant is carbon dioxide or $CO_2$ (0.037%). Water vapor is not included in the dry air percentages because it varies with humidity, from 0.3% to 4%.

Clouds consist of huge numbers of condensed water droplets, or microscopic aerosols. Clouds are important to climate, not only as the sources of precipitation, but also as reflectors of sunlight. Globally, clouds reflect about 30% of sunlight back into space.

The atmosphere has four layers:

1. **Troposphere:** the lowest layer, about 15 km high (varies with latitude and seasons). Weather takes place in the troposphere, and almost all clouds are in the troposphere. Temperature decreases with height in the troposphere.
2. **Stratosphere:** next layer, up to about 50 km (between troposphere and stratosphere is a thin transition zone called the **tropopause**). Temperature increases with height in the stratosphere, primarily because in the upper regions the ozone ($O_3$) layer absorbs much of the ultraviolet energy in the sun's spectrum.
3. **Mesosphere:** layer up to about 80 km (between stratosphere and mesosphere is a transition zone called the **stratopause**). Temperatures again drop with increasing altitude.

**4. Thermosphere:** in this layer, temperatures rise with altitude. The air in this zone is extremely thin.

Air pressure drops exponentially with altitude. For example, at the top of Mount Everest, air pressure is only about 40% that of the pressure at sea level. If one were to compress the atmosphere to a uniform pressure equal to that at sea level, the atmosphere would only be about 10 km thick (6 miles).

The winds, which move air from surface regions of high pressure to regions of low pressure, mix the entire atmosphere, even between northern and southern hemispheres, in about a year.

The spinning of Earth creates the **Coriolis effect**, which makes winds around low pressure systems in the northern hemisphere turn counterclockwise and winds around high pressure systems turn clockwise. The directions are reversed in the southern hemisphere.

## b. Hydrosphere

The oceans are also mixed by surface currents, which are moved by the winds and tides. Large-scale, ocean-wide gyres (circular ocean currents) turn the water, and in places near certain western coasts of the ocean, the flow intensifies to true currents: the Gulf Stream off the American Atlantic coast, the Pacific's Kuroshio Current off Japan, and the South Atlantic's Brazil Current off Brazil.

The large, basin-wide ocean gyres circulate clockwise in the northern hemisphere (North Pacific, North Atlantic) and counterclockwise in the southern hemisphere (South Pacific, South Atlantic, Indian Ocean). Again, Earth's spin and the resulting Coriolis effect are the cause of these patterns.

The oceans have a second, different kind of circulation called **thermohaline circulation** ("temperature" (*thermo*) + "salt" (*haline*)—the factors that determine the density of water). When water gets cold, it becomes more dense and tends to sink. When sea ice forms, like in winter at high latitudes, the freezing of fresh water into ice leaves the remaining ocean water more salty. Saltier water is heavier water, which also tends to sink. These two factors create the densest water at certain high latitude regions, particularly in winter in the north Atlantic and around Antarctica. This dense water plunges downward, flooding the deep basins of the world's oceans with cold water. Thus, if one goes downward from the hot water at the surface of the equator, one will find near the ocean floor a thick layer of water that is just a couple degrees above freezing. This cold water has come from the polar regions.

Considering the surface gyres and the deep thermohaline circulation, the world's oceans circulate in about 1,000 years. In that time period, all is mixed from surface to deep.

Oceans cover about 71% of the Earth's surface.

The dominant ions in seawater are chloride (55% by weight), sodium (30%), sulfate (8%), magnesium (4%), and calcium (1%). When precipitated, the sodium and chloride form salt, though the other elements are present as well.

## c. Soil

Soil is derived from two factors: rock that has been physically weathered into small particles, and biological material such as dead leaves. The amount of organic matter in the soil (from leaves and parts of organisms, for example) decreases with depth. Soil is typically about a meter thick, but this varies tremendously from place to place.

The amount of organic matter in the soil depends on the vegetation and, most crucially, on the temperature. Bacteria and fungi in the soil feed upon, and thus break down, the organic matter. This rate of breakdown changes with temperature. At higher temperatures, the bacteria are more active, and at lower temperatures, less so. Because of this, some soils in cold areas, like northern Canada and Siberia, are very thick and have a high percentage of organic matter. Tropical soils, however, have very little organic matter because the breakdown (decomposition) by microbes is rapid. Organic matter plays a large role in making soils fertile, so maintaining organic matter is crucial for maintaining soil fertility and enabling plants to grow. The widespread cutting down of trees and removal of vegetation in tropical areas robs the area of the vital organic material needed to maintain high-nutrient soils.

Soils hold water, to greater or lesser degrees. This water dissolves elements from the mineral grains in the soil (the material that came from parent rocks). The resulting dissolved ions serve as new sources of nutrients for plants. The dissolved ions can also move away from the soil and into groundwater. These ions are carried by the flow of groundwater into streams and then rivers, which eventually deposit them into the ocean.

The soil is key in the recycling of elements from vegetation to ions and then back to vegetation. As bacteria and fungi feed on the detritus from vegetation (leaves, dead roots, branches), they return elements to their ionic forms in the soil water, making these nutrients again available for the plants.

Organisms in the soil must breathe. They can do so because air circulates between the atmosphere and soil via pores in the soil.

### d. Life

Life is an active part of the biosphere, and it makes a huge difference to the surface state of the planet—in fact, to soil, ocean, and atmosphere.

Without life, there would be no soil—only sand piles here and there between large zones of bedrock. The roots of plants and the organic matter from the detritus of plants create a matrix that holds soil together and can retain water. Furthermore, the acids put forth by certain forms of soil life increase the rate of chemical weathering of soil minerals.

Regarding the oceans, algae photosynthesize at the surface where the sunlight hits. Other creatures feed on the algae. Their waste and the dead bodies of the algae sink downward. This removes elements from the surface of the ocean and places them into deep water. The elements circulate back up to the surface via currents and the thermohaline circulation. Life, therefore, affects the chemistry of the ocean.

Life also affects the atmosphere. Oxygen would be virtually nonexistent without photosynthesis. Other gases, such as carbon dioxide and methane, are also altered by the presence of life. Compared to the $CO_2$-rich atmospheres of Mars and Venus (with hardly any oxygen), Earth's atmosphere is low in $CO_2$ and high in $O_2$.

### You Should Review

- basic geological structure of Earth
- theory of plate tectonics
- geological time scale
- types of rocks
- structure and composition of atmosphere, ocean, and soil

## Questions

**41.** The Atlantic Ocean is
 a. growing at several kilometers per year.
 b. shrinking at several kilometers per year.
 c. shrinking at several centimeters per year.
 d. growing at several centimeters per year.

**42.** The San Andreas Fault in California is a
 a. subduction zone.
 b. spreading ridge.
 c. place of magnetic reversal.
 d. site of plate slippage.

**43.** Key evidence for the modern theory of plate tectonics came from
 a. the apparent fitting together of continents.
 b. mapping of depth contours on the ocean bottom.
 c. magnetic field stripes in the Atlantic Ocean's floor.
 d. chemical analysis of volcanoes.

**44.** Earth has layers because
  **a.** all planets have layers when they form.
  **b.** elements were in layers in the gas nebula that formed the solar system.
  **c.** it was once molten.
  **d.** plate tectonics causes geological shifts.

**45.** The Hawaiian Islands are in a chain because
  **a.** the volcanism that made them came from a long crack.
  **b.** they were made over millions of years.
  **c.** the Pacific Plate has moved over a hotspot.
  **d.** they are part of the East Pacific rise.

**46.** Which type of rock emerges from a volcano?
  **a.** igneous
  **b.** sedimentary
  **c.** metamorphic
  **d.** hadean

**47.** What kind of rock is marble?
  **a.** igneous
  **b.** sedimentary
  **c.** metamorphic
  **d.** hadean

**48.** When magma cools slowly,
  **a.** its mineral crystals are small.
  **b.** it has streaks.
  **c.** its mineral crystals grow large.
  **d.** it has bubbles.

**49.** Which is the second most abundant gas in Earth's atmosphere?
  **a.** carbon dioxide
  **b.** oxygen
  **c.** nitrogen
  **d.** water vapor

**50.** The thermohaline circulation is
  **a.** the way the polar atmosphere mixes.
  **b.** the way the deep ocean mixes.
  **c.** the way the lithosphere mixes.
  **d.** the way the soil mixes.

## Answers

**41. d.** The Atlantic Ocean is growing in width, as magma at the mid-ocean ridge spreads the ocean floor at a very slow rate.

**42. d.** At the San Andreas Fault, two continental plates are slipping past each other. This happens in occasional jolts, causing earthquakes in that region.

**43. c.** Magnetic field stripes in the Atlantic Ocean's floor show that the floor is growing in size, spreading away from the Mid-Atlantic Ridge.

**44. c.** Earth, in its early "years," was molten, which caused heavier materials to sink toward the center, segregating Earth into layers.

**45. c.** The chain of Hawaiian Islands demonstrates what happens when a tectonic plate moves over a stationary plume of magma (a hotspot) in the underlying mantle.

**46. a.** Rock that solidifies from the molten state is igneous rock. Hadean (choice **d**) does not apply here.

**47. c.** Marble is a classic metamorphic rock, having been transformed from limestone.

**48. c.** The crystals grow relatively large when the magma cools slowly. Whether it has streaks or bubbles cannot be determined from the information given.

**49. b.** At about 21%, oxygen is number two, after nitrogen. Even under moist conditions, water vapor does not become as highly concentrated as oxygen.

**50. b.** The thermohaline (referring to temperature and salt) creates dense water that sinks in the polar regions of the ocean, thereby mixing the deep ocean.

## F. Biodiversity and Ecology

### 1. Species and Biodiversity

One can note biodiversity on a number of scales, from genes to ecosystems. But the focus at some point always comes down to the species.

### a. What Is a Species?

In its classic sense, a **species** is a group of genetically related organisms with the potential for mating and producing offspring who are themselves capable of successfully mating. For example, robins can only reproduce with other robins. A species is thus reproductively isolated.

Reproductive isolation is brought about by any number of evolved mechanisms: physical mating apparatus, mating rituals, genetic compatibility. Geographical separation often plays a role in allowing different populations of a species to genetically diverge and separate over time into two different species.

A **subspecies** is a taxonomic level within a species that is genetically distinct but not reproductively isolated. In other words, members of different subspecies can reproduce. For example, the Florida panther is a subspecies of the mountain lion, which lives in the western United States (but formerly lived across the entire United States).

In 1973, the Endangered Species Act was passed to protect any species whose population is declining to such a level that the existence of the species is threatened.

### b. How Many Species?

Today, we have catalogued and defined about 1.6 million non-bacterial species. Total species estimates range from 3 to 30 million. Most ecologists think the number is somewhere in between, perhaps ten or more million. Occasionally, a new primate is discovered (for example, a new monkey species was discovered recently in South America), but most undiscovered species are insects.

Estimates are made by surveying regions where new species are found. One technique kills all the insects on a specific tree. The insects are surveyed for new species that seem to be specific for that tree. Then, knowing how many trees are in the area, one can estimate the number of unknown insects in that area.

Here are some different groups of organisms and the number of species currently known: plants (320,000), insects (900,000), fungi (75,000), mammals (5,500), and birds (10,000).

### c. Classification

Organisms are classified according to a nested hierarchy of named groups. Each species has a double scientific name of genus and species. Humans are *Homo sapiens*. The word **species** gets applied in two different ways: the species is *Homo sapiens*, which consists of a genus (*Homo*) and species name (*sapiens*). Within any genus, there can be many species. The ancient Neanderthals, *Homo neanderthalensis*, are in the same genus as modern humans but are a different species.

Levels of classification (in increasing levels of inclusivity):

species
genus
family
order
class
phylum
kingdom

### d. Tropical Biodiversity

The tropics, and in particular their rain forests, are famed for their biodiversity. Maps of the numbers of species, from poles to tropics, for amphibians, trees, and others show species diversity increasing toward the tropics in almost all cases. A single forest plot in South America could have as many species of butterfly or tree as all of England. There are many possible reasons for the high diversity in the tropics.

The high amount of sun in the tropics supplies energy to plants, which, in turn, supports more animals. The larger the amount of mass that can be supported, the larger the potential number of species.

The stability of climate in the tropics allows species to enter into highly specific arrangements with each other. Species of fig tree, for instance, are pollinated by a single species of fig wasp. Both depend on each other. Also, during the recent ice ages, the tropical rain forests might have dried up into zones called **refugia**, where pressures to evolve produced many new species.

The high latitudes experience large seasonal changes, which makes those species more adapted to wide geographical ranges, creating less diversity.

### e. Biomes

Biomes are large geographic regions within which are relatively similar basic types of plant and animals. A biome is larger than an ecosystem. The main determining factors that give shape to biomes are temperature and rainfall.

**Tundra** is characterized by polar regions with tiny plants produced during short summer growing seasons. It has thick soils of peat because of slow decomposition.

**Boreal forest** is characterized by evergreen trees such as spruce and fir across Canada and Russia. It has cold winters but warm summers.

**Temperate deciduous forest** is characterized by trees that lose their leaves each winter, such as maple, birch, and oak. It has cold winters and hot summers with adequate rainfall for trees. Despite the loss of their leaves, deciduous trees in these regions fare better than evergreen trees because flat leaves are more efficient solar energy collectors than needles.

**Prairies and grasslands** are characterized by warmer summers than areas of deciduous forests, but less rainfall. Hot dry summers create conditions for fires, which are an important part of the structure of these biomes. Clearing native grasslands has created some of the great "breadbasket" farmlands of the world.

**Deserts** are very dry biomes with little rain. Plants and animals have special adaptations to survive in this biome. Many plants are bulbous (cacti) to store water in their bodies for times of extended drought.

**Tropical seasonal forests and rain forests** have wet and dry seasons. In these areas, many trees can also be deciduous because they lose their leaves during the dry seasons. In the rain forests, large amounts of rainfall support green vegetation all year. Species diversity is at a maximum in this biome.

## 2. Principles of Biodiversity

### a. Island Biogeography

In the 1960s, MacArthur and Wilson developed the theory of island biogeography by studying the relationship between numbers of species and areas of islands. They found that larger islands held a greater number of species when specific groups were examined, such as birds or amphibians.

The theorists went farther. What determines the number of species on islands? Species die (go locally extinct), and species originate (they migrate from the mainland, fly over in the case of insects and birds, are blown over by the winds in the case of small insects, and come aboard from floating logs and other debris in the case of lizards).

For islands of the same size, islands closer to the mainland have a greater number of species because the immigration rate is higher. Islands with diverse habitats (such as mountains and swamps) have a high number of species. All else being equal, smaller islands have a greater rate of extinction than large islands because the smaller populations are more susceptible to environmental stressors or disease, which lead to a smaller number of species.

For example, in the Caribbean, Cuba is the largest island and has the greatest number of reptile and amphibian species. Furthermore, plotting the sizes of islands versus their numbers of species shows a mathematical law, allowing scientists to count on some theory behind the distributions.

Data compatible with the theory of island biogeography have been collected from other regions on continents and shows that the theory has some applicability to what will happen to species as humans fragment the landscape more and more. The theory will help in the design of nature preserves. For example, butterfly populations increase in English woodlands as the sizes of the woodlands increase.

### b. Predators and Prey

A key kind of interaction in nature is the **food chain**, or the chain of eating: mouse eats seed, snake eats mouse, hawk eats snake. In real nature, we find not simple chains but webs, which are more complex networks because predators often feed upon many different kinds of prey, and prey often can be fed upon by many different kinds of predators. Are there principles to the food webs?

**Trophic levels** describe the position that an organism occupies in a food chain. There are generally four or five trophic levels in any given food chain:

Level 1—**autotrophs** can be distinguished because they turn sunlight, carbon dioxide, and nutrients into the biomass and organic compounds upon which all other terrestrial life depends.
Level 2—herbivores are creatures such as deer and many insects that feed on plants
Level 3—carnivores that prey on the herbivores
Level 4—also carnivores, which, in the idealized situation, feed on the carnivores of level 3

As food passes from trophic level to trophic level (from gut to gut), it is converted into new biomass with an efficiency that is typically about 10%. In other words, it might take 10 kg of plant matter to make 1 kilogram of herbivore, and then 10 kg of herbivore to make 1 kg of carnivore. This is why the apex predators of ecosystems are rare and why there will always be far fewer eagles, for example, than mice.

### c. Sex

Many creatures reproduce without sex between males and females. Bacteria, for instance, can reproduce by cell splitting, creating two clones in a process called **binary fission**. Each daughter cell has the same DNA as the mother cell.

Many plants can reproduce by **vegetative propagation** (for example, taking a cutting from a houseplant, rooting it in water, and then planting it in soil), making a clone of the original plant. Some trees, such as aspens, reproduce with underground runners. So what looks like a patch of individual trees is actually a family of clones. Certain invertebrates, such as hydra, can also reproduce asexually by budding off small replicas, which fall off or swim away to form new individuals. Some insects and even some vertebrates (several species of lizards, for example) are capable of asexual reproduction in which the females lay unfertilized eggs that are capable of growing into new adults.

For the individual of an asexual species, reproduction is more efficient than in the sexual mode because in sex, each parent is only putting half its genes into the offspring. In the asexual mode, the sole parent is putting one hundred percent of its genes into each offspring.

However, sexual reproduction has the benefit of mixing genes and creating variation, which is one of the requirements in the recipe for evolution. Asexual reproduction relies on mutations for variation (except in some cases when bacteria exchange genes, called conjugation), but sexual reproduction creates variation by its very nature. Parasites and diseases can evolve quickly, putting populations of clones at risk. But when sex mixes genes, the offspring are all different. There is good evidence that populations of sexual species have lower susceptibility to parasites and other diseases than populations of asexual clones. What is gained in producing lots of genetic variation seems to make up for what is lost in efficiency of gene transfer for each individual during sex.

In higher organisms, such as plants and animals, sex cells (pollen and egg in plants, sperm and egg in animals) have half the chromosomes, and therefore half the genes, of the cells of the adults they derive from, due to a special process of cell division called **meiosis**.

### d. Keystone, Umbrella, and Invasive Species

**Keystone species** are species that play a key role (like the keystone in an arch) by holding the structure of the ecosystem together. Many top predators are keystone species because they affect the populations of their prey, which affects the populations of lower trophic levels. For example, the starfish along rocky coastlines are a keystone species because starfish affect the populations of many species of mollusks and barnacles.

**Umbrella species** are species that play an exaggerated role in conservation. Preserving an umbrella species that needs a particular habitat will automatically act like an umbrella to save many other species that also use that habitat. A classic example is the northern spotted owl of the old growth forests of the Pacific Northwest. (An old growth forest is forest that has never been cut.) The owl requires holes in old growth trees for its nests and will not nest elsewhere, so protecting the owl will protect the old growth forest and, as a result, all other plant and animal species in the forest.

A **poster** or **flagship species** is a particularly charismatic species that people tend to naturally rally around for its preservation. The giant panda of China is an example.

**Invasive species** are also called **alien** or **introduced species** because they come from other regions of the world and are usually transported by humans. The introduction could have been intentional (such as European starlings into Central Park in New York City), but it is often unintentional, as species can hitch rides on ships or even in airplane wheel cases. A classic example is the zebra mussel, originally from waters in Russia, which were intro-

duced in 1988 and can now be found all over the Great Lakes of the United States and even up stretches of the Missouri River. Its huge, dense populations clog pipes of factories and power plants and cause billions of dollars of damage each year.

Introduced species can be successful invaders when they come into an area with no natural predators and where the prey lacks evolved defenses against them. Invasive species are a serious problem for the world's healthy maintenance of biodiversity and economies.

**Extinct species** are a natural part of Earth's past. But humans are causing extinctions at a far greater rate than the "background" rate of nature (not counting mass extinctions from impacts like the one that took out the dinosaurs). The passenger pigeon and the dodo bird are two bird species that humans (or the animals that humans introduced) caused to go extinct.

**Endemic species** are species that occur in a specific region and nowhere else. Islands often have large numbers of endemic species. Lemurs, for example, are endemic to the island of Madagascar. Special regions where there are a large number of endemic species under threat (and which are unusually rich in overall biodiversity) are called biodiversity hotspots.

## 3. Basics of Ecology

Ecology is the study of the interactions of organisms with each other and with their physical and chemical environments.

### a. Definitions

A **population** is the system of locally interacting members of the same species. When individuals in a local population have substantial interaction among themselves (say, as potential mates) but only occasional links to other populations (say, in another valley), the two populations are said to be **metapopulations** in the context of the larger, more loosely linked species system.

A **community** is the locally interacting system of organisms of different species, usually considered as the plants, animals, and fungi. But there can also be soil communities that include species of bacteria.

An **ecosystem** consists of the community of creatures and the nonliving parts of the environment they are in contact with, such as water and soil. It usually does not have defined boundaries and can be a pond, swamp, local area of prairie, local woods, and so forth.

Ecosystems can become disturbed by natural events such as volcanoes or by humans. If left to restore themselves, they undergo a process of succession. Colonizing species come in first, followed by later species that often require the conditions created by the earlier species. Eventually, a stable endpoint community of organisms, called a **climax community**, is reached.

**Carrying capacity** is the maximum number of organisms of a particular species that an ecosystem can support.

**Reserves** are parts of nature set aside by humans for the preservation of species or wilderness in general. Reserves include National Parks and National Wildlife Refuges in the United States and various regions with different names in other countries.

**Fragmentation** occurs when a force (primarily human) fragments the natural landscape into patches (examples: construction of interstate highways and other roads, housing and urban developments, draining parts of wetlands, or cutting down parts of forests for farmlands). Habitat fragmentation can be harmful to a species because it may disrupt migration routes, leave individuals with fewer opportunities for mating and reproduction, and cut a population off from food and water sources.

A **watershed** is a region that includes all of the drainage of tributaries that feed a larger stream or river. For example, the very large Mississippi watershed would include the watershed of the Missouri River because the Missouri River empties into the Mississippi.

### b. Soil Ecology

When leaves die from trees in autumn or grasses die in winter, they fall to the ground. This material contains carbon and other elements that start to decompose and become part of the soil.

The new material is called **detritus**. Organisms in the soil that perform decomposition are called **detritus feeders** and include various insects, worms, fungi, and bacteria. Though we mainly know fungi as their visible forms of mushrooms (reproductive bodies), they normally occur as invisible threads (called **hyphae**) throughout the soil.

Organisms in the soil breathe because air enters and leaves the soil through openings between its grains. The deeper one goes in the soil, the less oxygen there is because the oxygen has been used by soil organisms.

Soil has layers. The uppermost, rich layer is called topsoil, which is important to preserve in farmlands. Farmers must beware of losing topsoil to erosion by wind and water.

### c. Marine Ecology

The continental shelf regions of oceans tend to be richer in life because they obtain increased nutrients from rivers and from the winds and tides that stir the shallow water, thereby mixing nutrients from below up to the surface. The open ocean is sometimes considered a marine desert because life is more sparse there.

At the top of the ocean is a zone called the **mixed layer**, which varies in depth but is usually about 100 meters thick. It is well mixed, having been stirred by the winds. The upper part that receives light is called the **pelagic zone**, which varies in depth depending on how far light penetrates down. The deep parts are called the **benthos**. Thus, marine biologists distinguish organisms as pelagic species and benthic species.

Special areas called **upwelling zones** occur off certain coasts, such as Chile and the coast of northwest Africa. Here, deep, nutrient-rich waters are brought up and fish are hugely abundant.

Tiny organisms in the ocean constitute the **plankton**, which generally drift with the currents. There are **phytoplankton**, which are green because they have chlorophyll and perform photosynthesis (eukaryotic algae and prokaryotic cyanobacteria), and **zooplankton** ("animal-plankton"). Zooplankton include tiny multicellular swimming crustaceans as well as the swimming larvae of creatures that will grow to adult sizes out of the plankton range, such as jellyfish and mollusks. Zooplankton feed on phytoplankton, and all are fed upon by a variety of fish and other organisms, making a marine food web.

A **fishery** is a commercial entity engaged in harvesting fish in a particular region (examples: northwest salmon fishery, the New England cod fishery). Many fisheries are in decline as the stocks of fish have been depleted.

**Aquaculture** is the commercial raising and farming of aquatic organisms in tanks or fenced-off areas of the ocean.

### d. Ecology and Energy

Sunlight is captured by plants using the pigment molecule chlorophyll. Plants are green because chlorophyll absorbs the red and blue wavelengths of light, reflecting some of the green. The energy captured is used to drive the process of photosynthesis, which creates simple sugar molecules from carbon dioxide and water. Plants get water from the soil (through their **xylem**) and carbon dioxide from the air, through pores in their leaves called **stomata** (or stomates). Marine algae are also green because of chlorophyll, but they get carbon dioxide from the water.

Terrestrial plants and marine algae are called **autotrophs**, or "self-feeders," because they create their own food, in a sense, from inorganic molecules. Insects and humans are **heterotrophs**, requiring autotrophs for food.

The molecules of organisms are high energy molecules because they can be burned by the metabolisms of organisms to maintain their bodies and exert force upon the environment for movement and food capture. The energy ultimately comes from the sun. Thus, when we walk, we are using transformed and stored solar energy. Life runs on solar energy.

The mass of a living thing or a collection of living things is called **biomass**, or biological mass. One can ask about the biomass of trees in a forest or the insect biomass of an ecosystem.

When plants convert their simple sugars made by photosynthesis into the more complex organic molecules that they need, such as proteins and starches, they use some of the sugar as a source of carbon for this next generation of organic molecules. They also burn some of the sugar for energy to drive the chemical reactions inside their cells that create the next generations of molecules. This burning uses up some of the sugars and requires oxygen, and it results in the chemical products of carbon dioxide and water, thus reversing the process of photosynthesis. This is called **respiration**. Heterotrophs also perform respiration (but not photosynthesis).

The amount of biomass created by the photosynthesis in a plant is called **gross primary production (GPP)**. It is usually expressed in terms of carbon. The carbon that actually goes into the full metabolism of molecules inside a plant is less—called **net primary production (NPP)**.

NPP = GPP – respiration

NPP can be calculated at the level of ecosystem and biome, as well. It varies across ecosystems and biomes, being highest in tropical rain forests and lowest in deserts.

Limiting factors control the amount of net primary production. Depending on the ecosystem or biome, limiting factors could include water, nitrate, phosphate, and other nutrients. Farmers overcome limiting factors—in particular, in soils—by adding fertilizers.

## 4. Biogeochemical Cycles

Biogeochemical cycles are the cycles of elements essential to life. These cycles are thus biological (*bio*) and include geological processes (*geo*) and chemical reactions (*chemical*).

### a. Carbon on Land

The most important biogeochemical cycle is that of carbon, the essential element in the organic molecules of life. Carbon moves in and out of various forms. Photosynthesis and respiration form a coupled pair of processes that convert carbon dioxide into organic molecules and back again. Most respiration takes place in the soil, as respiration from bacteria and fungi releases carbon dioxide. The cycle is more complex with other forms of carbon as well. Some bacteria release waste carbon in the form of methane ($CH_4$). Other types of bacteria consume methane.

### b. Carbon in the Biosphere

The atmosphere contains about 700 billion tons of carbon, primarily in the form of carbon dioxide. The amount of carbon in all biomass is roughly equal. The carbon in the world's soils is about three times that amount. The oceans contain the largest pool, or reservoir, of carbon because seawater also has carbon in other forms: bicarbonate and carbonate ions. Atmosphere, plants, algae, soil, and ocean are all considered **pools**, between which carbon is shuffled in and out of various forms in amounts known as **fluxes**. Global net primary productivity is the flux of carbon from the atmosphere into all photosynthesizers, for example.

### c. Nitrogen in the Biosphere

Nitrogen, which is important in protein synthesis, is another element that has a biogeochemical cycle. Like carbon, there are pools (or reservoirs) of nitrogen in the atmosphere (as $N_2$ gas), in organisms (primarily in proteins), in the soil (in the detritus), and in water (as nitrate and ammonium ions). Fluxes describe the conversion of nitrogen from one form to another.

**Nitrogen fixation** occurs when soil or marine bacteria take in nitrogen gas and convert it into the useful ammonium ion for their bodies. Some ecologically and agriculturally important soil bacteria live within the roots of plants in a symbiotic relationship. When we say that bean plants or clover can fix nitrogen, it is really the bacteria in the nodules on their roots that perform that function, not the plants themselves.

**Ammonification** is also done by bacteria in the soil, as the bacteria process proteins in detritus and convert the organic nitrogen into ammonium ions.

**Nitrogen assimilation** occurs when organisms take up nitrogen as ammonium ions or nitrate ions from the environment in soil or water.

In **denitrification**, other kinds of bacterial specialists convert nitrate ions in soil or water into nitrogen gas. Denitrifiers live in places of no or little oxygen. Finally, nitrifying bacteria take ammonium ions and convert them into nitrate ions.

### d. Phosphorus in the Biosphere

Phosphorus is another crucial element for all living things. It also has a cycle, which is relatively simpler than the cycles of carbon and nitrogen because phosphorus does not have a gaseous form. It primarily cycles between its ion (phosphate ions in soil and water) and its form in life (various molecules inside cells). Phosphorus is used as part of the ladder of DNA and is essential for energy molecules inside cells, such as ATP.

### e. Bioessential Elements

All of the dozen or so elements that are essential to living things have biogeochemical cycles. The major elements and their approximate mass percentages in a typical plant are: carbon (C, 45%), oxygen (O, 45%), hydrogen (H, 6%), nitrogen (N, 1.6%), sulfur

(S, 0.1%), phosphorus (P, 0.2%), potassium (K, 1%), calcium (Ca, 0.5%), magnesium (Mg, 0.2%), and iron (Fe, 0.01%). The elements N, S, P, K, Ca, and Mg are macronutrients because they occur in relatively large amounts. Iron and other elements not listed, such as manganese, molybdenum, and copper, are micronutrients. Hydrogen and oxygen, though essential elements, are not considered nutrients because they occur abundantly in water. In humans, the percentages change somewhat but not drastically (not so much that iron is larger than phosphorus, for example). More protein in humans means more nitrogen, to cite one element's differences between humans and plants.

### You Should Review

- principles of biodiversity and ecology
- numbers of species
- classification system
- biome types
- food webs in ocean and on land
- interaction of predators and prey
- asexual versus sexual reproduction
- biogeochemical cycles of carbon and nitrogen

## Questions

**51.** Which category contains the fewest number of species?
  a. birds
  b. primates
  c. mammals
  d. fungi

**52.** Which one is NOT one of the possible theories that at least partially explains the high diversity in the tropics, such as rain forests?
  a. high solar energy
  b. Pleistocene refugia
  c. low seasonal variability
  d. Permian-Triassic extinction

**53.** Fire can be an important part of the structure of an ecosystem. This is particularly true in which of the following biomes?
  a. tundra
  b. chaparral
  c. boreal forest
  d. prairie

**54.** Food chains are parts of food webs, in which we go from plants at the first trophic level (primary producers) to a second trophic level, and so on. Why do food chains in nature rarely exceed 4 or 5 levels?
  a. because evolution has not yet created that degree of complexity
  b. because organisms die more easily at the higher levels
  c. because of inefficiencies, the available energy becomes less and less at higher levels
  d. because food chains limit the levels of food webs

**55.** The California sea otter, native to the coast, controls the populations of starfish, which control the populations of many other marine creatures among the kelp beds. The otter is an example of a(n)
  a. umbrellate species.
  b. invasive species.
  c. keystone species.
  d. mammal species.

**56.** Consider the following food web: oak seedlings eaten by rabbits; rabbits eaten by wolves. What happens to the oak seedlings if the wolf population suddenly declines from a disease?
  a. Seedlings decrease.
  b. Seedlings are eaten by something else.
  c. Seedlings increase.
  d. Seedlings are also hit by a disease.

**57.** Which is NOT true about marine ecology?
  **a.** Phytoplankton are functionally equal to land plants.
  **b.** Fish eat zooplankton.
  **c.** Zooplankton grow up into plankton.
  **d.** Fish are part of the food web.

**58.** The term *fragmentation* refers to which of the following?
  **a.** invasive species that divide the structure of ecosystems
  **b.** the dispersed nature of marine food webs
  **c.** successive waves of species as an ecosystem develops
  **d.** humans segregating nature into chunks

**59.** In considering the pools of the biogeochemical carbon cycle, which has the most carbon in it?
  **a.** ocean
  **b.** soil
  **c.** plants
  **d.** atmosphere

**60.** Which bacteria thrive in places in the ocean with low oxygen?
  **a.** nitrogen fixers
  **b.** denitrifiers
  **c.** nitrifiers
  **d.** ammoniaficators

## Answers

**51. b.** Compared to birds and fungi, mammals have the fewest species. Because only a small fraction of all mammals are primates, primates have the fewest number of species on the list.

**52. d.** The Permian-Triassic extinction occurred 250 million years ago and has nothing to do with the differences today between tropical and high-latitude biodiversity. The other answer choices are all possible contributing reasons to the diversity pattern.

**53. d.** Prairies have dense vegetation and often long intervals of summer drought. Fires started by lightning are a natural part of these grasslands, and many plants have even become evolutionarily adapted by developing seeds that germinate after a fire.

**54. c.** Typically, each level only converts 10% of the energy of the previous level into biomass. As the levels progress, the energy available is very small, thus limiting the number of levels reached.

**55. c.** The otter is a keystone species because, like the top stone in an arch, it holds much of the rest of the ecosystem in its structure.

**56. a.** If the wolves decline, the rabbits increase in population. If the rabbits increase, they eat more seedlings, so the seedlings decline.

**57. c.** Zooplankton are a type of plankton; they do not grow up into plankton.

**58. d.** Human activities fragment nature.

**59. a.** The ocean has about 10 to 50 times more carbon than any of the other pools. In the ocean, carbon is found mostly in the form of the bicarbonate ion (with the carbonate ion second).

**60. b.** Denitrifiers live in places of low oxygen, and use nitrate as a source of oxygen, creating nitrogen gas.

## G. Global Environmental Challenges

### 1. Population and Land Use

#### a. Population

Prior to the invention of agriculture approximately 10,000 years ago, humans in their hunting and gathering phase were limited to about ten million people worldwide. But by the pyramid days of ancient Egypt 5,000 years ago, global population had grown tenfold, to about 100 million due to agriculture.

By 1830, the population had reached its first billion.

By the late 1950s, the world held two billion people.

The third, fourth, and fifth billion marks were reached by the late 1950s, the early 1970s, and the mid-1980s, respectively.

The six billion mark was reached in the late 1990s, and seven billion in 2011, due to a worldwide growth rate of about 85 million people a year (ten times the population of New York or Los Angeles). However, while the population continues to grow, the growth rate is starting to decline. Factors that cause the growth rate to decline include a higher standard of living and better education (for women, in particular). Scientists expect the world population to reach at least eight billion, but many variables may influence how high the population ultimately climbs.

#### b. Land Use

Global land = 140 million square kilometers = 14 billion hectares (about five acres per person).

**Usable land:** 31% of the world's land (4.4 billion hectares) is unusable because it is rock, ice, tundra, or desert, leaving 9.6 billion hectares for potential human use.

**Agricultural use:** The major human land use is for agricultural production, which currently covers 4.7 billion hectares. Of that, 70% is permanent pasture and 30% is crop land. So agriculture (pasture + crops) takes 34% of the world's land.

**Urbanized land:** Globally, only about 1% of land (about 140 million hectares) is considered urbanized, including highways. In some local areas, the urbanized land approaches 100% coverage.

Therefore, 14 billion hectares – 4.4 (unusable) – 4.7 (agriculture) – 0.14 (urbanized) = 4.8 billion hectares of potential usable land remains.

This is about 34% of the total land, or about as much as humans currently use for all agriculture. However, much of the prime land for agriculture has already been used, so what remains is not as high in quality.

### 2. Humans Alter the Biosphere

Unlike other species, humans deploy vast arrays of chemical processes (factories, residences, and forms of transportation). In our use of energy and in the ways we process matter, we create substances that alter the chemistry of the biosphere.

#### a. Carbon Dioxide and the Greenhouse Effect

Carbon dioxide ($CO_2$) is typically measured in units of ppm (parts per million) because there are only small amounts of it in the atmosphere. *Million* refers to a million randomly selected molecules of air. Today, $CO_2$ is present in a concentration of somewhat more than 370 ppm (which is equal to 0.037%).

$CO_2$, though present in such a small amount of the atmosphere, is of critical importance because it is a greenhouse gas. Oxygen and nitrogen gas are not. A greenhouse gas lets in visible radiation (light, short-wave radiation) from the sun, which enters the atmosphere and passes directly through to the ground (therefore we can't see the $CO_2$). But a greenhouse gas absorbs infrared radiation. Infrared radiation (long-wave radiation) is what Earth uses to cool to space and to balance the energy received from the sun. Greenhouse gases are like one-way insulation, letting light in but blocking the escape of infrared radiation. Earth's surface will warm up to compensate for any extra insulation in the atmosphere.

Without $CO_2$, Earth would be very cold, below the freezing point of water. So present conditions require $CO_2$.

But there can also be too much: $CO_2$, emitted as a waste gas from the combustion of fossil fuels (coal, oil, natural gas), is rising. Data from bubbles trapped in Antarctic ice show that for 10,000 years prior to the industrial revolution, $CO_2$ was fairly constant at about 280 ppm. Now it is above 370 ppm and rising from human activities at the rate of 1.5 to 2 ppm per year.

## b. Ozone and Ultraviolet Radiation

Ozone is a molecule with three oxygen atoms ($O_3$), unlike the regular oxygen ($O_2$) that makes up 21% of Earth's atmosphere. Ozone is made naturally by cosmic rays that cause chemical reactions in Earth's stratosphere. Ozone readily absorbs the ultraviolet portions of the sun's spectrum that enter Earth's atmosphere. This absorption also destroys some of the ozone, so a balance is reached between creation and destruction that results in a natural amount of ozone that is constantly present.

Without this protective ozone layer, biologically damaging ultraviolet (UV) rays would reach the surface of the planet. UV exposure is a main cause of skin cancer.

Until recently, ozone was on a worrisome decline. Human-made gases called **chlorofluorocarbons** (CFCs, containing chlorine, fluorine, and carbon) used in refrigerators, air-conditioners, and some aerosol cans, when released, travel up into the stratosphere. There, the CFCs act as a catalyst to destroy the ozone at a rate much faster than its natural rate of destruction. Humans had altered the balance, and global ozone levels started dropping, particularly in the area above Antarctica, endangering people in Australia and New Zealand.

In 1987, many nations signed the Montreal Protocol, a global agreement to phase out the production and use of CFCs. Substitute gases were invented to replace CFCs. As a result, the ozone decline has been halted. Over the coming decades, the ozone layer should be able to repair itself and return to its natural level.

## c. Acid Rain

Acid rain is yet another human perturbation to the atmosphere and is related to the combustion of fossil fuels, particularly coal. Coal, the remains of ancient plants from hundreds of millions of years ago, contains sulfur, one of the bio-essential elements. When the coal is burned in power plants to obtain energy (most of which comes from converting carbon to $CO_2$), the sulfur also combines with oxygen to create sulfur dioxide ($SO_2$) gas, which then enters the atmosphere. The $SO_2$ further combines with water vapor and ultimately becomes sulfuric acid ($H_2SO_4$) in cloud droplets. The rain that falls from these clouds is acidic—acid rain.

Nitrogen also contributes to acid rain as nitric acid, which is derived from nitrogen oxides created from the high temperature reactions with air in power plants and automobiles.

Acid rain falls mostly in the regions downwind of power plants. It has been responsible for ecological damage to many streams and lakes.

Laws governing the release of acids from power plants are in place, but could be strengthened further. Acid rain is a problem that potentially could be controlled with adequate environmental regulation. Emissions of pollutants from automobiles have been improved, for example, with better technology.

## d. Toxins

**Primary pollutants** are chemicals released directly into the atmosphere.

Besides some of the gases already discussed, primary pollutants include the following:

- *Suspended particulate matter* (PM) consists of all kinds of tiny particles from smog stacks and even metals.

- *Volatile organic compounds* (VOC, hydrocarbons) are organic gases from a variety of sources, such as leaks that you smell when you fill your car with gasoline and even gases from lighter fluids used to start barbeques.
- *Carbon monoxide* (CO) derives from the incomplete combustion of fossil fuels (organic carbon is oxidized to CO, rather than $CO_2$, during complete combustion); CO is odorless and the leading annual cause of death by poisoning in the United States.

Primary pollutants can be altered chemically by interactions with sunlight and become **photochemical pollutants**.

- **Tropospheric ozone** is one such pollutant. Different from the natural, stratospheric ozone, tropospheric ozone is ozone or pollution in an urban area.
- **Photochemical smog**, another secondary pollutant, is created when car exhaust is acted upon by sunlight to form a brown haze that is highly irritating to the lungs. Smog is particularly troublesome in cities that lie in valleys and are subject to air inversions, in which a lid of air sits over the city and does not move for a long period of time.

After cigarette smoke, **radon gas** is the second leading cause of lung cancer. Radon, a daughter product of uranium in Earth's rocks, is a radioactive gas that leaks from particular kinds of soils. It can accumulate indoors, as in basements. When breathed in, radon gas follows a nuclear decay pathway within the lungs, releasing radiation and ultimately leaving lead trapped within.

Scrap rocks from uranium mining are a form of radioactive waste. Of even more concern are the waste byproducts from nuclear power plants. These are daughter products of controlled nuclear fission, which uses uranium but creates radioactive iodine, cesium, plutonium, and other elements as waste. This material is secured and stored on the site of the nuclear power plants, but plans are being created for long-term, permanent storage. Many communities oppose nuclear waste storage in their areas due to fears of radioactive contamination.

## 3. Energy Systems

Our lives are dependent on external sources of energy as we burn fossil fuels at a total rate that is many times greater than the metabolisms of all humans.

### a. Energy versus Power
**Power** is the rate of energy flow; unit is kilowatts (kW, 1 kW = 1 kilojoule/second).
**Energy** is the summation of power over time; measured in kilowatt-hours or BTU (for British thermal unit, the energy it takes to raise 1 pound of water by 1°F).

### b. Fossil Fuel Combustion
All fossil fuels contain carbon and hydrogen. When a fossil fuel is reacted (burned) with oxygen from the air, the chemical products are carbon dioxide and water vapor. Because the produced $CO_2$ and $H_2O$ together have a lower molecular energy than the reactants of fossil fuel and oxygen, energy is released in the reaction. Fossil fuels are the main source of energy for all the processes of civilization.

Types of fossil fuels differ in their relative amounts of carbon and hydrogen. The more carbon a fossil fuel has, the more carbon dioxide it releases for a given amount of energy. In this regard, coal is the worst fuel and natural gas (which is primarily methane, $CH_4$) is the best fuel, with oil rating somewhere in the middle.

Fossil fuels come from biological sources that lived many millions of years ago. Oil is from marine algae, buried and transformed. Coal is from terrestrial plants that lived in vast swampy environments, buried and transformed. Natural gas is mostly derived as a breakdown product of either coal or oil. All occur underground and must be dug up or piped to the surface, transported, and processed for human use.

A significant factor in world politics is the uneven distribution of fossil fuels, especially oil. This shows how geological processes from hundreds of millions of years ago affect human life today.

### c. Energy Today

The global primary energy supply consists of the following (total is 99% because numbers are rounded off):

- oil (35%)
- coal (23%)
- natural gas (21%)
- wood and combustible wastes (11%)
- nuclear (7%)
- hydroelectric (2%)

How is energy used? Roughly one-third of it is used for industry, one-third for transportation, and one-third for residential (this varies by country).

Hydroelectric energy utilizes vertical drops in rivers. Water is diverted, usually from behind dams, into turbines, which turn generators to produce electricity. (All mechanical electricity-generating power plants turn turbines to make electricity.)

Nuclear power plants generate intense heat from the controlled splitting (fission) of uranium atoms. The heat creates steam, which turns turbines to make electricity.

Fossil fuel power plants work the same way, except that the source of heat is the combustion of the fuel.

### d. Efficiency from Supply to Use

**Efficiency** is output of useful work divided by the input energy, measured in percent. For example, how much of the energy in oil goes into making the automobile travel, and how much is wasted as heat in the exhaust system and from cooling the engine?

For fossil fuel power plants, a typical efficiency is about 33%. Although better engineering can improve this number, it cannot and will not ever be 100% because the Second Law of Thermodynamics limits how much of one kind of energy can be converted into a different kind of energy.

All devices, from refrigerators to light bulbs to cars, can be quantified in terms of efficiency. Improvements in energy efficiency can cut down on pollutants and the use of fossil fuels, which not only are limited but produce the greenhouse gas carbon dioxide.

### e. Future Energy Technologies

Research continues on future energy technologies, sources of energy that do not emit carbon dioxide and are renewable.

**Hydrogen** can be burned with oxygen to produce harmless water vapor. However, hydrogen does not occur naturally. To have a hydrogen economy in the future, we need to make hydrogen from the splitting of water, which requires an energy source, like fossil fuel or solar energy. (Hydrogen can also be made from natural gas, but this creates $CO_2$, so to avoid the emission of $CO_2$, it would have to be sequestered—see the next page.)

**Wind energy** uses the pressure of moving air to turn turbines to make electricity. Many large wind turbines are going up all over the world, particularly in northern Europe. These have blades 100 feet or more in length. Wind energy is site-specific. In the United States, for example, states such as the Dakotas and the western part of Texas have particular potential for wind development. If set up in farm fields, only a small percent of the land is used, and farmers can still grow their crops under the turbines; the land would do double duty.

**Solar energy** has two main types: **solar thermal energy** that uses sunlight to heat water or air for direct use, mainly for domestic water heating or wintertime home heating, but also for heating water to steam to turn turbines and generate electricity; and **solar photovoltaic energy** that uses solar cells (silicon cells, originally perfected by NASA for space use) to create electricity directly from the photons of the sun. Like wind electricity, photovoltaic electricity's use is increasing, but not as much because the costs are still quite high relative to conventional energy sources.

**Nuclear fusion** uses the energy released from fusing hydrogen into helium (which is the process that takes place in the center of the sun). Fusion requires enormous temperatures and pressures in the fusion reactor's center, which will probably use incredibly high-tech magnetic "bottles" to hold the reactants (because nothing material could withstand those conditions). Fusion has been accomplished in high-energy physics labs, but no fusion energy plants exist yet.

**Carbon sequestration** is a technology that stops the emission of $CO_2$ by trapping and disposing of carbon dioxide waste, which would allow humans to continue burning fossil fuels, depending on supply. One possibility is to pipe carbon dioxide deep into the ocean, but this might make conditions intolerably acidic for some benthic marine life. Another possibility is to pipe it into deep aquifers of salty, unusable water far beneath the land surface. But would the $CO_2$ leak back up into the atmosphere? A small industrial project off the shores of Scandinavia is currently injecting $CO_2$ into the ocean. Much remains to be tested with these technologies.

## 4. Systems of Matter and Life

The biosphere is an interacting system of matter and energy, of humans and nature.

### a. Waste Disposal

**Municipal solid waste** describes general garbage. Disposal methods include landfills, combustion, recycling, and the composting of organics.

**Sewage** describes liquid and solid body wastes treated in sewage treatment plants. A number of steps are involved: Preliminary and primary treatments remove debris and organic particles, respectively. Secondary treatment involves bacteria in aqueous slurries. The bacteria consume the dissolved organics in the sewage. Before the treated waste water is put back into a natural water system, it is disinfected. Many variations exist, and new technologies, often using more advanced biological processes to help, are being explored. In sewage treatment, we are mimicking (and using) the natural recycling capabilities of bacteria in nature, in the soil, and in the deep ocean.

### b. Deforestation

**Deforestation** is the cutting of areas of forest. This occurs at a rate of ten million hectares per year. Deforestation occurs to supply raw material for the lumber and paper industries, or it can also take place when trees are burned to create open land for pasture or crops.

**Clear-cutting** is the term used when patches of forest are completely cut for industrial use. The other approach is **selective cutting**, when only certain trees (say large trees or a certain species) are harvested, leaving the rest to grow for future harvests or just remain as forest.

Certain regions, such as the New England states, are undergoing **reforestation**. Farming, which was a strong part of their economy up to a hundred years ago, eventually could not compete with the midwestern and western farms. Through reforestation, much of the land in New England is returning to forest.

Deforestation usually releases $CO_2$. If trees are burned, $CO_2$ goes into the atmosphere. Even if the trees are to be used for paper or lumber, the twigs and dead roots decay rapidly, and thus are a lesser, though still important, source of $CO_2$ from these areas of deforestation. Reforestation, on the other hand, removes $CO_2$ from the atmosphere because it puts living plants back into the environment. Through the process of photosynthesis, the plants take $CO_2$ from the atmosphere and use it to make their food. This can help mitigate the rising threat of a greenhouse effect.

### c. Nature's Services

**Nonrenewable resources** are resources that cannot be renewed in anywhere close to the time in which we are depleting them. For example, though oil is formed continuously during the geological ages, the rate is infinitesimal compared to our rate of extraction and burning. Minerals are also nonrenewable resources, as are the fossil fuels oil, coal, and gas, as they all take millions of years to form.

**Renewable resources**, on the other hand, can be regenerated by natural processes. For example, fresh water is reformed by the water cycle, in which water from the ocean is evaporated (leaving the salt behind) and then forms droplets in clouds, which in turn rain over land. Thus, the fresh water in rivers is renewed. Of course, humans can still exert stress upon the water systems when deep, underground aquifers are pumped faster than they are being renewed, or when water is drawn from watersheds at rates that do not allow enough water for the fish in the natural stream to survive.

Trees would be considered a renewable resource because they can regrow. However, old-growth forests are nonrenewable because they take many hundreds of years to develop to their full climax state.

Nature is our basic life support system. It is important to preserve the services of nature. Much is not yet understood, but it is clear that biodiversity is crucial for the healthy continuation of most natural systems.

### You Should Review

- human population
- land use
- greenhouse effect
- acid rain
- toxins
- ozone depletion
- energy technologies
- waste disposal and deforestation
- renewable versus nonrenewable resources

## Questions

**61.** What is the global human population today?
  a. between seven and eight billion
  b. between four and five billion
  c. between five and six billion
  d. between six and seven billion

**62.** Which of the following statements about global land use is NOT true?
  a. Cropland is increasing.
  b. Old-growth forest is decreasing.
  c. Unusable land (rock, ice, desert) is greater than urbanized land area.
  d. Pasture is less common than cropland.

**63.** Considering the unit *ppm* as parts per million, how many ppm is oxygen in Earth's atmosphere?
  a. 21 ppm
  b. 21,000 ppm
  c. 210,000 ppm
  d. 2,100 ppm

**64.** Stratospheric ozone absorbs
  a. infrared radiation.
  b. visible light.
  c. ultraviolet radiation.
  d. green radiation.

**65.** The Montreal Protocol limited
  a. the production of carbon dioxide.
  b. the production of acid rain.
  c. the production of dimethyl sulfide.
  d. the production of chlorofluorocarbons.

**66.** Which of the following requires storage for thousands of years to be safe?
   a. radon
   b. radioactive waste
   c. photochemical waste
   d. greenhouse poisons

**67.** Which is mostly methane?
   a. oil
   b. natural gas
   c. coal waste
   d. propane

**68.** Which is not a future possibility as a primary source of energy?
   a. fusion
   b. hydrogen
   c. wind
   d. photovoltaic

**69.** A good future source of energy for farmers to consider as a source of profit is
   a. fission.
   b. fusion.
   c. wind.
   d. hydrogen.

**70.** The systems in nature that help purify water do not include
   a. solar energy.
   b. infrared radiation.
   c. clouds.
   d. the ocean.

## Answers

**61. a.** The global human population reached seven billion in late 2011 and will not be at eight billion until about 2025.

**62. d.** Pasture is about twice the area of cropland, for the world average. The other statements are true.

**63. c.** Oxygen gas is 21% of Earth's atmosphere, which converts to 210,000 ppm; ($\frac{210,000}{1,000,000} = 0.21 = 21\%$).

**64. c.** Stratospheric ozone is a natural protective shield because it absorbs the ultraviolet wavelengths of solar radiation that would otherwise cause great damage to living things at the surface.

**65. d.** The Montreal Protocol was a global agreement to phase out the production and release of ozone-destroying chlorofluoro-carbons.

**66. b.** Radioactive waste from weapons production and nuclear power plants requires very long-term storage to allow the radioactivity to decrease to safe levels.

**67. b.** Natural gas is predominantly methane, piped up from underground reservoirs and sometimes from gas domes at the top of oil pools under Earth.

**68. b.** Hydrogen cannot be a primary source of energy because there are no natural supplies of hydrogen. Hydrogen must be made by splitting water (or using methane) via a primary energy source. Hydrogen is therefore best considered a possible energy storage material.

**69. c.** Wind energy could be particularly attractive to farmers because the wind turbines take up little space, and the land can still be used for farming. Thus, the land does double duty.

**70. b.** Infrared radiation is how Earth cools itself to space, which of all the answers has least to do with the water cycle, whereby solar energy evaporates water from the ocean. The water vapor forms clouds, which shower purified water onto the land as rain.

## III. Suggested Sources for Further Study

Bryson, Bill. A *Short History of Nearly Everything* (New York: Broadway, 2004). Bryson is a simply fabulous writer. This book focuses on the history of major discoveries, from physics to geology and evolution. You learn about the characters who made history at the same time that you learn much of the science.

Mathez, Edmond A., and James D. Webster. *The Earth Machine: The Science of a Dynamic Planet* (New York: Columbia University Press, 2007). An excellent book about geology and plate tectonics.

Trefil, James. *The Nature of Science: An A-Z Guide to the Laws and Principles Governing our Universe* (Boston: Houghton Mifflin, 2003). Trefil is an accomplished science writer as well as scientist. This book contains many key concepts of science, including how science works.

There are many textbooks on environmental science, and they all cover much of the same material relevant to general science: some chemistry evolution, biodiversity, the chemical cycles, human impacts, some geology, and the science of the atmosphere and ocean. They are fairly expensive, but you should be able to find used books or earlier editions for a fraction of the new book price. Slightly older editions will be fine for your needs. Some popular texts include the following.

Botkin, Daniel B., and Edward A. Keller. *Environmental Science: Earth as a Living Planet, 8th Edition* (Hoboken, NJ: John Wiley & Sons, 2010).

Raven, Peter H., and Linda R. Berg. *Environment, 8th Edition.* (Hoboken, NJ: John Wiley & Sons, 2011).

Skinner, Brian J., and Barbara W. Murck. *The Blue Planet: An Introduction to Earth System Science, 3rd Edition.* (Hoboken, NJ: John Wiley & Sons, 2011).

Wright, Richard T., and Dorothy Boorse. *Environmental Science: Toward a Sustainable Future, 11th Edition.* (Boston: Addison-Wesley, 2010).

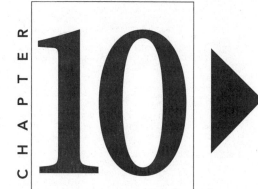

# PRACTICE EXAM II

### CHAPTER SUMMARY

This is the second of three practice exams based on actual nursing school entrance exams used today. Take this test to see how much you have improved since you took the first exam.

The practice test that follows is closely modeled on real entrance exams used to admit candidates to nursing programs throughout the country. This test will help prepare you for admissions tests like the NET, the APNE, the RNSAE, and other entrance tests. As with the first practice test in Chapter 3, it covers four essential topics—Verbal Ability, Math, Science, and Reading Comprehension—and uses a multiple-choice format with four answer choices, **a** through **d**. Although the practice tests in this book will prepare you for any nursing school entrance exam, be sure to learn the specifics for the exam that you are facing—it may vary somewhat in content and format (number of questions or sections) from this practice test.

For this second exam, simulate an actual test-taking experience as much as possible. First, find a quiet place where you can work undisturbed for three hours. Keep a timer or alarm clock on hand to observe the time limits specified in the directions. Time each section separately, according to the directions set out at the beginning of each segment. Stop working when the alarm goes off even if you have not completed the section. Between sections, take five minutes to clear your mind, and take a 15-minute break after Section 3. These breaks, and the time limits given for each section, approximate the testing schedule of commonly used entrance exams for nursing programs.

Using a number 2 pencil, mark your answers on the answer sheet on the following page. The answer key is located on page 323—of course, you should not refer to it until you have completed the test. A section on how to score your test follows the answer key.

## Section 1: Verbal Ability

| | | | | | | | | | | | | | | | | | |
|---|---|---|---|---|---|---|---|---|---|---|---|---|---|---|---|---|---|
| 1. | ⓐ | ⓑ | ⓒ | ⓓ | 18. | ⓐ | ⓑ | ⓒ | ⓓ | 35. | ⓐ | ⓑ | ⓒ | ⓓ |
| 2. | ⓐ | ⓑ | ⓒ | ⓓ | 19. | ⓐ | ⓑ | ⓒ | ⓓ | 36. | ⓐ | ⓑ | ⓒ | ⓓ |
| 3. | ⓐ | ⓑ | ⓒ | ⓓ | 20. | ⓐ | ⓑ | ⓒ | ⓓ | 37. | ⓐ | ⓑ | ⓒ | ⓓ |
| 4. | ⓐ | ⓑ | ⓒ | ⓓ | 21. | ⓐ | ⓑ | ⓒ | ⓓ | 38. | ⓐ | ⓑ | ⓒ | ⓓ |
| 5. | ⓐ | ⓑ | ⓒ | ⓓ | 22. | ⓐ | ⓑ | ⓒ | ⓓ | 39. | ⓐ | ⓑ | ⓒ | ⓓ |
| 6. | ⓐ | ⓑ | ⓒ | ⓓ | 23. | ⓐ | ⓑ | ⓒ | ⓓ | 40. | ⓐ | ⓑ | ⓒ | ⓓ |
| 7. | ⓐ | ⓑ | ⓒ | ⓓ | 24. | ⓐ | ⓑ | ⓒ | ⓓ | 41. | ⓐ | ⓑ | ⓒ | ⓓ |
| 8. | ⓐ | ⓑ | ⓒ | ⓓ | 25. | ⓐ | ⓑ | ⓒ | ⓓ | 42. | ⓐ | ⓑ | ⓒ | ⓓ |
| 9. | ⓐ | ⓑ | ⓒ | ⓓ | 26. | ⓐ | ⓑ | ⓒ | ⓓ | 43. | ⓐ | ⓑ | ⓒ | ⓓ |
| 10. | ⓐ | ⓑ | ⓒ | ⓓ | 27. | ⓐ | ⓑ | ⓒ | ⓓ | 44. | ⓐ | ⓑ | ⓒ | ⓓ |
| 11. | ⓐ | ⓑ | ⓒ | ⓓ | 28. | ⓐ | ⓑ | ⓒ | ⓓ | 45. | ⓐ | ⓑ | ⓒ | ⓓ |
| 12. | ⓐ | ⓑ | ⓒ | ⓓ | 29. | ⓐ | ⓑ | ⓒ | ⓓ | 46. | ⓐ | ⓑ | ⓒ | ⓓ |
| 13. | ⓐ | ⓑ | ⓒ | ⓓ | 30. | ⓐ | ⓑ | ⓒ | ⓓ | 47. | ⓐ | ⓑ | ⓒ | ⓓ |
| 14. | ⓐ | ⓑ | ⓒ | ⓓ | 31. | ⓐ | ⓑ | ⓒ | ⓓ | 48. | ⓐ | ⓑ | ⓒ | ⓓ |
| 15. | ⓐ | ⓑ | ⓒ | ⓓ | 32. | ⓐ | ⓑ | ⓒ | ⓓ | 49. | ⓐ | ⓑ | ⓒ | ⓓ |
| 16. | ⓐ | ⓑ | ⓒ | ⓓ | 33. | ⓐ | ⓑ | ⓒ | ⓓ | 50. | ⓐ | ⓑ | ⓒ | ⓓ |
| 17. | ⓐ | ⓑ | ⓒ | ⓓ | 34. | ⓐ | ⓑ | ⓒ | ⓓ | | | | | |

## Section 2: Reading Comprehension

| | | | | | | | | | | | | | | | | | |
|---|---|---|---|---|---|---|---|---|---|---|---|---|---|---|---|---|---|
| 1. | ⓐ | ⓑ | ⓒ | ⓓ | 16. | ⓐ | ⓑ | ⓒ | ⓓ | 31. | ⓐ | ⓑ | ⓒ | ⓓ |
| 2. | ⓐ | ⓑ | ⓒ | ⓓ | 17. | ⓐ | ⓑ | ⓒ | ⓓ | 32. | ⓐ | ⓑ | ⓒ | ⓓ |
| 3. | ⓐ | ⓑ | ⓒ | ⓓ | 18. | ⓐ | ⓑ | ⓒ | ⓓ | 33. | ⓐ | ⓑ | ⓒ | ⓓ |
| 4. | ⓐ | ⓑ | ⓒ | ⓓ | 19. | ⓐ | ⓑ | ⓒ | ⓓ | 34. | ⓐ | ⓑ | ⓒ | ⓓ |
| 5. | ⓐ | ⓑ | ⓒ | ⓓ | 20. | ⓐ | ⓑ | ⓒ | ⓓ | 35. | ⓐ | ⓑ | ⓒ | ⓓ |
| 6. | ⓐ | ⓑ | ⓒ | ⓓ | 21. | ⓐ | ⓑ | ⓒ | ⓓ | 36. | ⓐ | ⓑ | ⓒ | ⓓ |
| 7. | ⓐ | ⓑ | ⓒ | ⓓ | 22. | ⓐ | ⓑ | ⓒ | ⓓ | 37. | ⓐ | ⓑ | ⓒ | ⓓ |
| 8. | ⓐ | ⓑ | ⓒ | ⓓ | 23. | ⓐ | ⓑ | ⓒ | ⓓ | 38. | ⓐ | ⓑ | ⓒ | ⓓ |
| 9. | ⓐ | ⓑ | ⓒ | ⓓ | 24. | ⓐ | ⓑ | ⓒ | ⓓ | 39. | ⓐ | ⓑ | ⓒ | ⓓ |
| 10. | ⓐ | ⓑ | ⓒ | ⓓ | 25. | ⓐ | ⓑ | ⓒ | ⓓ | 40. | ⓐ | ⓑ | ⓒ | ⓓ |
| 11. | ⓐ | ⓑ | ⓒ | ⓓ | 26. | ⓐ | ⓑ | ⓒ | ⓓ | 41. | ⓐ | ⓑ | ⓒ | ⓓ |
| 12. | ⓐ | ⓑ | ⓒ | ⓓ | 27. | ⓐ | ⓑ | ⓒ | ⓓ | 42. | ⓐ | ⓑ | ⓒ | ⓓ |
| 13. | ⓐ | ⓑ | ⓒ | ⓓ | 28. | ⓐ | ⓑ | ⓒ | ⓓ | 43. | ⓐ | ⓑ | ⓒ | ⓓ |
| 14. | ⓐ | ⓑ | ⓒ | ⓓ | 29. | ⓐ | ⓑ | ⓒ | ⓓ | 44. | ⓐ | ⓑ | ⓒ | ⓓ |
| 15. | ⓐ | ⓑ | ⓒ | ⓓ | 30. | ⓐ | ⓑ | ⓒ | ⓓ | 45. | ⓐ | ⓑ | ⓒ | ⓓ |

## Section 3: Quantitative Ability

| | | | | | | | | | | | | | | | |
|---|---|---|---|---|---|---|---|---|---|---|---|---|---|---|---|
| 1. | ⓐ | ⓑ | ⓒ | ⓓ | 18. | ⓐ | ⓑ | ⓒ | ⓓ | 35. | ⓐ | ⓑ | ⓒ | ⓓ |
| 2. | ⓐ | ⓑ | ⓒ | ⓓ | 19. | ⓐ | ⓑ | ⓒ | ⓓ | 36. | ⓐ | ⓑ | ⓒ | ⓓ |
| 3. | ⓐ | ⓑ | ⓒ | ⓓ | 20. | ⓐ | ⓑ | ⓒ | ⓓ | 37. | ⓐ | ⓑ | ⓒ | ⓓ |
| 4. | ⓐ | ⓑ | ⓒ | ⓓ | 21. | ⓐ | ⓑ | ⓒ | ⓓ | 38. | ⓐ | ⓑ | ⓒ | ⓓ |
| 5. | ⓐ | ⓑ | ⓒ | ⓓ | 22. | ⓐ | ⓑ | ⓒ | ⓓ | 39. | ⓐ | ⓑ | ⓒ | ⓓ |
| 6. | ⓐ | ⓑ | ⓒ | ⓓ | 23. | ⓐ | ⓑ | ⓒ | ⓓ | 40. | ⓐ | ⓑ | ⓒ | ⓓ |
| 7. | ⓐ | ⓑ | ⓒ | ⓓ | 24. | ⓐ | ⓑ | ⓒ | ⓓ | 41. | ⓐ | ⓑ | ⓒ | ⓓ |
| 8. | ⓐ | ⓑ | ⓒ | ⓓ | 25. | ⓐ | ⓑ | ⓒ | ⓓ | 42. | ⓐ | ⓑ | ⓒ | ⓓ |
| 9. | ⓐ | ⓑ | ⓒ | ⓓ | 26. | ⓐ | ⓑ | ⓒ | ⓓ | 43. | ⓐ | ⓑ | ⓒ | ⓓ |
| 10. | ⓐ | ⓑ | ⓒ | ⓓ | 27. | ⓐ | ⓑ | ⓒ | ⓓ | 44. | ⓐ | ⓑ | ⓒ | ⓓ |
| 11. | ⓐ | ⓑ | ⓒ | ⓓ | 28. | ⓐ | ⓑ | ⓒ | ⓓ | 45. | ⓐ | ⓑ | ⓒ | ⓓ |
| 12. | ⓐ | ⓑ | ⓒ | ⓓ | 29. | ⓐ | ⓑ | ⓒ | ⓓ | 46. | ⓐ | ⓑ | ⓒ | ⓓ |
| 13. | ⓐ | ⓑ | ⓒ | ⓓ | 30. | ⓐ | ⓑ | ⓒ | ⓓ | 47. | ⓐ | ⓑ | ⓒ | ⓓ |
| 14. | ⓐ | ⓑ | ⓒ | ⓓ | 31. | ⓐ | ⓑ | ⓒ | ⓓ | 48. | ⓐ | ⓑ | ⓒ | ⓓ |
| 15. | ⓐ | ⓑ | ⓒ | ⓓ | 32. | ⓐ | ⓑ | ⓒ | ⓓ | 49. | ⓐ | ⓑ | ⓒ | ⓓ |
| 16. | ⓐ | ⓑ | ⓒ | ⓓ | 33. | ⓐ | ⓑ | ⓒ | ⓓ | 50. | ⓐ | ⓑ | ⓒ | ⓓ |
| 17. | ⓐ | ⓑ | ⓒ | ⓓ | 34. | ⓐ | ⓑ | ⓒ | ⓓ | | | | | |

## Section 4: General Science

| | | | | | | | | | | | | | | | |
|---|---|---|---|---|---|---|---|---|---|---|---|---|---|---|---|
| 1. | ⓐ | ⓑ | ⓒ | ⓓ | 18. | ⓐ | ⓑ | ⓒ | ⓓ | 35. | ⓐ | ⓑ | ⓒ | ⓓ |
| 2. | ⓐ | ⓑ | ⓒ | ⓓ | 19. | ⓐ | ⓑ | ⓒ | ⓓ | 36. | ⓐ | ⓑ | ⓒ | ⓓ |
| 3. | ⓐ | ⓑ | ⓒ | ⓓ | 20. | ⓐ | ⓑ | ⓒ | ⓓ | 37. | ⓐ | ⓑ | ⓒ | ⓓ |
| 4. | ⓐ | ⓑ | ⓒ | ⓓ | 21. | ⓐ | ⓑ | ⓒ | ⓓ | 38. | ⓐ | ⓑ | ⓒ | ⓓ |
| 5. | ⓐ | ⓑ | ⓒ | ⓓ | 22. | ⓐ | ⓑ | ⓒ | ⓓ | 39. | ⓐ | ⓑ | ⓒ | ⓓ |
| 6. | ⓐ | ⓑ | ⓒ | ⓓ | 23. | ⓐ | ⓑ | ⓒ | ⓓ | 40. | ⓐ | ⓑ | ⓒ | ⓓ |
| 7. | ⓐ | ⓑ | ⓒ | ⓓ | 24. | ⓐ | ⓑ | ⓒ | ⓓ | 41. | ⓐ | ⓑ | ⓒ | ⓓ |
| 8. | ⓐ | ⓑ | ⓒ | ⓓ | 25. | ⓐ | ⓑ | ⓒ | ⓓ | 42. | ⓐ | ⓑ | ⓒ | ⓓ |
| 9. | ⓐ | ⓑ | ⓒ | ⓓ | 26. | ⓐ | ⓑ | ⓒ | ⓓ | 43. | ⓐ | ⓑ | ⓒ | ⓓ |
| 10. | ⓐ | ⓑ | ⓒ | ⓓ | 27. | ⓐ | ⓑ | ⓒ | ⓓ | 44. | ⓐ | ⓑ | ⓒ | ⓓ |
| 11. | ⓐ | ⓑ | ⓒ | ⓓ | 28. | ⓐ | ⓑ | ⓒ | ⓓ | 45. | ⓐ | ⓑ | ⓒ | ⓓ |
| 12. | ⓐ | ⓑ | ⓒ | ⓓ | 29. | ⓐ | ⓑ | ⓒ | ⓓ | 46. | ⓐ | ⓑ | ⓒ | ⓓ |
| 13. | ⓐ | ⓑ | ⓒ | ⓓ | 30. | ⓐ | ⓑ | ⓒ | ⓓ | 47. | ⓐ | ⓑ | ⓒ | ⓓ |
| 14. | ⓐ | ⓑ | ⓒ | ⓓ | 31. | ⓐ | ⓑ | ⓒ | ⓓ | 48. | ⓐ | ⓑ | ⓒ | ⓓ |
| 15. | ⓐ | ⓑ | ⓒ | ⓓ | 32. | ⓐ | ⓑ | ⓒ | ⓓ | 49. | ⓐ | ⓑ | ⓒ | ⓓ |
| 16. | ⓐ | ⓑ | ⓒ | ⓓ | 33. | ⓐ | ⓑ | ⓒ | ⓓ | 50. | ⓐ | ⓑ | ⓒ | ⓓ |
| 17. | ⓐ | ⓑ | ⓒ | ⓓ | 34. | ⓐ | ⓑ | ⓒ | ⓓ | | | | | |

## Section 5: Biology

1. ⓐ ⓑ ⓒ ⓓ
2. ⓐ ⓑ ⓒ ⓓ
3. ⓐ ⓑ ⓒ ⓓ
4. ⓐ ⓑ ⓒ ⓓ
5. ⓐ ⓑ ⓒ ⓓ
6. ⓐ ⓑ ⓒ ⓓ
7. ⓐ ⓑ ⓒ ⓓ
8. ⓐ ⓑ ⓒ ⓓ
9. ⓐ ⓑ ⓒ ⓓ
10. ⓐ ⓑ ⓒ ⓓ
11. ⓐ ⓑ ⓒ ⓓ
12. ⓐ ⓑ ⓒ ⓓ
13. ⓐ ⓑ ⓒ ⓓ
14. ⓐ ⓑ ⓒ ⓓ
15. ⓐ ⓑ ⓒ ⓓ
16. ⓐ ⓑ ⓒ ⓓ
17. ⓐ ⓑ ⓒ ⓓ
18. ⓐ ⓑ ⓒ ⓓ
19. ⓐ ⓑ ⓒ ⓓ
20. ⓐ ⓑ ⓒ ⓓ
21. ⓐ ⓑ ⓒ ⓓ
22. ⓐ ⓑ ⓒ ⓓ
23. ⓐ ⓑ ⓒ ⓓ
24. ⓐ ⓑ ⓒ ⓓ
25. ⓐ ⓑ ⓒ ⓓ
26. ⓐ ⓑ ⓒ ⓓ
27. ⓐ ⓑ ⓒ ⓓ
28. ⓐ ⓑ ⓒ ⓓ
29. ⓐ ⓑ ⓒ ⓓ
30. ⓐ ⓑ ⓒ ⓓ
31. ⓐ ⓑ ⓒ ⓓ
32. ⓐ ⓑ ⓒ ⓓ
33. ⓐ ⓑ ⓒ ⓓ
34. ⓐ ⓑ ⓒ ⓓ
35. ⓐ ⓑ ⓒ ⓓ
36. ⓐ ⓑ ⓒ ⓓ
37. ⓐ ⓑ ⓒ ⓓ
38. ⓐ ⓑ ⓒ ⓓ
39. ⓐ ⓑ ⓒ ⓓ
40. ⓐ ⓑ ⓒ ⓓ
41. ⓐ ⓑ ⓒ ⓓ
42. ⓐ ⓑ ⓒ ⓓ
43. ⓐ ⓑ ⓒ ⓓ
44. ⓐ ⓑ ⓒ ⓓ
45. ⓐ ⓑ ⓒ ⓓ
46. ⓐ ⓑ ⓒ ⓓ
47. ⓐ ⓑ ⓒ ⓓ
48. ⓐ ⓑ ⓒ ⓓ
49. ⓐ ⓑ ⓒ ⓓ
50. ⓐ ⓑ ⓒ ⓓ

## Section 6: Chemistry

1. ⓐ ⓑ ⓒ ⓓ
2. ⓐ ⓑ ⓒ ⓓ
3. ⓐ ⓑ ⓒ ⓓ
4. ⓐ ⓑ ⓒ ⓓ
5. ⓐ ⓑ ⓒ ⓓ
6. ⓐ ⓑ ⓒ ⓓ
7. ⓐ ⓑ ⓒ ⓓ
8. ⓐ ⓑ ⓒ ⓓ
9. ⓐ ⓑ ⓒ ⓓ
10. ⓐ ⓑ ⓒ ⓓ
11. ⓐ ⓑ ⓒ ⓓ
12. ⓐ ⓑ ⓒ ⓓ
13. ⓐ ⓑ ⓒ ⓓ
14. ⓐ ⓑ ⓒ ⓓ
15. ⓐ ⓑ ⓒ ⓓ
16. ⓐ ⓑ ⓒ ⓓ
17. ⓐ ⓑ ⓒ ⓓ
18. ⓐ ⓑ ⓒ ⓓ
19. ⓐ ⓑ ⓒ ⓓ
20. ⓐ ⓑ ⓒ ⓓ
21. ⓐ ⓑ ⓒ ⓓ
22. ⓐ ⓑ ⓒ ⓓ
23. ⓐ ⓑ ⓒ ⓓ
24. ⓐ ⓑ ⓒ ⓓ
25. ⓐ ⓑ ⓒ ⓓ
26. ⓐ ⓑ ⓒ ⓓ
27. ⓐ ⓑ ⓒ ⓓ
28. ⓐ ⓑ ⓒ ⓓ
29. ⓐ ⓑ ⓒ ⓓ
30. ⓐ ⓑ ⓒ ⓓ
31. ⓐ ⓑ ⓒ ⓓ
32. ⓐ ⓑ ⓒ ⓓ
33. ⓐ ⓑ ⓒ ⓓ
34. ⓐ ⓑ ⓒ ⓓ
35. ⓐ ⓑ ⓒ ⓓ
36. ⓐ ⓑ ⓒ ⓓ
37. ⓐ ⓑ ⓒ ⓓ
38. ⓐ ⓑ ⓒ ⓓ
39. ⓐ ⓑ ⓒ ⓓ
40. ⓐ ⓑ ⓒ ⓓ
41. ⓐ ⓑ ⓒ ⓓ
42. ⓐ ⓑ ⓒ ⓓ
43. ⓐ ⓑ ⓒ ⓓ
44. ⓐ ⓑ ⓒ ⓓ
45. ⓐ ⓑ ⓒ ⓓ
46. ⓐ ⓑ ⓒ ⓓ
47. ⓐ ⓑ ⓒ ⓓ
48. ⓐ ⓑ ⓒ ⓓ
49. ⓐ ⓑ ⓒ ⓓ
50. ⓐ ⓑ ⓒ ⓓ

## Section 1: Verbal Ability

Find the correctly spelled word in the following questions. You have 15 minutes to answer the 50 questions in this section.

1. a. worrying
   b. worying
   c. worreying
   d. worriing

2. a. impeed
   b. impeede
   c. impied
   d. impede

3. a. weery
   b. wearey
   c. weary
   d. waery

4. a. foxes
   b. foxs
   c. foxxs
   d. foxen

5. a. openning
   b. oppening
   c. opening
   d. oppenning

6. a. admitted
   b. admited
   c. addmitted
   d. addmited

7. a. spear
   b. speer
   c. spier
   d. speir

8. a. concede
   b. conceed
   c. consede
   d. conseed

9. a. encouredging
   b. encouraging
   c. incurraging
   d. incouraging

10. a. phenomina
    b. phenominna
    c. phenomena
    d. phinomina

11. a. compatibel
    b. compatable
    c. compatible
    d. commpatible

12. a. receptacal
    b. receptacle
    c. recepticle
    d. receptacel

13. a. pronounnced
    b. pronounsed
    c. pronouncd
    d. pronounced

14. a. superviser
    b. supervizer
    c. supervizor
    d. supervisor

15. a. neumonia
    b. pneumonia
    c. pnumonia
    d. newmonia

**16.** **a.** annoid
**b.** anoyed
**c.** annoyed
**d.** annoyd

**17.** **a.** apperatus
**b.** aparatus
**c.** apparatus
**d.** aparratus

**18.** **a.** coedeine
**b.** codine
**c.** codeine
**d.** codiene

**19.** **a.** acompany
**b.** acommpany
**c.** accompeny
**d.** accompany

**20.** **a.** consistant
**b.** consistent
**c.** consistint
**d.** concistent

**21.** **a.** assinement
**b.** asignment
**c.** assignment
**d.** assignmant

**22.** **a.** eficient
**b.** eficeint
**c.** efficient
**d.** efficeint

**23.** **a.** ameliorate
**b.** amiliorate
**c.** amieliorate
**d.** amielierate

**24.** **a.** viewpoint
**b.** veiwpoint
**c.** viewpointe
**d.** veiupoint

**25.** **a.** agravated
**b.** agravaeted
**c.** aggravated
**d.** aggravatid

Find the misspelled word in the following questions.

**26.** **a.** panicking
**b.** licking
**c.** mimicing
**d.** no mistakes

**27.** **a.** relys
**b.** toys
**c.** lies
**d.** no mistakes

**28.** **a.** immensly
**b.** animosity
**c.** confound
**d.** no mistakes

**29.** **a.** tribes
**b.** curiosity
**c.** spectacle
**d.** no mistakes

**30.** **a.** wreckage
**b.** ilegible
**c.** united
**d.** no mistakes

**31.** **a.** pianos
**b.** heros
**c.** banjos
**d.** no mistakes

**32.** a. cried
b. busier
c. toyed
d. no mistakes

**33.** a. lattitude
b. attitude
c. rattled
d. no mistakes

**34.** a. intrigued
b. hypnotized
c. fasinated
d. no mistakes

**35.** a. amendment
b. phisique
c. melancholy
d. no mistakes

**36.** a. dissatisfied
b. disrespect
c. discrete
d. no mistakes

**37.** a. illuminate
b. enlighten
c. clarify
d. no mistakes

**38.** a. abolish
b. forfit
c. negate
d. no mistakes

**39.** a. zoology
b. meterology
c. anthropology
d. no mistakes

**40.** a. ajournment
b. tournament
c. confinement
d. no mistakes

**41.** a. vague
b. trepidation
c. vengence
d. no mistakes

**42.** a. tuition
b. mediocre
c. tramendous
d. no mistakes

**43.** a. manufacture
b. meander
c. masage
d. no mistakes

**44.** a. terrice
b. reference
c. vigilant
d. no mistakes

**45.** a. skien
b. knobby
c. blemished
d. no mistakes

**46.** a. brackets
b. parenthisis
c. ellipsis
d. no mistakes

**47.** a. visionary
b. virtuoso
c. wierd
d. no mistakes

**48.** **a.** language
**b.** philosophy
**c.** sonet
**d.** no mistakes

**49.** **a.** depo
**b.** aisle
**c.** knight
**d.** no mistakes

**50.** **a.** perscribe
**b.** deviate
**c.** plausible
**d.** no mistakes

# Section 2: Reading Comprehension

Read each passage and answer the accompanying questions based solely on the information found in the passage. You have 45 minutes to complete this section.

Millions of people in the United States are affected by eating disorders. More than 90% of those afflicted are adolescent or young adult women. While all eating disorders share some common manifestations, anorexia nervosa, bulimia nervosa, and binge eating each have distinctive symptoms and risks.

People who intentionally starve themselves, even while experiencing severe hunger pains, suffer from *anorexia nervosa*. The disorder, which usually begins around the time of puberty, involves extreme weight loss to at least 15% below the individual's normal body weight. Many people with the disorder look emaciated but are convinced they are overweight. In patients with anorexia nervosa, starvation can damage vital organs such as the heart and brain. To protect itself, the body shifts into slow gear: menstrual periods stop,

blood pressure rates drop, and thyroid function slows. Excessive thirst and frequent urination may occur. Dehydration contributes to constipation, and reduced body fat leads to lowered body temperature and the inability to withstand cold. Mild anemia, swollen joints, reduced muscle mass, and light-headedness also commonly occur in those having anorexia nervosa.

Anorexia nervosa sufferers can exhibit sudden angry outbursts or become socially withdrawn. One in ten cases of anorexia nervosa leads to death from starvation, cardiac arrest, other medical complications, or suicide. Clinical depression and anxiety place many individuals with eating disorders at risk for suicidal behavior.

People with *bulimia nervosa* consume large amounts of food and then rid their bodies of the excess calories by vomiting, abusing laxatives or diuretics, taking enemas, or exercising obsessively. Some use a combination of all these forms of purging. Individuals with bulimia who use drugs to stimulate vomiting, bowel movements, or urination may be in considerable danger, as this practice increases the risk of heart failure. Dieting heavily between episodes of binging and purging is common.

Because many individuals with bulimia binge and purge in secret and maintain normal or above normal body weight, they can often successfully hide their problem for years. But bulimia nervosa patients—even those of normal weight—can severely damage their bodies by frequent binge eating and purging. In rare instances, binge eating causes the stomach to rupture; purging may result in heart failure due to loss of vital minerals such as potassium. Vomiting can cause the esophagus to become inflamed and glands near the cheeks to become swollen. As in anorexia nervosa, bulimia may lead to irregular menstrual periods. Psychological effects include compulsive stealing as well as possible indications of obsessive-compulsive disorder, an illness characterized by repetitive thoughts and behaviors. Obsessive-compulsive disorder can also accompany anorexia nervosa. As with anorexia nervosa, bulimia typically begins during adolescence. Eventually, half of those with anorexia nervosa will develop bulimia. The condition occurs most often in women but is also found in men.

*Binge-eating disorder* is found in about 2% of the general population. As many as one-third of this group are men. It also affects older women, though with less frequency. Recent research shows that binge-eating disorder occurs in about 30% of people participating in medically supervised weight control programs. This disorder differs from bulimia because its sufferers do not purge. Individuals with binge-eating disorder feel that they lose control of themselves when eating. They eat large quantities of food and do not stop until they are uncomfortably full. Most sufferers are overweight or obese and have a history of weight fluctuations. As a result, they are prone to the serious medical problems associated with obesity, such as high cholesterol, high blood pressure, and diabetes. Obese individuals also have a higher risk for gallbladder disease, heart disease, and some types of cancer. Usually, they have more difficulty losing weight and keeping it off than do people with other serious weight problems. Like anorexics and bulimics who exhibit psychological problems, individuals with binge-eating disorder have high rates of simultaneously occurring psychiatric illnesses—especially depression.

1. Fatalities occur in what percent of people with anorexia nervosa?
   a. 2%
   b. 10%
   c. 15%
   d. 30%

2. Which of the following consequences do all the eating disorders mentioned in the passage have in common?
   a. heart ailments
   b. stomach rupture
   c. swollen joints
   d. diabetes

3. People with binge-eating disorder are prone to all of the following EXCEPT
   a. loss of control.
   b. depression.
   c. low blood pressure.
   d. high cholesterol.

4. Which of the following is NOT a true statement about people with anorexia nervosa?
   a. People with anorexia nervosa tend to be more socially withdrawn.
   b. People with anorexia nervosa can be prone to anger.
   c. People with anorexia nervosa always end their own lives.
   d. People with anorexia nervosa suffer from anemia.

5. People who have an eating disorder but nevertheless appear to be of normal weight are most likely to have
   a. obsessive-compulsive disorder.
   b. bulimia nervosa.
   c. binge-eating disorder.
   d. anorexia nervosa.

6. Glandular functions of anorexia patients slow down as a result of
   a. lowering body temperatures.
   b. excessive thirst and urination.
   c. protective measures taken by the body.
   d. the loss of essential minerals.

**7.** The inability to eliminate body waste is related to

    **a.** dehydration.

    **b.** an inflamed esophagus.

    **c.** the abuse of laxatives.

    **d.** weight control programs.

**8.** Which of the following is true of binge-eating disorder patients?

    **a.** They feel discomfort after eating.

    **b.** They binge to avoid obesity.

    **c.** They should try weight control programs.

    **d.** They are in danger of brain damage.

**9.** Which of the following represents up to two-thirds of the binge-eating disorder population?

    **a.** older males

    **b.** older females

    **c.** younger males

    **d.** younger females

The U.S. population is going gray. A rising demographic tide of aging baby boomers—those born between 1946 and 1964—and increased longevity have made adults age 65 and older the fastest growing segment of today's population. In 30 years, this segment of the population will be nearly twice as large as it is today. By then, an estimated 70 million people will be over age 65. The number of "oldest old"—those age 85 and older—is 34 times greater than in 1900 and likely to expand five-fold by 2050.

This unprecedented "elder boom" will have a profound effect on American society, particularly the field of healthcare. Is the U.S. health system equipped to deal with the demands of an aging population? Although we have adequate physicians and nurses, many of them are not trained to handle the multiple needs of older patients. Today, we have about 9,000 *geriatricians*, or physicians who are

experts in aging-related issues. Some studies estimate a need for 36,000 geriatricians by 2030.

Many doctors today treat a patient of 75 the same way they would treat a 40-year-old patient. However, although seniors are healthier than ever, physical challenges often increase with age. By age 75, adults often have two to three medical conditions. Diagnosing multiple health problems and knowing how they interact is crucial for effectively treating older patients. Healthcare professionals—often pressed for time in hectic daily practices—must be diligent about asking questions and collecting information from their elderly patients. Finding out about a patient's over-the-counter medications or living conditions could reveal an underlying problem.

Lack of training in geriatric issues can result in healthcare providers overlooking illnesses or conditions that may lead to illness. Inadequate nutrition is a common, but often unrecognized, problem among frail seniors. An elderly patient who has difficulty preparing meals at home may become vulnerable to malnutrition or another medical condition. Healthcare providers with training in aging issues may be able to address this problem without the costly solution of admitting a patient to a nursing home.

Depression, a treatable condition that affects nearly five million seniors, also goes undetected by some healthcare providers. Some healthcare professionals view depression as "just part of getting old." Untreated, this illness can have serious, even fatal consequences. According to the National Institute of Mental Health, older Americans account for a disproportionate share of suicide deaths, making up 18% of suicide deaths in 2000. Healthcare providers could play a vital role in preventing this outcome—several studies have shown that up to 75% of seniors who die by suicide visited a primary care physician within a month of their deaths.

Healthcare providers face additional challenges to providing high-quality care to the aging population. Because the numbers of ethnic minority elders are growing faster than the aging population as a whole, providers must train to care for a more racially and ethnically diverse population of elderly. Respect and understanding of diverse cultural beliefs is necessary to provide the most effective healthcare to all patients. Providers must also be able to communicate complicated medical conditions or treatments to older patients who may have a visual, hearing, or cognitive impairment.

As older adults make up an increasing proportion of the healthcare caseload, the demand for aging specialists must expand as well. Healthcare providers who work with the elderly must understand and address not only the physical but also the mental, emotional, and social changes involved in the aging process. They need to be able to distinguish between "normal" characteristics associated with aging and illness. Most crucially, they should look beyond symptoms and consider ways that will help a senior maintain and improve his or her quality of life.

**10.** The author uses the phrase *going gray* in order to
   **a.** maintain that everyone's hair loses its color eventually.
   **b.** suggest the social phenomenon of an aging population.
   **c.** depict older Americans in a positive light.
   **d.** demonstrate the normal changes of aging.

**11.** In the third paragraph, the author implies that doctors who treat elderly patients as they would a 40-year-old patient
   **a.** provide equitable, high-quality care.
   **b.** avoid detrimental stereotypes about older patients.
   **c.** encourage middle-age adults to think about the long-term effects of their habits.
   **d.** do not offer the most effective care to their older patients.

**12.** In the fifth paragraph, the word *vital* most nearly means
   **a.** lively.
   **b.** animated.
   **c.** heavy.
   **d.** crucial.

**13.** In the fifth paragraph, the author cites the example of untreated depression in elderly people in order to
   **a.** prove that mental illness can affect people of all ages.
   **b.** undermine the perception that mental illness only affects young people.
   **c.** support the claim that healthcare providers need age-related training.
   **d.** show how mental illness is a natural consequence of growing old.

**14.** According to the passage, which of the following is NOT a possible benefit of geriatric training for healthcare providers?
   **a.** Improved ability to explain a medical treatment to a person with a cognitive problem
   **b.** Knowledge of how heart disease and diabetes may act upon each other in an elderly patient
   **c.** Improved ability to attribute disease symptoms to the natural changes of aging
   **d.** More consideration for ways to improve the quality of life for seniors

Anthrax is an infectious disease caused by spores of the bacterium *Bacillus anthracis*. *B. anthracis* spores are highly resistant to inactivation and may be present in the soil for decades, occasionally infecting grazing animals that ingest the spores. Goats, sheep, and cattle are examples of animals that may become infected. Human infection may occur by three routes of exposure to anthrax spores: cutaneous (through the skin), gastrointestinal (by ingestion), and pulmonary (inhalation). In North America, human cases of anthrax are infrequent. However, the United States military views anthrax as a potential biological terrorism threat because the spores are so resistant to destruction and can be easily spread by release into the air. The development of anthrax as a biological weapon by several foreign countries has been documented.

Human anthrax cases can occur in three forms. Cutaneous infection is the most common manifestation of anthrax in humans, accounting for more than 95% of cases. Ingestion of undercooked or raw, infected meat can cause gastrointestinal anthrax infection. Breathing in airborne spores may lead to inhalation anthrax. The mortality rates from anthrax vary depending on exposure and are approximately 20% for cutaneous anthrax without antibiotics and 25% to 75% for gastrointestinal anthrax; inhalation anthrax has a fatality rate of 80% or higher. Cutaneous anthrax can usually be successfully treated with antibiotics, and some antibiotics have also been approved for postexposure prophylaxis.

The only known effective preexposure prevention against anthrax is the anthrax vaccine. The vaccine was developed from a strain of *B. anthracis*. The vaccine derives from the cell-free culture filtrate of this strain and, in its final formulation, is absorbed onto an aluminum salt. A well-controlled clinical trial using an anthrax vaccine similar to the licensed anthrax vaccine was conducted in U.S. millworkers processing imported animal hair. During the trial, 26 cases of anthrax were reported at the mills—five inhalation and 21 cutaneous cases. Of the five inhalation cases, two individuals had received the placebo, while three individuals were just in the observational group. Four of the five people who developed inhalation anthrax died. No cases of inhalation anthrax occurred in vaccine recipients. Based upon a comparison between the anthrax vaccine and placebo recipients, the authors calculated a vaccine efficacy level of 92.5 percent.

The licensed anthrax vaccine, termed Anthrax Vaccine Adsorbed (AVA), is recommended for individuals who may come in contact with animal products that may be contaminated with anthrax spores, as well as for individuals engaged in diagnostic or investigational activities that may bring them in contact with anthrax spores. It is also recommended for persons at high risk, such as veterinarians and others handling potentially infected animals. There is only a single anthrax vaccine licensed in the United States. New vaccines using current technology are under development.

15. Why did the author write this passage?
    a. To scare readers into getting tested for anthrax poisoning frequently
    b. To persuade the government to be more active about promoting AVA
    c. To inform about anthrax, its causes, and its possible prevention
    d. To scientifically prove the potential danger of anthrax poisoning when working with animals

**16.** Which of the following is NOT true, according to the passage?
- **a.** The most fatal type of anthrax is gastrointestinal anthrax.
- **b.** *Bacillus anthracis* spores can be transmitted through eating meat.
- **c.** Pulmonary anthrax can usually be treated with medicine.
- **d.** Animals are often infected through tainted soil.

**17.** Based on paragraph three, what was a finding in the clinical trial of the millworkers?
- **a.** The vaccine had no effect on the health of the millworkers.
- **b.** The vaccine was effective in preventing inhalation anthrax.
- **c.** The vaccine was effective in preventing gastrointestinal anthrax.
- **d.** The vaccine was just as effective as the placebo in preventing cutaneous anthrax.

**18.** What does the word *strain* mean as it is used in the passage?
- **a.** subgroup
- **b.** stress
- **c.** injury
- **d.** exertion

**19.** According to the second paragraph, which of the following is true?
- **a.** Gastrointestinal anthrax can result from both ingestion and inhalation.
- **b.** Postexposure prophylaxis is easily treated with antibiotics.
- **c.** Inhalation anthrax is considerably more dangerous than cutaneous anthrax.
- **d.** Cutaneous anthrax accounts for about half of anthrax cases.

**20.** Which of the following people should use Anthrax Vaccine Adsorbed (AVA)?
- **a.** A woman who works on a farm with animals that have not been tested for anthrax
- **b.** A police officer who has received a call about a possibly contaminated package
- **c.** A man who is afraid he might become infected with cutaneous anthrax
- **d.** An FBI agent who has inspected a package found to be contaminated with anthrax

**21.** What is the purpose of the third paragraph of the passage?
- **a.** To further prove the fatality of inhalation anthrax
- **b.** To demonstrate how a controlled clinical trial is set up to test new drugs
- **c.** To introduce a possible prevention for anthrax and prove its effectiveness
- **d.** To explain the widespread search for an anthrax cure

The *dystonias* are movement disorders in which sustained muscle contractions cause twisting and repetitive movements or abnormal postures. The movements, which are involuntary and sometimes painful, may affect a single muscle; a group of muscles such as those in the arms, legs, or neck; or the entire body. Diminished intelligence and emotional imbalance are not usually features of the dystonias.

*Generalized dystonia* affects most or all of the body. *Focal dystonia* is localized to a specific body part. *Multifocal dystonia* involves two or more unrelated body parts. *Segmental dystonia* affects two or more adjacent parts of the body. *Hemidystonia* involves the arm and leg on the same side of the body.

Early symptoms may include a deterioration in handwriting after writing several lines, foot cramps, and a tendency of one foot to pull up or drag after running or walking some distance. The neck may turn or pull involuntarily, especially when the person is tired. Other possible symptoms are tremor and voice or speech difficulties. The initial symptoms can be very mild and may be noticeable only after prolonged exertion, stress, or fatigue. Over a period of time, the symptoms may become more noticeable and widespread and may be unrelenting; however, sometimes there is little or no progression.

*Torsion dystonia*, previously called *dystonia musculum deformans* or DMD, is a rare, generalized dystonia that may be inherited, usually begins in childhood, and becomes progressively worse. It can leave individuals seriously disabled and confined to a wheelchair.

*Spasmodic torticollis*, or *torticollis*, is the most common of the focal dystonias. In torticollis, the muscles in the neck that control the position of the head are affected, causing the head to twist and turn to one side. In addition, the head may be pulled forward or backward. Torticollis can occur at any age, although most individuals first experience symptoms in middle age. It often begins slowly and usually reaches a plateau. About 10% to 20% of those with torticollis experience a spontaneous remission; however, the remission may not be lasting.

*Blepharospasm*, the second most common focal dystonia, is the involuntary, forcible closure of the eyelids. The first symptoms may be uncontrollable blinking. Only one eye may be affected initially, but eventually both eyes are usually involved. The spasms may leave the eyelids completely closed, causing functional blindness even though the eyes and vision are normal.

*Cranial dystonia* is a term used to describe dystonia that affects the muscles of the head, face, and neck. *Oromandibular dystonia* affects the muscles of the jaw, lips, and tongue. The jaw may be pulled either open or shut, and speech and swallowing can be difficult. *Spas-*

*modic dysphonia* involves the muscles of the throat that control speech. Also called *spastic dysphonia* or *laryngeal dystonia*, it causes strained and difficult speaking or breathy and effortful speech. *Meige's syndrome* is the combination of blepharospasm and oromandibular dystonia, and sometimes spasmodic dysphonia.

*Dopa-responsive dystonia* (DRD) is a condition successfully treated with drugs. Typically, DRD begins in childhood or adolescence with progressive difficulty in walking and, in some cases, spasticity. In *Segawa's dystonia*, the symptoms fluctuate during the day from relative mobility in the morning to increasingly worse disability in the afternoon and evening as well as after exercise. Some scientists feel DRD is not only rare but also rarely diagnosed since it mimics many of the symptoms of cerebral palsy.

22. A person who experiences contractions of the face, arms, and legs likely suffers from
    a. multifocal dystonia.
    b. focal dystonia.
    c. segmental dystonia.
    d. hemidystonia.

23. An early symptom of blepharospasm might be
    a. blindness.
    b. involuntary winking.
    c. the urge to blink.
    d. difficulty swallowing.

24. Genetics may be implicated in
    a. torsion dystonia.
    b. torticollis.
    c. oromandibular dystonia.
    d. DRD.

25. Meige's syndrome directly affects both
    a. speech and mobility.
    b. mobility and vision.
    c. vision and speech.
    d. hearing and vision.

**26.** The symptoms of torticollis are most similar to those of
   **a.** cranial dystonia.
   **b.** DRD.
   **c.** blepharospasm.
   **d.** oromandibular dystonia.

**27.** A person with DRD usually
   **a.** has difficulty verbalizing.
   **b.** experiences writer's cramp.
   **c.** improves following exercise.
   **d.** responds well to medication.

**28.** All dystonia patients experience
   **a.** uncontrolled movement.
   **b.** progressive deterioration.
   **c.** symptoms at an early age.
   **d.** incessant discomfort.

**29.** Cranial dystonia is an example of a
   **a.** hemidystonia.
   **b.** multifocal dystonia.
   **c.** segmental dystonia.
   **d.** generalized dystonia.

**30.** The least common forms of dystonia mentioned in the passage are
   **a.** spasmodic and torsion dystonia.
   **b.** dopa-responsive and cranial dystonia.
   **c.** oromandibular and spasmodic dystonia.
   **d.** torsion and dopa-responsive dystonia.

Lyme disease is sometimes called the "great imitator" because its many symptoms mimic those of other illnesses. When treated, this disease usually presents few or no lingering effects. Left untreated, it can be extremely debilitating and sometimes fatal.

Lyme disease is caused by a bacterium carried and transmitted by the *Ixodes dammini* tick. In 1982, the damaging microorganism was identified as *Borrelia burgdorferi*. Ticks are parasites that require blood for sustenance. They feed three times (in the larva, nymph, and adult stages) during a two-year life cycle, and feedings can last up to several days. As many as 3,000 eggs hatch into larvae, which is the first stage of the life cycle. The larvae then attach to host organisms, such as mice. Human infection by a tick at this stage is a rare occurrence.

Following the first blood meal, larvae molt into nymphs. These transformed organisms are about the size of a bread crumb. During this and subsequent stages of the life cycle, the tick chooses larger hosts on which to feed, including humans. Because of their tiny size, nymphs present the greatest danger to humans. Some studies indicate that as many as 80% of humans are infected by nymphs. As the life cycle progresses, nymphs engorged with blood become adults. During this stage, adults will mate, assuring continuance of the life cycle. Ticks generally rely on humid conditions and temperatures above 40° Fahrenheit to survive.

Human infection occurs when the tick attaches itself to the body, feeding on blood while transmitting bacteria. Since this process can take up to 48 hours, it is possible for an individual to remove the tick before infection occurs. When infection does occur, one of the early visible signs is a rash called *erythema migrans*, although in some cases, there is no rash at all. The mark left by the tick, often taking a bull's-eye shape, can range from the size of a quarter to one foot across. Some rashes disappear temporarily and then return. This inconsistent symptom adds to the perplexing nature of the disease.

Symptoms can materialize within a few days to a few weeks following bacterial transmission and include flu-like aches and pains, fever, and weakness. As the illness progresses, problems such as respiratory distress, irregular heartbeat, liver infection, bladder discomfort, and double vision can occur. Infected individuals may experience all, none, or a combination of symptoms.

Early diagnosis and antibiotic treatment of the earliest acute stage of Lyme disease generally leads to rapid recovery. An inaccurate diagnosis or lack of early treatment can lead to health problems such as heart muscle damage, severe joint pain, and meningitis. Lyme disease that reaches a chronic stage can lead to severe arthritis, paralysis, brain infection, and nervous system disorders; however, symptoms of chronic Lyme disease, despite lasting six months or longer, are generally treatable with antibiotics, and long-term illness is rare. Researchers are working on a vaccine, but its completion remains uncertain.

**31.** Lyme disease infection occurs
   **a.** 48 hours after a tick attaches itself to the human body.
   **b.** while ticks consume blood.
   **c.** after the *erythema migrans* rash appears.
   **d.** when flu-like symptoms begin.

**32.** Lyme disease that reaches the chronic stage tends to exhibit symptoms for
   **a.** 48 hours or less.
   **b.** a few days.
   **c.** six months or more.
   **d.** at least two years.

**33.** It can be inferred from the passage that *Ixodes dammini* ticks are LEAST likely to infect people in temperate zones during the
   **a.** spring.
   **b.** summer.
   **c.** fall.
   **d.** winter.

**34.** Diagnosis of Lyme disease is made difficult by the
   **a.** similarities between it and other ailments.
   **b.** changing shape of the erythema migrans.
   **c.** unpredictable life cycle of the tick.
   **d.** lack of prolonged effects produced.

**35.** Transmission of *Borrelia burgdorferi* to humans during the larva stage
   **a.** accounts for the majority of infections.
   **b.** is a relatively infrequent phenomenon.
   **c.** generally occurs at temperatures below 40°F.
   **d.** lasts up to several days.

**36.** One early symptom of Lyme disease is
   **a.** arthritis.
   **b.** meningitis.
   **c.** fever.
   **d.** difficulty breathing.

Tai chi developed in China in about the twelfth century A.D. It started as a martial art, or a practice for fighting or self-defense, usually without weapons. Over time, people began to use tai chi for health purposes as well. Many different styles of tai chi, and variations of each style, developed. The term *tai chi* has been translated in various ways, including "internal martial art," "supreme ultimate boxing," "boundless fist," and "balance of the opposing forces of nature." While accounts of tai chi's history often differ, the most consistently important figure is a Taoist monk (and semi-legendary figure) in twelfth-century China named Chang San-Feng. Chang is said to have observed five animals—the tiger, dragon, leopard, snake, and crane—and to have concluded that the snake and the crane, through their movements, were the ones most able to overcome strong, unyielding opponents. Chang developed an initial set of exercises that imitated the movements of animals. He also brought flexibility and suppleness in place of strength to the martial arts, as well as some key philosophical concepts.

A person practicing tai chi moves his or her body in a slow, relaxed, and graceful series of movements. One can practice on one's own or in a group. The movements make up what are called forms or routines. Some movements are named for animals or birds, such as "White Crane Spreads Its Wings." The simplest style of tai chi uses 13 movements; more complex styles can have dozens.

In tai chi, each movement flows into the next. The entire body is always in motion, with the movements performed gently and at uniform speed. It is considered important to keep the body upright, especially the upper body—many tai chi practitioners mimic the image of a string that goes from the top of the head into the heavens—and to let the body's weight sink to the soles of the feet.

In addition to movement, two other important elements in tai chi are breathing and meditation. In tai chi practice, it is considered important to concentrate; put aside distracting thoughts; and breathe in a deep, relaxed, and focused manner. Practitioners believe that this breathing and meditation have many benefits, such as massaging the internal organs, aiding the exchange of gases in the lungs, helping the digestive system work better, increasing calmness and awareness, and improving balance.

Another concept in tai chi is that the forces of yin and yang should be in balance. In Chinese philosophy, yin and yang are two opposing principles or elements that make up the universe and everything in it. Yin is believed to have the qualities of water—such as coolness, darkness, stillness, and inward and downward directions—and to be feminine in character. Yang is believed to have the qualities of fire—such as heat, light, action, and upward and outward movement—and to be masculine in character. In this belief system, an individual's yin and yang need to be in balance in order for him or her to be healthy, and tai chi is a practice that supports this balance.

**37.** From the passage it can be inferred that tai chi
   **a.** is a very personal meditative act that is best performed alone.
   **b.** is the ideal form of self-protection for women who are not very strong.
   **c.** is a simple practice that does not take a lot of study to pick up.
   **d.** helps maintain inner equilibrium for those who practice.

**38.** Which of the following is NOT true, according to paragraph four?
   **a.** Meditation might be recommended for someone with stomach problems.
   **b.** Tai chi is best done in a quiet setting.
   **c.** Snakes and cranes are highly meditative animals.
   **d.** Breathing exercises are a good idea for someone in a high-stress job.

**39.** What is the main idea of this passage?
   **a.** Tai chi is an ideal way to lose weight while honing self-defense skills.
   **b.** Tai chi is a method through which people can balance their yin and yang.
   **c.** Tai chi is a practice through which participants enjoy both physical and mental benefits.
   **d.** Tai chi is an ancient martial art used to combat many health problems.

**40.** What is the best definition of the word *elements* in paragraph four?
   **a.** forces of nature
   **b.** principles
   **c.** chemical building blocks
   **d.** simple substances

**41.** Which of the following is NOT an accepted translation of *tai chi*?
   **a.** boundless fist
   **b.** internal martial art
   **c.** supreme ultimate boxing
   **d.** self-defense without weapons

**42.** Chang San-Feng derived the movements of tai chi from a snake and a crane because
 a. their graceful style was effective in besting their enemies.
 b. they had the strongest and most powerful upper bodies of all the animals he studied.
 c. they were the most flexible of the animals he studied.
 d. their temperament was an ideal balance of yin and yang.

**43.** Which of the following is most likely true about those who are longtime devotees to tai chi?
 a. They are Chinese.
 b. They are vegetarians.
 c. They pay attention to their posture.
 d. They are either very masculine or very feminine.

**44.** Which of the following is not a characteristic of tai chi teachings?
 a. balance
 b. a kind personality
 c. flexibility
 d. grace

**45.** Which of the following is not one of the bene-fits that practitioners of tai chi get from breathing and meditation?
 a. more efficient exchange of gases in the lungs
 b. better functioning digestive systems
 c. increased calmness and awareness
 d. higher blood glucose levels

# Section 3: Quantitative Ability

There are 50 questions in this section. You have 45 minutes to complete this section.

**1.** $4\frac{2}{5} + 3\frac{1}{2} + \frac{3}{8}$ is equal to
 a. $7\frac{3}{20}$
 b. $7\frac{2}{5}$
 c. $8\frac{11}{40}$
 d. $8\frac{7}{8}$

**2.** The area of a rectangular examination table that is 150 cm long and 70 cm wide is
 a. 1.05 square m.
 b. 105 square m.
 c. 1,050 square m.
 d. 10,500 square m.

**3.** A licensed practical nurse has to lift four patients during his eight-hour shift. The patients weigh 152 pounds, 168 pounds, 182 pounds, and 201 pounds. Approximately how many pounds will the nurse have to lift during his shift?
 a. 690 pounds
 b. 700 pounds
 c. 710 pounds
 d. 750 pounds

**4.** If $x = 6$, $y = -2$, and $z = 3$, what is the value of the following expression?
 $\frac{xz - xy}{z^2}$
 a. 5
 b. $3\frac{1}{3}$
 c. $\frac{2}{3}$
 d. $-\frac{2}{3}$

**5.** What is the area of a triangle with a height of 10 inches and a base of 2 inches?
 **a.** 10 square inches
 **b.** 12 square inches
 **c.** 20 square inches
 **d.** 22 square inches

**6.** In a hospital emergency room last week, the staff treated 33 patients on Sunday, 27 on Monday, 13 on Tuesday, 22 on Wednesday, 18 on Thursday, 24 on Friday, and 31 on Saturday. During this week, what was the average number of patients treated per day?
 **a.** 20
 **b.** 24
 **c.** 27
 **d.** 30

**7.** There are only nine empty spots on a university bowling team. If 60 people try out, what percentage of those who try out will not make the team?
 **a.** 15%
 **b.** 16%
 **c.** 17%
 **d.** 85%

**8.** 75 is 60% of what number?
 **a.** 45
 **b.** 80
 **c.** 125
 **d.** 135

**9.** 33.33 + 3.3 + 0.333 + 333 is equal to
 **a.** 69.963
 **b.** 339.963
 **c.** 366.933
 **d.** 369.963

**10.** The track at a local high school is $\frac{1}{4}$ of a mile around. For a training run for a 10-mile race, a competitor wants to run half the total distance of the upcoming race. How many laps will she have to run?
 **a.** 10
 **b.** 20
 **c.** 30
 **d.** 40

**11.** What is the area of the following figure?

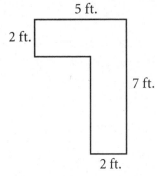

 **a.** 19 sq. ft.
 **b.** 20 sq. ft.
 **c.** 24 sq. ft.
 **d.** 38 sq. ft.

**12.** What is $7\frac{1}{5}\%$ of 465, rounded to the nearest tenth?
 **a.** 32.5
 **b.** 33
 **c.** 33.5
 **d.** 34

**13.** $3\frac{7}{10} - 2\frac{3}{8}$ is equal to
 **a.** $1\frac{13}{40}$
 **b.** $1\frac{7}{20}$
 **c.** $1\frac{11}{18}$
 **d.** $2\frac{1}{80}$

**14.** On the following number line, point $L$ is to be located halfway between points $M$ and $N$. What number will correspond to point $L$?

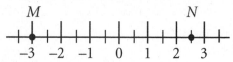

a. $-\frac{1}{4}$

b. $-\frac{1}{2}$

c. $-1\frac{1}{4}$

d. 0

**15.** If two angles of a triangle measure 47° and 86°, what is the measure of the third angle?

a. 39°

b. 43°

c. 47°

d. 86°

**16.** Which of the following is equivalent to $2y^2$?

a. $2y(y)$

b. $2(y + y)$

c. $y^2 + 2$

d. $y + y + y + y$

**17.** $367.08 \times 0.15$ is equal to

a. 22.0248

b. 55.051

c. 55.062

d. 540.62

**18.** $(-10) + (-4) + (\frac{1}{2}) - (-\frac{1}{4})$ is equal to

a. $-5\frac{3}{4}$

b. $-6\frac{1}{4}$

c. $-13\frac{1}{4}$

d. $-13\frac{3}{4}$

**19.** At a carnival, a merry-go-round ride costs 2 tickets and a roller coaster ride costs 3 tickets. If you have 24 tickets and spend them on only one type of ride, how many more merry-go-round rides than roller coaster rides can you get?

a. 1

b. 2

c. 3

d. 4

**20.** Serena planted $\frac{1}{4}$ of the tulip seeds in the packet. Her mother planted $\frac{1}{3}$ of the remaining seeds. If there are 30 seeds left in the packet, how many were there to begin with?

a. 40

b. 60

c. 90

d. 180

**21.** There are 25 students in a first-grade class. If $\frac{2}{5}$ of the class is in Reading Group A and 20% of the class is in Reading Group B, how many total students are in Groups A and B combined?

a. 10

b. 15

c. 18

d. 20

**22.** Mary's average time to run a mile is 9 minutes 36 seconds. How long will it take her to run 10 miles?

a. 1 hour 6 minutes

b. 1 hour 32 minutes

c. 1 hour 36 minutes

d. 1 hour 46 minutes

**23.** Forty-eight cookies are provided at a meeting. During the meeting, $\frac{5}{8}$ of the cookies are eaten. Andrew takes $\frac{1}{3}$ of the remaining cookies to share with his department. Lia takes 5 cookies for her officemates. How many cookies are left?
 a. 1
 b. 4
 c. 6
 d. 7

**24.** Dried mango costs $6.30 per pound at the local market. If Kendra wants to buy 2.5 pounds and has only a $20 bill, how much change will she receive?
 a. $4.25
 b. $5.00
 c. $5.45
 d. $15.75

**25.** Of the 1,125 nurses who work in the hospital, 135 speak fluent Spanish. What percentage of the nursing staff speaks fluent Spanish?
 a. 7.3%
 b. 8.3%
 c. 12%
 d. 14%

**26.** A hospital emergency room receives an admission on August 3 at 10:42 P.M. and another admission at 1:19 A.M. on August 4. How much time has elapsed between admissions?
 a. 1 hour 37 minutes
 b. 2 hours 23 minutes
 c. 2 hours 37 minutes
 d. 3 hours 23 minutes

**27.** A first-year family medicine resident earns $50,000 a year. In her second year of residency, her salary increases to $51,500 a year. By what percent does her salary increase?
 a. 3%
 b. 10%
 c. 15%
 d. 30%

**28.** Which of the following hospital rooms has the greatest perimeter?
 a. a rectangular room 12 feet $\times$ 8 feet
 b. a rectangular room 14 feet $\times$ 7 feet
 c. a square room 10 feet $\times$ 10 feet
 d. a square room 11 feet $\times$ 11 feet

**29.** A person can be scalded by hot water at a temperature of about 122°F. At about what temperature Centigrade could a person be scalded? $C = \frac{5}{9}(F - 32)$
 a. 35.5°C
 b. 50°C
 c. 55°C
 d. 216°C

**30.** New nursing staff have to buy shoes to wear on duty at the full price of $84.50, but nurses who have worked in the hospital at least a year can get a 15% discount at a local shoe store, and nurses who have worked at least three years get an additional 10% off the discounted price. How much does a nurse who has worked at least three years have to pay for shoes?
 a. $63.78
 b. $64.65
 c. $71.83
 d. $72.05

**31.** In the medical-surgical unit of a hospital, the ratio of certified nurse assistants (CNAs) to nurses during a shift cannot be less than 3 to 2. During the day shift, 6 nurses are on duty. For this shift, which of the following is an acceptable number of CNAs on duty?

a. 3
b. 6
c. 8
d. 10

**32.** Body mass index (BMI) is equal to weight in kg divided by (height in m)$^2$. A man who weighs 64.8 kg has a BMI of 20. How tall is he?

a. 0.9 m
b. 1.8 m
c. 2.16 m
d. 3.24 m

**33.** A patient's hospice stay costs one-fourth as much as his visit to the emergency room. His home nursing costs twice as much as his hospice stay. If his total health care bill was $140,000, how much did his home nursing cost?

a. $10,000
b. $20,000
c. $40,000
d. $80,000

**34.** An insurance policy pays 80% of the first $20,000 of a certain patient's medical expenses, 60% of the next $40,000, and 40% of the $40,000 after that. If the patient's total medical bill is $92,000, how much will the policy pay?

a. $36,800
b. $49,600
c. $52,800
d. $73,600

**35.** A doctor can treat four Alzheimer's patients per hour; however, stroke patients need three times as much of the doctor's time. If the doctor treats patients six hours per day and has already treated ten Alzheimer's patients and three stroke patients today, how many more stroke patients will she have time to treat today?

a. one
b. two
c. three
d. five

**36.** A medical evacuation helicopter can transport a patient 100 miles to the hospital in 37.5 minutes. What is the speed of the helicopter in miles per hour?

a. 100
b. 160
c. 225
d. 267

**37.** What is the value of $x$ in the following figure?

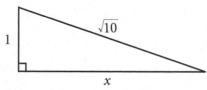

a. 2
b. 3
c. 5
d. 9

**38.** $\dfrac{3\frac{1}{9}}{1\frac{1}{6}}$ is equal to

a. $\frac{4}{9}$
b. $\frac{2}{3}$
c. $1\frac{1}{3}$
d. $2\frac{2}{3}$

**39.** Ron is half as old as Sam, who is three times as old as Ted. The sum of their ages is 55. How old is Ron?

a. 5
b. 10
c. 15
d. 30

**40.** At a certain school, one-half of the students are female and one-twelfth of the students are from outside the state. If there are equal numbers of male and female students from outside the state, what proportion of the students would you expect to be females from outside the state?

a. $\frac{1}{24}$
b. $\frac{1}{12}$
c. $\frac{1}{6}$
d. $\frac{1}{3}$

**41.** $54\frac{1}{2}\%$ is equal to

a. 0.545
b. 5.45
c. 54.5
d. 545

**42.** If $\sqrt{(2x+2)} = 4$, what does $x$ equal?

a. 1
b. 2
c. 7
d. 10

**43.** A man turns on his daughter's nightlight at 7:15 P.M., right before he puts her to bed. When he wakes her up at 8 A.M., he turns off the nightlight. In total, how many minutes was the light on?

a. 720 minutes
b. 735 minutes
c. 765 minutes
d. 775 minutes

**44.** What is the value of $x$ in the following figure?

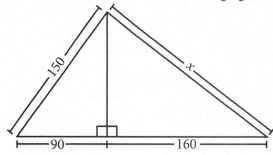

a. 200
b. 210
c. 240
d. 270

**45.** Angle $k$ is complementary to angle $j$. If angle $j$ measures 72°, what is the measure of angle $k$?

a. 18°
b. 81°
c. 108°
d. 180°

**46.** Based on the following information, estimate the weight of a person who is 5'5" tall.

| HEIGHT | WEIGHT |
| --- | --- |
| 5' | 110 lbs. |
| 6' | 170 lbs. |

a. 125 lbs.
b. 130 lbs.
c. 135 lbs.
d. 140 lbs.

**47.** Alena has $10 and wants to buy 12 oranges at $0.40 each and 11 apples at $0.60 each. If there is no sales tax, how much more money does she need?

a. $1.40
b. $1.60
c. $11.40
d. $13.00

**48.** What is the value of $3xy$ when $y = \frac{2}{x}$ and $x = 34$?
   a. 5
   b. 6
   c. 51
   d. 204

**49.** To lower a fever of 105°, ice packs are applied for 1 minute and then removed for 5 minutes before being applied again. Each application lowers the fever by half a degree. How long will it take to lower the fever to 99°?
   a. 1 hour
   b. 1 hour 12 minutes
   c. 1 hour 15 minutes
   d. 1 hour 30 minutes

**50.** Fifteen milliliters of a solution separates into two liquids as shown in the following figure. The lighter liquid makes up what percentage of the total solution?

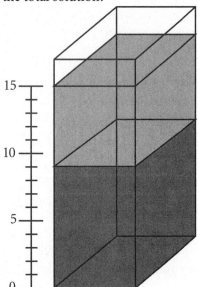

   a. 33%
   b. 40%
   c. 60%
   d. 66%

# Section 4: General Science

There are 50 questions in this section. You have 45 minutes to complete this section.

**1.** Considering the four fundamental forces of physics, this one governs beta decay of radioactive atoms.
   a. strong nuclear force
   b. electromagnetism
   c. gravity
   d. weak nuclear force

**2.** What important event happened in 1957?
   a. first human to orbit Earth
   b. first landing a rover on Mars
   c. first human landing on the Moon
   d. first satellite to be put in orbit

**3.** What table would you set not with plates and forks but with rows of types of atoms?
   a. periodic table
   b. molecular table
   c. valence table
   d. bonding table

**4.** The parts of an atom that create the chemical bonds with other atoms are
   a. valence shells.
   b. nuclei.
   c. quark triplets.
   d. isotopes.

**5.** In what kind of atomic bond between atoms are electrons shared in pairs?
   a. ionic
   b. hydrogen
   c. van der Waals
   d. covalent

**6.** Consider the chemical reaction for photosynthesis: $6CO_2 + 6H_2O \rightarrow C_6H_{12}O_6 + \underline{\quad} O_2$. How many molecules of oxygen ($O_2$) are made on the right-hand side (what number goes in the blank space)?
   **a.** 6
   **b.** 1
   **c.** 12
   **d.** 4

**7.** In photosynthesis, the charge on the carbon in the reactant carbon dioxide is +4, and the charge on the carbon in the resulting carbohydrate product is –4. In this reaction, the carbon is said to have been
   **a.** stripped.
   **b.** oxidized.
   **c.** neutralized.
   **d.** reduced.

**8.** Applying an amount of energy less than the heat of fusion to a liquid at the melting point of a particular substance does what?
   **a.** settles the liquid
   **b.** warms the liquid
   **c.** starts to solidify the liquid
   **d.** evaporates the liquid

**9.** The basic building blocks of proteins are
   **a.** amino acids.
   **b.** nucleic acids.
   **c.** carbohydrates.
   **d.** lipids.

**10.** Which is an example of an inorganic compound?
   **a.** blood hemoglobin
   **b.** quartz
   **c.** DNA
   **d.** wood

**11.** The idea that Earth's continents were once all joined together and later drifted apart in a "continental drift" was first proposed by
   **a.** Alfred Wegener.
   **b.** Niels Bohr.
   **c.** James Watson.
   **d.** Erwin Schrodinger.

**12.** In a scientific investigation, which variable is the one you consciously manipulate or change over time?
   **a.** control
   **b.** dependent
   **c.** independent
   **d.** analytical

**13.** Crude oil originates from
   **a.** ancient fossilized organic materials.
   **b.** the natural metabolic processes of plants and organisms.
   **c.** minerals subjected to high temperatures and pressures.
   **d.** coal deposits that have liquefied.

**14.** Albert Einstein developed the
   **a.** wave theory of light.
   **b.** general theory of relativity.
   **c.** three laws of motion.
   **d.** theory of universal gravitation.

**15.** Which of the following is a drawback of using hydrogen gas as an alternative fuel source?
   **a.** It cannot be made from any natural product.
   **b.** It is extremely polluting.
   **c.** It is not found naturally.
   **d.** It is too heavy to use in cars.

**16.** All forms of energy can be converted at maximum efficiency into
   **a.** mechanical motion.
   **b.** electricity.
   **c.** potential energy.
   **d.** heat.

**17.** When entropy decreases, what else must be true?
   **a.** Entropy must increase on some larger scale.
   **b.** The decrease must be at the level of the universe.
   **c.** A mistake was made in the calculation.
   **d.** Entropy is adjusted to a flow of heat.

**18.** Which scientist, often called the "Father of Modern Science," was tried for heresy by the Roman Inquisition and forced to spend the rest of his life under house arrest?
   **a.** Sir Isaac Newton
   **b.** Johannes Kepler
   **c.** Galileo Galilei
   **d.** Nikola Tesla

**19.** When a crane at a building site lifts a beam to its top height, what type of energy is created?
   **a.** kinetic energy
   **b.** potential energy
   **c.** chemical energy
   **d.** electrical energy

**20.** Your body operates with
   **a.** gravitational potential energy.
   **b.** electrical energy.
   **c.** chemical potential energy.
   **d.** nuclear energy.

**21.** Entomology is the study of
   **a.** birds.
   **b.** plants.
   **c.** insects.
   **d.** mammals.

**22.** Approximately when did life begin?
   **a.** 3.7 million years ago
   **b.** 37 million years ago
   **c.** 370 million years ago
   **d.** 3,700 million years ago

**23.** Penicillin is a group of antibiotics derived from
   **a.** bacteria.
   **b.** fungi.
   **c.** plants.
   **d.** animals.

**24.** In the ribosomes, which all cells have, what important cell process occurs?
   **a.** DNA is duplicated.
   **b.** Proteins are assembled.
   **c.** Cell membranes are synthesized.
   **d.** Cell nuclei are degraded.

**25.** Groups of DNA bases that code for types of amino acids occur as
   **a.** quintuplets.
   **b.** doublets.
   **c.** triplets.
   **d.** quadruplets.

**26.** In the universal tree of life, derived from comparing the rRNA possessed by all living forms, what does the r stand for?
   **a.** rhizocyclic
   **b.** retrospiral
   **c.** recentible
   **d.** ribosomal

**27.** Liposomes formed from lipids might be naturally occurring structures that formed the precursors for what later structure of cells?
   **a.** immune systems
   **b.** enzymes
   **c.** nuclei
   **d.** membranes

**28.** Which of the following modern-day life forms is most closely related to Tyrannosaurus rex, in terms of closeness in the evolutionary sense?
   **a.** rattlesnakes
   **b.** pigeons
   **c.** lobsters
   **d.** frogs

**29.** If a cell has an organelle called a chloroplast, which type of cell is it?
   **a.** bikaryotic
   **b.** prokaryotic
   **c.** eukaryotic
   **d.** postkaryotic

**30.** The scientific study of bones is called
   **a.** osteology.
   **b.** ornithology.
   **c.** entomology.
   **d.** histology.

**31.** Sodium chloride is commonly known as
   **a.** baking powder.
   **b.** table salt.
   **c.** baking soda.
   **d.** bleach.

**32.** Burmese pythons are a type of snake not normally found in Florida, but pet owners have brought them to the state and sometimes set them free in the wild. Once in the wild, the snakes reproduce and cause harm to the natural Florida ecosystem. In Florida, Burmese pythons are an example of a(n)
   **a.** keystone species.
   **b.** invasive species.
   **c.** umbrella species.
   **d.** flagship species.

**33.** The bifocal lens was invented by
   **a.** Thomas Edison.
   **b.** Benjamin Franklin.
   **c.** Albert Einstein.
   **d.** John Isaac Hawkins.

**34.** The type of rock that is formed by changes to another rock through extreme heat and/or pressure is known as
   **a.** igneous.
   **b.** sedimentary.
   **c.** metamorphic.
   **d.** biogenic.

**35.** During which era did single-celled life originate?
   **a.** Archean
   **b.** Hadean
   **c.** Paleozoic
   **d.** Holocene

**36.** In plants, which type of vascular tissue takes food made in the leaves down to the roots?
   **a.** xylem
   **b.** trachea
   **c.** capillaries
   **d.** phloem

**37.** We know that the Cretaceous-Tertiary mass extinction, which killed off the dinosaurs and many other species, including many species of ocean algae, was caused by the impact of a giant object from space because of
   **a.** a worldwide clay layer that contains unnaturally high levels of the element iridium.
   **b.** charcoal evidence of worldwide forest fires.
   **c.** chemical signatures of massive amounts of sulfuric acid aerosols in the atmosphere.
   **d.** mutations in the surviving organisms caused by UV radiation after the ozone layer was destroyed.

**38.** The acid used in car batteries is
   **a.** sulfuric acid.
   **b.** ferulic acid.
   **c.** citric acid.
   **d.** hydrochloric acid.

**39.** The intensity of an earthquake is measured by what instrument?
   **a.** altimeter
   **b.** electrometer
   **c.** seismometer
   **d.** spectrometer

**40.** What was the mass extinction that came just prior to the evolution of the dinosaurs?
a. Cretaceous-Tertiary
b. Permian-Triassic
c. Triassic-Jurassic
d. Carboniferous-Permian

**41.** The first American to orbit the Earth was
a. John Glenn.
b. Neil Armstrong.
c. Buzz Aldrin.
d. Mike Adams.

**42.** If you were a scientist investigating the origin of human social bonding, you would be in the field of
a. evolutionary psychology.
b. reversible geology.
c. physical anthropology.
d. revolutionary biology.

**43.** Of the organisms listed, which is the most recent, in terms of evolution?
a. Australopithecus
b. Cyanobacteria
c. Fungi
d. Lichen

**44.** Considering human ancestry, which one of the following is farthest from humans, in terms of how long ago the lineage that led to us diverged from the lineage that led to this ape?
a. bonobo
b. chimp
c. gorilla
d. orangutan

**45.** If an aqueous solution is alkaline, it is
a. acidic.
b. basic.
c. neutral.
d. ionic.

**46.** Which of the following was the first to evolve?
a. reptiles
b. mammals
c. amphibians
d. dinosaurs

**47.** Electricity is the movement of
a. heat.
b. electrons.
c. light.
d. protons.

**48.** Which of the following drives electrical current?
a. voltage
b. resistance
c. amperage
d. gravity

**49.** Which of the following best represents velocity?
a. distance per unit force
b. force per unit distance
c. distance per unit time
d. distance times force

**50.** If emission spectra from a distant galaxy are shifted toward the red, then they must have
a. shorter wavelengths.
b. longer wavelengths.
c. no electromagnetic radiation.
d. fewer light photons.

# Section 5: Biology

There are 50 questions in this section. You have 45 minutes to complete this section.

1. Autotrophs are most likely to have which organelle?
   a. Golgi apparatus
   b. chloroplasts
   c. lysosomes
   d. mitochondria

2. In most flowering plants, water moves upward from the roots via which of the following structures?
   a. sieve tubes
   b. phloem
   c. stomata
   d. xylem

3. A third copy of a chromosome is an example of
   a. haploidy.
   b. diplody.
   c. polyploidy.
   d. aneuploidy.

4. The reproductive organ of a plant that is responsible for pollen production is known as the
   a. carpel.
   b. pistil.
   c. stamen.
   d. stigma.

5. In mammals, which of the following are cell fragments that play a key role in blood clotting?
   a. platelets
   b. neutrophils
   c. red blood cells
   d. monocytes

6. Swelling that is due to excess fluid accumulating in interstitial spaces is known as
   a. effusion.
   b. erythema.
   c. edema.
   d. progenesis.

7. Pyruvate is converted to carbon dioxide and ethanol during which of the following processes?
   a. photosynthesis
   b. glycolysis
   c. alcohol fermentation
   d. oxidation

8. Self-fertilization may also be referred to as
   a. syngamy.
   b. autogamy.
   c. allogamy.
   d. incompatibility.

9. The embryological process by which a fertilized ovum divides is known as
   a. the $G_2$ phase.
   b. the M phase.
   c. cleavage.
   d. cytokinesis.

10. What diatomic molecule is important in biological processes, including neurotransmission, vasodilation, and the immune response?
    a. $O_2$
    b. $N_2$
    c. NO
    d. $N_2O$

11. Which of the following does not encourage natural selection?
    a. traits learned by parents
    b. traits helpful to survival
    c. harsh climates
    d. competition for limited resources

**12.** If a cell lacks energy to transport material through its cell membrane, which process would it NOT use?
 **a.** osmosis
 **b.** active transport
 **c.** filtration
 **d.** diffusion

**13.** In a cell with 16 chromosomes, how many gametes with how many chromosomes each would be present after meiosis?
 **a.** 2 with 8 chromosomes each
 **b.** 2 with 16 chromosomes each
 **c.** 4 with 4 chromosomes each
 **d.** 4 with 8 chromosomes each

**14.** Essential amino acids
 **a.** must be supplied by diet.
 **b.** are not endogenously synthesized.
 **c.** include phenylalanine, threonine, and valine.
 **d.** all of the above

**15.** Membranes in cells are used for all of the following EXCEPT
 **a.** providing rigid support.
 **b.** regulating transport of substances.
 **c.** containing cytoplasm.
 **d.** containing DNA.

**16.** About how much blood does the average person have in his or her body?
 **a.** 2.5 to 3 liters
 **b.** 4.5 to 5 liters
 **c.** 6 to 7 liters
 **d.** 8 to 9.5 liters

**17.** Blood from the lungs travels to the left atrium of the heart through the
 **a.** aorta.
 **b.** superior vena cava.
 **c.** pulmonary artery.
 **d.** pulmonary veins.

**18.** A person with phenylketonuria should limit intake of what amino acid?
 **a.** tyrosine
 **b.** phenylalanine
 **c.** histidine
 **d.** asparagine

**19.** Transfusion of incorrect blood types results in
 **a.** excess production.
 **b.** chemical reduction of hemoglobin.
 **c.** agglutination of erythrocytes.
 **d.** lymphocytosis.

**20.** Which of the following is not an aromatic amino acid?
 **a.** tyrosine
 **b.** tryptophan
 **c.** threonine
 **d.** phenylalanine

**21.** In an organism, the allele Q is dominant over q. If one parent is homozygous dominant (QQ) and the other is homozygous recessive (qq), what percentage of their offspring will express the recessive trait?
 **a.** 0%
 **b.** 25%
 **c.** 50%
 **d.** 100%

**22.** A bacteriophage can be described as
   a. a bacterium that causes illness.
   b. a virus that infects bacteria.
   c. a bacteria-fighting organelle.
   d. an inner membrane of bacteria.

**23.** A gene expressed more in males than in females is
   a. linked to the Y chromosome.
   b. linked to non-sex chromosomes.
   c. linked to the gene for testosterone.
   d. not possible to determine the chromosome link.

**24.** What is the codon responsible for the third amino acid in the sequence represented in the genetic code UAUUUCGCUGCA?
   a. U
   b. UAU
   c. UUC
   d. GCU

**25.** Secondary consumers interact with primary consumers through
   a. commensalism.
   b. trophic levels.
   c. mutualism.
   d. natural selection.

**26.** What is the main function of the cerebellum?
   a. to control respiration and heartbeat
   b. to coordinate skeletal movements
   c. to determine personality
   d. to act as a relay center between the cerebrum and the medulla

**27.** The myelin sheath covers
   a. the lungs.
   b. the retina of the eye.
   c. tendons.
   d. the axons of neurons.

**28.** A cell experiences a genetic mutation and is unable to deliver the appropriate amino acids according to the genetic code. Which of the following is affected?
   a. DNA
   b. mRNA
   c. rRNA
   d. tRNA

**29.** Which of the following glands make up part of the exocrine system?
   a. thyroid
   b. pituitary gland
   c. hypothalamus
   d. sweat gland

**30.** More than 90% of dietary fat is in the form of
   a. triglycerides.
   b. phospholipids.
   c. cholesterol.
   d. lipase.

**31.** The ventricles are actively filled during which phase of the cardiac cycle?
   a. atrial systole
   b. atrial diastole
   c. ventricular systole
   d. valvular stenosis

**32.** In humans, which of the following is the only layer of skin that contains actively dividing cells?
   a. subcutaneous cuticle
   b. basement membrane
   c. stratum corneum
   d. stratum basale

**33.** Which of the following is the site of protein synthesis within a eukaryotic cell?
   a. the ribosomes
   b. the nucleus
   c. the mitochondria
   d. the Golgi apparatus

**34.** Hypertension is commonly known as
  **a.** high blood pressure.
  **b.** diabetes.
  **c.** high cholesterol.
  **d.** arthritis.

**35.** Nutrients, wastes, and gases are exchanged between maternal and fetal blood via the
  **a.** placenta.
  **b.** amnion.
  **c.** yolk sac.
  **d.** fallopian tube.

**36.** The gene for blue eyes is recessive. If your mother has blue eyes and your brown-eyed father has one gene for blue eyes and one for brown eyes, what are your chances of having blue eyes?
  **a.** 100%
  **b.** 75%
  **c.** 50%
  **d.** 25%

**37.** On some invertebrates, which of the following are the bristle-like, hollow, or chitinous outgrowths of the epidermis?
  **a.** the setae
  **b.** the cilia
  **c.** the hair
  **d.** the whiskers

**38.** A low hematocrit is a symptom of
  **a.** anemia.
  **b.** atherosclerosis.
  **c.** type I diabetes.
  **d.** arthritis.

**39.** What are the tiny air sacs where exchange of respiratory gases occurs in mammals and reptiles?
  **a.** the bronchioles
  **b.** the bronchi
  **c.** the sinuses
  **d.** the alveoli

**40.** Bioluminescence, which occurs in deep-sea fish, bacteria, and fireflies, occurs during the oxidation of which of the following substances?
  **a.** chlorophyll
  **b.** hemoglobin
  **c.** luciferin
  **d.** melanin

**41.** Which of the following is the bony material perforated by tiny canals containing nerve cells in human teeth?
  **a.** gingiva
  **b.** pulp
  **c.** enamel
  **d.** dentin

**42.** Macular degeneration is a condition affecting what organ?
  **a.** the kidney
  **b.** the liver
  **c.** the eye
  **d.** the brain

**43.** Which of the following is an attribute of prokaryotes?
  **a.** They have a defined nucleus.
  **b.** Their DNA is formed into chromosomes.
  **c.** They have membrane-enclosed mitochondria.
  **d.** They are unicellular.

**44.** Which of the following is considered an accessory organ in the digestive system?
   **a.** the anus
   **b.** the liver
   **c.** the esophagus
   **d.** the pharynx

**45.** Which of the following would be considered an acquired characteristic?
   **a.** the large muscles of a weight lifter
   **b.** the appendix of a human being
   **c.** the nocturnal vision of an owl
   **d.** the large ears of a rabbit

**46.** If a plant is in an environment that depletes all available oxygen, how will it get its energy?
   **a.** photosynthesis
   **b.** transpiration
   **c.** fermentation
   **d.** cellular respiration

**47.** In the following pedigree, the recessive trait is shaded and is not sex-linked. What is the probability that children 3 and 4 carry the recessive allele?

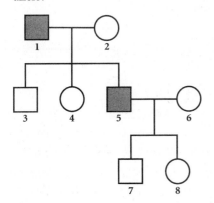

   **a.** 0%
   **b.** 50%
   **c.** 100%
   **d.** not possible to determine

**48.** Which adaptation do protists and plants share that separate them from fungi?
   **a.** chloroplasts
   **b.** cell walls
   **c.** specialized tissue
   **d.** nucleus

**49.** Groups of three nucleotides that specify a particular amino acid to be added in a protein sequence are known as
   **a.** base pairs.
   **b.** chromosomes.
   **c.** genes.
   **d.** codons.

**50.** One parent has genotype nn for a recessive trait, and the other parent has an unknown genotype and does not show the recessive trait. What is the genotype of their offspring that do NOT show the recessive trait?
   **a.** NN
   **b.** Nn
   **c.** nn
   **d.** cannot be determined

## Section 6: Chemistry

There are 50 questions in this section. You have 45 minutes to complete this section. Use the periodic table on the next page when necessary to help you answer the following questions.

| IA | | | | | | | | | | | | | | | | | VIIA | VIIIA |
|---|---|---|---|---|---|---|---|---|---|---|---|---|---|---|---|---|---|---|
| 1 H 1.00794 | IIA | | | | | | | | | | | | | | | | 1 H 1.00794 | 2 He 4.002602 |
| 3 Li 6.941 | 4 Be 9.012182 | | | | | | | | | | | IIIA | IVA | VA | VIA | | 5 B 10.811 ... | |

(Periodic table of elements)

**1.** The best example of a strong acid is
   a. KOH.
   b. $HNO_2$.
   c. $H_2SO_4$.
   d. $Ca(OH)_2$.

**2.** $CuO + H_2SO_4 \rightarrow CuSO_4 + H_2O$
The reaction shown here is best described by which of the following?
   a. base + acid → salt + water
   b. metal + acid → salt + hydrogen
   c. metal oxide + acid → salt + water
   d. metal carbonate + acid → salt + carbonate acid (unstable)

**3.** How many moles of hydrogen are in 18.0 g of $H_2O$?
   a. 1
   b. 2
   c. 9
   d. 18

**4.** The reaction $Fe_2O_3 + 2Al \rightarrow 2Fe + Al_2O_3$ is best classified as what type of reaction?
   a. double displacement reaction
   b. oxidation-reduction reaction
   c. acid-base reaction
   d. decomposition reaction

**5.** Balance the following reaction:
$AlBr_3 + K_2SO_4 \rightarrow KBr + Al_2(SO_4)_3$.
   a. $2AlBr_3 + 2K_2SO_4 \rightarrow 4KBr + Al_2(SO_4)_2$
   b. $2AlBr_3 + 3K_2SO_4 \rightarrow 4KBr + Al_2(SO_4)_3$
   c. $2AlBr_3 + 2K_2SO_4 \rightarrow 6KBr + Al_2(SO_4)_3$
   d. $2AlBr_3 + 3K_2SO_4 \rightarrow 6KBr + Al_2(SO_4)_3$

**6.** Which of the following functional groups is found in all aldehydes?
   a. $NH_2$
   b. COOH
   c. C=O
   d. OH

**7.** What is the formula for cobalt (II) phosphate?
 **a.** $CoPO_4$
 **b.** $Co_2PO_4$
 **c.** $Co_3(PO_4)_2$
 **d.** $Co_2(PO_4)_3$

**8.** Which of the following choices best describes the structure of the class of molecules that is the major constituent of cell membranes?
 **a.** a carboxylic acid bonded to an amino group
 **b.** one molecule of glycerol bonded to three fatty acids
 **c.** one molecule of glycerol bonded to two fatty acids and one phosphate group
 **d.** one molecule of glycerol bonded to one fatty acid and two hydroxyl groups

**9.** Osmotic pressure is defined as
 **a.** the change in pressure of a liquid undergoing osmosis.
 **b.** pressure that must be applied to prevent net diffusion of pure solvent through a semipermeable membrane into solution.
 **c.** the combined pressure of gases in the external atmosphere of a system undergoing osmosis.
 **d.** pressure that is proportional to osmotic potential.

**10.** Which of the following is classified as an aldehyde?
 **a.** $CH_4$
 **b.** $CH_2Cl_2$
 **c.** $CH_3C(O)CH_3$
 **d.** $CH_3CH_2C(O)H$

**11.** The nuclear process $^{238}_{92}U \rightarrow {}^{234}_{90}Th + {}^{4}_{2}He$ is an example of
 **a.** $\alpha$ decay.
 **b.** $\beta$ decay.
 **c.** $\gamma$ emission.
 **d.** nuclear fusion.

**12.** What is the formula for bismuth (III) hydroxide?
 **a.** $Bi_3OH$
 **b.** $Bi(OH)_3$
 **c.** $Bi(OH)_2$
 **d.** $BiOH$

**13.** What are the products of the reaction between sodium metal and water?
 **a.** $NaH^+_{(aq)} + OH^-_{(aq)}$
 **b.** $NaOH_{(aq)} + H_{2(g)}$
 **c.** $Na_{(s)} + H_{2(g)} + O_{2(g)}$
 **d.** $NaOH_{(aq)} + H_{2(g)} + O_{2(g)}$

**14.** Which best describes the following redox reaction: $Br^-_{(aq)} + MnO^-_{4(aq)} \rightarrow Br_{2(l)} + Mn^{+2}_{(aq)}$?
 **a.** Br and Mn are both reduced.
 **b.** Br is oxidized and Mn is reduced.
 **c.** Br is oxidized and O is reduced.
 **d.** Br is reduced and Mn is oxidized.

**15.** Rank the following atoms in order of increasing atomic size: Cs, F, Li, N.
 **a.** Li < Cs < N < F
 **b.** F < N < Li < Cs
 **c.** F < Li < Cs < N
 **d.** Cs < F < N < Li

**16.** Which of the following is a weak acid?
 **a.** HCl
 **b.** $HNO_3$
 **c.** $H_2SO_4$
 **d.** $H_2CO_3$

**17.** What is the molecular formula of a compound with empirical formula $CH_2O$ and molar mass 90 g?
 **a.** $CH_2O$
 **b.** $C_3H_3O_3$
 **c.** $C_3H_6O_3$
 **d.** $C_6H_{14}O$

18. Which of the following has the largest atomic radius?
    a. K
    b. Rb
    c. Ca
    d. Sr

19. In which of the following states of matter are molecules most likely to move freely?
    a. solid
    b. liquid
    c. gas
    d. All have similar freedom of movement.

20. Which of the following species is being oxidized in this redox reaction?
    $Zn_{(s)} + Cu^{2+}_{(aq)} \rightarrow Zn^{2+}_{(aq)} + Cu_{(s)}$
    a. $Zn_{(s)}$
    b. $Cu^{2+}_{(aq)}$
    c. $Zn^{2+}_{(aq)}$
    d. $Cu_{(s)}$

21. Which of the following is the strongest acid?
    a. $H_2PO_4^-$
    b. KOH
    c. $NH_4^+$
    d. $H_3PO_4$

22. In which of the following solutions is $Ag_2CO_3$ most soluble?
    a. 0.2 M $Na_2CO_3$
    b. 0.3 M KCl
    c. 0.1 M $Na_2CO_3$
    d. 0.01 M $AgNO_3$

23. β decay results in the emission of a(n) _____ from a heavy atom.
    a. helium nucleus
    b. electron
    c. proton
    d. high energy photon

24. A trans fat describes fatty acids that contain
    a. no C–C double bonds.
    b. multiple C–C double bonds and some C–C single bonds.
    c. at least one C–C double bond with a trans geometry.
    d. only C–C double bonds.

25. Which of the following are the general products of a combustion reaction?
    a. $C_{(s)}$, $O_2$, and $H_2$
    b. $C_{(s)}$, $H_2O$, and $O_2$
    c. $CO_2$ and $H_2$
    d. $CO_2$ and $H_2O$

26. Compounds have a set volume but an unset shape when they are
    a. solid.
    b. liquid.
    c. gas.
    d. Molecules always behave this way.

27. For every three moles of $P_2O_5$ produced by the following reaction, how many molecules of P are required?
    $4P + 5O_2 \rightarrow 2P_2O_5$
    a. $6.02 \times 10^{23}$
    b. $1.20 \times 10^{24}$
    c. $3.01 \times 10^{23}$
    d. $3.61 \times 10^{24}$

28. $LiOH + HBr \rightarrow LiBr + H_2O$
    How many grams of lithium hydroxide will you need to add to your reaction to produce exactly 72.6 grams of lithium bromide?
    a. 10
    b. 20
    c. 30
    d. 40

**29.** Which of the following is a transition metal?
  **a.** Lithium
  **b.** Iron
  **c.** Aluminum
  **d.** Tin

**30.** Give the number of valence electrons for a sulfur atom (S).
  **a.** 2
  **b.** 4
  **c.** 6
  **d.** 16

**31.** Which of the following is the electron configuration of a neutral atom of Ca?
  **a.** [Ar] $3s^2$
  **b.** [Ar] $3d^2$
  **c.** [Ar] $4p^2$
  **d.** [Ar] $4s^2$

**32.** Which of the following bonds is the most polar?
  **a.** $Cl_2$
  **b.** NaCl
  **c.** $F_2$
  **d.** HF

**33.** Which of the following is the correct name for $Li_2SO_3$?
  **a.** lithium sulfite
  **b.** lithium sulfide
  **c.** lithium sulfate
  **d.** lithium disulfate

**34.** What is the oxidation number of sodium in the following reaction?
  $$Pb(NO_3)_{2(aq)} + 2NaI_{(aq)} \rightarrow PbI_{2(s)} + 2NaNO_{3(aq)}$$
  **a.** +1
  **b.** +2
  **c.** −1
  **d.** −2

**35.** Carbon dating involves the decay of a carbon-14 isotope with a beta particle. Which of the following equations describes this decay?
  **a.** $^{14}_6C \rightarrow {}^{13}_5B + {}^1_1H$
  **b.** $^{14}_6C \rightarrow {}^{14}_7N + {}^0_{-1}\beta$
  **c.** $^{14}_6C \rightarrow {}^{13}_5B + {}^1_0n$
  **d.** $^{14}_7N + {}^1_0n \rightarrow {}^{14}_6C + {}^1_1H$

**36.** A dating technique involves electron capture by potassium-40 isotope according to the following equation: $^{40}_{19}K + {}^0_{-1}e \rightarrow {}^{40}_{18}Ar$. If the half-life of potassium-40 is $1.2 \times 10^9$ years, how long does it take for only 10 g to remain of the original 40 g of potassium-40 in a rock sample?
  **a.** $1.2 \times 10^9$ years
  **b.** $0.6 \times 10^9$ years
  **c.** $2.4 \times 10^9$ years
  **d.** $1.8 \times 10^9$ years

**37.** Which of the following elements is a member of the actinide series?
  **a.** Uranium
  **b.** Terbium
  **c.** Tellurium
  **d.** Radon

**38.** Which of the following is the symbol for the isotope with 18 protons and 22 neutrons?
  **a.** $^{40}_{18}Ar$
  **b.** $^{22}_{18}Ar$
  **c.** $^{40}_{22}Ti$
  **d.** $^{90}_{40}Zr$

**39.** Vanillin, the above molecule responsible for vanilla's taste and smell, possesses all of the following functional groups except
   **a.** aldehyde.
   **b.** ketone.
   **c.** alcohol.
   **d.** ether.

**40.** What is the effect of the addition of a catalyst to a reaction in equilibrium?
   **a.** The reaction favors the formation of the products.
   **b.** The reaction favors the formation of the reactants.
   **c.** There is no change in composition of the reaction.
   **d.** The rate of the reaction slows.

**41.** Which of the following pairs are allotropes?
   **a.** $O_2$ and $O_3$
   **b.** $Fe^{2+}$ and $Fe^{3+}$
   **c.** $OH^-$ and $H_3O^+$
   **d.** $H_2O_2$ and $H_2O$

**42.** A gas is held in a rigid 4 L container at 1 atm and 27°C. If the temperature is raised to 117°C, what will the pressure in the container be?
   **a.** 4.3 atm
   **b.** 0.77 atm
   **c.** 1.3 atm
   **d.** 0.23 atm

**43.** Which of the following is the name of the oxyacid $HClO_4$?
   **a.** perchloric acid
   **b.** chloric acid
   **c.** chlorous acid
   **d.** hypochlorous acid

**44.** Which of the following is an example of a decomposition reaction?
   **a.** $C_3H_{8(g)} + 5O_{2(g)} \rightarrow 3CO_{2(g)} + 4H_2O_{(l)}$
   **b.** $N_{2(g)} + 3H_{2(g)} \rightarrow 2NH_{3(g)}$
   **c.** $CaCO_{3(s)} \rightarrow CaO_{(s)} + CO_{2(g)}$
   **d.** $CaO_{(s)} + H_2O_{(l)} \rightarrow Ca(OH)_{2(s)}$

**45.** Which of the following does NOT have the electron configuration $[Ne]3s^23p^6$?
   **a.** Cl
   **b.** $S^{2-}$
   **c.** $K^+$
   **d.** $Ca^{2+}$

**46.** Which of the following classes of molecules does NOT have a carbonyl group?
   **a.** ester
   **b.** amide
   **c.** aldehyde
   **d.** amine

**47.** Write the correct answer, including correct significant figures, for the following calculation:
$4.12 \times 10^{-3} + 9.54 \times 10^{-5}$
   **a.** $4.22 \times 10^{-3}$
   **b.** $4.22 \times 10^{-8}$
   **c.** $1.37 \times 10^{-8}$
   **d.** $13.66 \times 10^{-2}$

**48.** What is the formula for thallium (III) hydroxide?

    **a.** $TlOH_3$

    **b.** $Tl(OH)_3$

    **c.** $Tl_3(OH)$

    **d.** $Tl_3(OH)_3$

**49.** $H_2PO_4^- + OH^- \leftarrow \rightarrow HPO_4^{-2} + H_2O$

Part of the blood's buffer system is shown above. What is the conjugate acid in this system?

    **a.** $H_2PO_4^-$

    **b.** $OH$

    **c.** $HPO_4^{-2}$

    **d.** $H_2O$

**50.** Balance the following reaction:

$C_3H_8 + O_2 \rightarrow CO_2 + H_2O$

    **a.** $C_3H_8 + 5O_2 \rightarrow 3CO_2 + 4H_2O$

    **b.** $C_3H_8 + 6O_2 \rightarrow 3CO_2 + 2H_2O$

    **c.** $C_3H_8 + 6O_2 \rightarrow 4CO_2 + 3H_2O$

    **d.** $C_3H_8 + 4O_2 \rightarrow 3CO_2 + 4H_2O$

## Answers

### Section 1: Verbal Ability

**1. a.** worrying

**2. d.** impede

**3. c.** weary

**4. a.** foxes

**5. c.** opening

**6. a.** admitted

**7. a.** spear

**8. a.** concede

**9. b.** encouraging

**10. c.** phenomena

**11. c.** compatible

**12. b.** receptacle

**13. d.** pronounced

**14. d.** supervisor

**15. b.** pneumonia

**16. c.** annoyed

**17. c.** apparatus

**18. c.** codeine

**19. d.** accompany

**20. b.** consistent

**21. c.** assignment

**22. c.** efficient

**23. a.** ameliorate

**24. a.** viewpoint

**25. c.** aggravated

**26. c.** The correct spelling is mimicking.

**27. a.** The correct spelling is relies.

**28. a.** The correct spelling is immensely.

**29. d.** no mistakes

**30. b.** The correct spelling is illegible.

**31. b.** The correct spelling is heroes.

**32. d.** no mistakes

**33. a.** The correct spelling is latitude.

**34. c.** The correct spelling is fascinated.

**35. b.** The correct spelling is physique.

**36. d.** no mistakes

**37. d.** no mistakes

**38. b.** The correct spelling is forfeit.

**39. b.** The correct spelling is meteorology.

**40. a.** The correct spelling is adjournment.
**41. c.** The correct spelling is vengeance.
**42. c.** The correct spelling is tremendous.
**43. c.** The correct spelling is massage.
**44. a.** The correct spelling is terrace.
**45. a.** The correct spelling is skein.
**46. b.** The correct spelling is parenthesis.
**47. c.** The correct spelling is weird.
**48. c.** The correct spelling is sonnet.
**49. a.** The correct spelling is depot.
**50. a.** The correct spelling is prescribe.

## Section 2: Reading Comprehension

**1. b.** See the third paragraph: *One in ten* (10% of) cases of anorexia end in death.

**2. a.** See the second and third paragraphs for reference to heart problems with anorexia, the fourth and fifth paragraphs for discussion of heart problems with bulimia, and the last paragraph, where heart disease is mentioned as a risk in obese people who suffer from binge-eating disorder.

**3. c.** Near the end of the last paragraph, the passage indicates that binge-eating disorder patients experience *high* blood pressure.

**4. c.** The final sentence of the third paragraph states that individuals with eating disorders are at risk for suicidal behavior, but not that people with anorexia always end their own lives.

**5. b.** The first sentence of the fifth paragraph tells us that bulimia sufferers are often able to keep their problem a secret, partly because they maintain a normal or above-normal weight.

**6. c.** In the second paragraph, the thyroid gland function is mentioned as slowing down—one effort on the part of the body to protect itself.

**7. a.** According to the second paragraph, dehydration contributes to constipation.

**8. a.** The final paragraph of the passage states that binge-eating disorder patients *eat large quantities of food and do not stop until they are uncomfortably full.*

**9. d.** See the second sentence of the sixth paragraph. If as many as one-third of the binge-eating disorder population are men, it stands to reason that up to two-thirds are younger women, given that about 90% of all eating disorder sufferers are adolescent and young adult women.

**10. b.** The author uses the phrase *going gray* as a metaphor for growing older. It describes the phenomenon of a large segment of a population growing older.

**11. d.** The passage emphasizes the need for age-specific care.

**12. d.** In this context, *vital* most nearly means critical or crucial. The sentence implies that healthcare providers will be very important in helping to avoid suicide deaths in older Americans, which is a growing issue.

**13. c.** Although choices **a** and **b** may be correct statements, they do not reflect the author's purpose in citing the example of untreated depression in the elderly. Choice **d** is incorrect.

**14. c.** According to the passage, geriatric training improves a healthcare provider's ability to *distinguish between "normal" characteristics associated with aging and illness.*

**15. c.** This is an informative passage, neutral in tone, which explains what anthrax is, what causes it, and what is being done to find a preventative vaccine.

**16. c.** According to paragraph two, pulmonary anthrax, or inhalation anthrax, has a fatality rate of 80% or higher. It is cutaneous anthrax that can usually be treated successfully with antibiotics.

**17. b.** According to paragraph three, although four of the five people who contracted inhalation anthrax died, *no cases of inhalation anthrax occurred in vaccine recipients.*

**18. a.** In paragraph three, *strain* is a noun that means a subgroup, breed, or type of the bacterium.

**19. c.** The second paragraph states that mortality rates are *approximately 20% for cutaneous anthrax without antibiotics, while inhalation anthrax has a fatality rate of 80% or higher.*

**20. d.** According to the final paragraph of the passage, *Anthrax Vaccine Adsorbed (AVA) is recommended for . . . individuals engaged in diagnostic or investigational activities that may bring them in contact with anthrax spores.* The police officer in choice **b** may not inspect the package her/himself, so AVA may not be necessary.

**21. c.** The introduction of the clinical trial is used to show that there is a vaccine available for anthrax and that it proved successful when tested.

**22. a.** The third sentence of the second paragraph states that multifocal dystonia *involves two or more unrelated body parts.*

**23. b.** The third sentence of paragraph six states that *only one eye may be affected initially* by blepharospasm. The passage does not suggest that blindness occurs in the early stages of blepharospasm (choice **a**), while the word "urge" suggests a conscious desire rather than an involuntary movement (choice **c**). Difficulty swallowing is a symptom of oromandibular dystonia (choice **d**).

**24. a.** According to the fourth paragraph, torsion dystonia may be inherited.

**25. c.** Meige's syndrome combines symptoms of blepharospasm (affecting the eyes) and oromandibular dystonia (affecting the lips and tongue).

**26. a.** Both torticollis and cranial dystonia affect the neck and head, as indicated in the fifth and seventh paragraphs.

**27. d.** The first sentence of the last paragraph states that DRD patients can be successfully treated with drugs.

**28. a.** The second sentence states that dystonia-related movements are involuntary.

**29. c.** Cranial dystonia affects muscles in the head, face, and neck. Since it affects two or more adjacent body parts, cranial dystonia is a segmental dystonia.

**30. d.** In the fourth paragraph, torsion dystonia is referred to as a *rare* ailment. Dopa-responsive dystonia is also labeled rare in the last sentence of the passage.

**31. b.** See the first sentence of paragraph four.

**32. c.** See the last paragraph of the passage.

**33. d.** The end of the third paragraph says that ticks prefer humid, relatively warm weather.

**34. a.** See the first sentence of the passage.

**35. b.** The end of the second paragraph says that larval infection of humans is a *rare occurrence.*

**36. c.** After the rash, which may or may not appear, the next symptoms are the flu-like symptoms listed in the fifth paragraph.

**37. d.** The passage states several times that tai chi is used to maintain balance through breathing, meditation, and concentration.

**38. c.** Paragraph four states that meditation helps the digestive system and increases calmness. It also states that in tai chi practice, it is important to concentrate and put aside distraction, so a quiet setting would be ideal. It says nothing about the temperament of animals.

**39. c.** The passage, when taken as a whole, introduces tai chi and talks about its influences on the minds and bodies of its participants.

**40. b.** Two important *elements* of tai chi, or *principles* that define it, are breathing and meditation.

**41. d.** The first paragraph states that *the term* tai chi *has been translated in various ways, including "internal martial art," "supreme ultimate boxing," "boundless fist," and "balance of the opposing forces of nature."*

**42. a.** According to the first paragraph, Chang concluded that *the snake and the crane, through their movements, were the ones most able to overcome strong, unyielding opponents.*

**43. c.** Paragraph three discusses the importance of posture in longtime tai chi devotees and how important it is to keep the body upright.

**44. b.** The passage mentions the importance of maintaining the balance of yin and yang, Chang's introduction of flexibility to martial arts, and the gracefulness of the sport. Nothing is mentioned about the personalities of tai chi participants.

**45. d.** According to paragraph four, practitioners of tai chi believe that *breathing and meditation have many benefits, such as massaging the internal organs, aiding the exchange of gases in the lungs, helping the digestive system work more efficiently, increasing calmness and awareness, and improving balance.*

## Section 3: Quantitative Ability

**1. c.** $4\frac{2}{5} + 3\frac{1}{2} + \frac{3}{8}$ can be rewritten: $4 + 3 + \frac{2}{5} + \frac{1}{2} + \frac{3}{8}$. To add the fractions, find the least common multiple of 5, 2, and 8, which is 40. Next, rewrite the problem: $7 + \frac{16}{40} + \frac{20}{40} + \frac{15}{40} = 7\frac{51}{40} = 8\frac{11}{40}$.

**2. a.** Be careful with the units in this problem, since the answer choices are given in meters, not centimeters as in the question. First, convert the dimensions of the examination table into meters: 150 cm × 1 m/100 cm = 1.5 m and 70 cm × 1 m/100 cm = 0.7 m. The area of a rectangle is *length × width*, so the area of the table is 1.5 m × 0.7 m = 1.05 square m.

**3. b.** Add all four weights for a total of 703; 703 rounded to the nearest ten is 700.

**4. b.** Substitute the values into the given expression: $\frac{6(3)-6(-2)}{(3)^2}$ then becomes $\frac{18-(-12)}{9} = \frac{30}{9}$, or $3\frac{1}{3}$.

**5. a.** The formula to use here is $A = \frac{1}{2}bh$ or $A = \frac{1}{2}(10)(2) = 10$ square inches.

**6. b.** To find the average number of patients treated per day, add up the patients treated during the week and divide by the number of days: $\frac{33+27+13+22+18+24+31}{7} = \frac{168}{7} = 24$.

**7. d.** If 60 people try out and only nine can make the team, then 60 − 9 = 51 people who will not make the team: $\frac{\%}{100} = \frac{51}{60}, \frac{5,100}{60} = 85$.

**8. c.** 60% of some number *n* equals 75, so $0.60n = 75$. Divide both sides by 0.60 to find the answer: $\frac{0.60n}{0.60} = \frac{75}{0.60}, n = 125$.

**9. d.** Line up your decimal points carefully when adding.

```
  33.330
   3.300
   0.333
 333.000
 369.963
```

**10. b.** If the runner wants to travel half the total distance, she wants to run five miles. In order to run one mile, she would have to run around the track four times around, so in order to run five miles, she would have to run 4(5) = 20 times around.

**11. b.** To solve this problem, find the area of two rectangles and then add the results. Use an imaginary line to block off the first rectangle at the top of the figure. This rectangle measures 5 feet by 2 feet. Using the formula $A = lw$, this comes to 10 square feet. The second rectangle is also 5 feet by 2 feet. Add the two together for a total of 20 square feet.

**12. c.** Change the percent to a decimal and then multiply: $0.072 \times 465 = 33.48$, which, rounded to the nearest tenth, is 33.5.

**13. a.** First, find the least common denominator, 40, and rewrite the problem as $3\frac{28}{40} - 2\frac{15}{40}$. Subtract the whole numbers, then the fractions, and then add the results to get $1\frac{13}{40}$.

**14. a.** The halfway point on the number line is between 0 and $-\frac{1}{2}$, which is $-\frac{1}{4}$.

**15. c.** The three angles of a triangle always add up to 180°, so the third angle of this triangle equals $180° - (47° + 86°) = 180° - 133° = 47°$.

**16. a.** To square $y$, multiply $y$ times $y$.

**17. c.** This is a simple multiplication problem as long as you keep the decimal values straight. First, ignore the decimal points and multiply the two numbers: $36708 \times 15 = 550620$. Because there are a total of four decimal digits in 367.08 and 0.15, count off four places from the right in 550620, placing the decimal point to the left of the last four digits to get the answer: 55.0620, or 55.062.

**18. c.** Do the operations in order from left to right: $-10 + (-4) = -14$. Next, $-14 + \frac{1}{2} = -13\frac{1}{2}$. Then, $-13\frac{1}{2} - (-\frac{1}{4}) = -13\frac{1}{2} + \frac{1}{4} = -13\frac{1}{4}$.

**19. d.** With 24 tickets, you can get $\frac{24}{2} = 12$ merry-go-round rides or $\frac{24}{3} = 8$ roller coaster rides. So, you can get $12 - 8 = 4$ more merry-go-round rides than roller coaster rides for 24 tickets.

**20. b.** Use the answers provided and work backward. Start with choice **c**. If there were 90 seeds and Serena planted $\frac{1}{4}$ of them, then she planted 22.5 Already, this answer doesn't make sense. Try choice **b**. If they started with 60 and Serena planted $\frac{1}{4}$, then $60 - \frac{60}{4}$ or $60 - 15$ or 45 remained. If her mother then planted $\frac{1}{3}$ of the remaining, then $45 - \frac{45}{3}$ or $45 - 15$ or 30 remained. This matches the question, so choice **b** is correct.

**21. b.** If $\frac{2}{5}$ of the students are in Group A, then $\frac{2}{5} \times 25 = 10$ are in Group A. If 20% of the class is in Group B, then $.20(25) = 5$ students are in Group B: $10 + 5 = 15$.

**22. c.** Multiply both parts of the time by 10, then fix your units: 9 minutes $\times 10 = 90$ minutes; 36 seconds $\times 10 = 360$ seconds. Next, change the seconds into minutes: 360 seconds $\div 60 = 6$ minutes; 90 minutes $+ 6$ minutes $= 96$ minutes; 96 minutes $= 1$ hour (60 of the minutes) 36 minutes.

**23. d.** During the meeting, $\frac{5}{8}(48) = 30$ cookies were eaten, leaving $48 - 30 = 18$ cookies. Andrew takes $\frac{1}{3}(8) = 6$ of these cookies, leaving $18 - 6 = 12$ cookies. Lia takes 5 cookies, leaving $12 - 5 = 7$ at the end.

**24. a.** If Kendra wants to buy 2.5 pounds and mango costs $6.30 per pound, her purchase will cost $6.30(2.5) = $15.75$. $20.00 - $15.75 = $4.25$.

**25. c.** Divide 135 (the number of Spanish-speaking nurses at the hospital) by 1,125 (the total numbers of nurses at the hospital) to arrive at 0.12 or 12%.

**26. c.** From 10:42 to 12:42, two hours have elapsed. From 12:42 to 1:00, another 18 minutes have elapsed ($60 - 42 = 18$). Next, between 1:00 and 1:19, there is another 19 minutes, for a total of 2 hours 37 minutes.

**27. a.** To find the percent increase, first subtract the original salary from the new salary: $51,500 − $50,000 = $1,500. The percent increase is the difference divided by the original amount: $\frac{\$1,500}{\$50,000} = 0.03 = 3\%$.

**28. d.** First, you have to determine the perimeters of all four rooms. This is done by using the formula for a square ($P = 4s$), or for a rectangle ($P = 2l + 2w$), as follows: $(2 \times 12) + (2 \times 8) = 40$ for choice **a**; $(2 \times 14) + (2 \times 7) = 42$ for choice **b**; $4 \times 10 = 40$ for choice **c**; $4 \times 11 = 44$ for the correct choice, **d**.

**29. b.** Convert Fahrenheit to Centigrade using the formula given: $C = \frac{5}{9}(122 - 32)$; that is, $C = \frac{5}{9} \times 90$; so $C = 50°$.

**30. b.** You cannot just take 25% off the original price, because the 10% discount after three years of service is taken off the price that has already been reduced by 15%. Figure the problem in two steps: After the 15% discount, the price is $71.83. Ninety percent of that—subtracting 10%—is $64.65.

**31. d.** Let $n$ be the number of CNAs that are present. Since the ratio of CNAs to nurses on a given shift has to be *at least* 3 to 2, $\frac{n}{6} \geq \frac{3}{2}$. Cross-multiply to get $2n \geq 18$. Divide both sides by 2 to see that $n \geq 9$. The only answer choice that is greater than or equal to 9 is **d**, so this is the correct answer.

**32. b.** Substituting known quantities into the BMI formula yields $20 = \frac{64.8}{x^2}$. Next, multiply both sides by $x^2$ to get $20x^2 = 64.8$, and then divide through by 20 to get $x^2 = 3.24$. Now take the square root of both sides to get $x = 1.8$.

**33. c.** Let $E$ = emergency room cost; $H$ = hospice cost; $N$ = home nursing cost; $H = \frac{1}{4}E$, and $N = 2H = 2(\frac{1}{4}E) = \frac{1}{2}E$. The total bill is $E + H + N = E + (\frac{1}{4})E + (\frac{2}{4})E = \$140,000$. So $(\frac{7}{4})E = \$140,000$. Multiplying both sides by $\frac{4}{7}$ yields $E = \$80,000$. Therefore, $N = \frac{1}{2}E = \$40,000$.

**34. c.** You must break the $92,000 into the amounts mentioned in the policy: $92,000 = $20,000 + $40,000 + $32,000. The amount the policy will pay is $(0.8)(\$20,000) + (0.6)(\$40,000) + (0.4)(\$32,000) = \$16,000 + \$24,000 + \$12,800 = \$52,800$.

**35. a.** Each Alzheimer's patient takes $\frac{1}{4}$ hour. Each stroke patient thus takes $\frac{3}{4}$ hour. The doctor has already spent $10(\frac{1}{4}) + 3(\frac{3}{4}) = \frac{10}{4} + \frac{9}{4} = \frac{19}{4} = 4\frac{3}{4}$ hours with patients today. Her six-hour schedule minus $4\frac{3}{4}$ hours leaves $1\frac{1}{4}$ hours left to see patients. Since each stroke patient takes $\frac{3}{4}$ hour, the doctor has time to treat only one more stroke patient in the $1\frac{1}{4}$ hours remaining.

**36. b.** The question asks for the speed in miles per hour, so first convert the time it takes to get to the hospital to hours: $37.5 \ \cancel{\text{min}} \times \frac{1 \ \text{hr}}{60 \ \cancel{\text{min}}} = 0.625$ hr. Then divide the number of miles traveled by the time to get the answer: $\frac{100 \ \text{miles}}{0.625 \ \text{hr}} = 160$ mph.

**37. b.** Use the Pythagorean theorem: $1^2 + x^2 = (\sqrt{10})^2$; $1 + x^2 = 10$, so $x^2 = 9$. Thus, $x = 3$.

**38. d.** First, convert the mixed numbers to improper fractions: $\frac{3\frac{1}{9}}{1\frac{1}{6}} = \frac{\frac{28}{9}}{\frac{7}{6}}$. Next, invert the denominator and multiply, canceling where possible: $\frac{28}{9} \times \frac{6}{7} = \frac{8}{3} = 2\frac{2}{3}$.

**39. c.** Let $T$ = Ted's age; $S$ = Sam's age = $3T$; $R$ = Ron's age = $\frac{S}{2} = \frac{3T}{2}$. The sum of the ages is $\frac{3T}{2} + 3T + T = \frac{3T}{2} + \frac{6T}{2} + \frac{2T}{2} = \frac{11T}{2}$, which is equal to 55. Now multiply both sides of the resulting equation, $55 = \frac{11T}{2}$, by 2 to get $110 = 11T$. Divide through by 11 to get $10 = T$. That is Ted's age, so Ron is $\frac{3T}{2} = \frac{30}{2}$ = 15 years old.

**40. a.** If half the students are female, then you would expect half of the out-of-state students to be female. One-half of $\frac{1}{12} = (\frac{1}{2})(\frac{1}{12}) = \frac{1}{24}$.

**41. a.** $54\frac{1}{2}\%$ is the same as 54.5%. Move the decimal point two places to the left to get 0.545.

**42. c.** First, get rid of the square root sign by squaring both sides of the equation: $2x + 2 = 16$. Subtract 2 from both sides to find that $2x = 14$. Divide both sides by 2 to find that $x = 7$.

**43. c.** Calculate the distance of both times from midnight, then add them together. 7:15 is 4 hours 45 minutes from midnight. 8 A.M. is 8 hours from midnight. The total is 12 hours 45 minutes: 12 hours = 12(60) minutes or 720 minutes; 720 + 45 = 765 minutes.

**44. a.** First, find the length of the side that is common to both of the right triangles in the figure. Call that side $y$. Apply the Pythagorean theorem to the triangle on the left: $90^2 + y^2 = 150^2$, so that $y^2 = 150^2 - 90^2 = 22,500 - 8,100 = 14,400$. If $y^2 = 14,400$, then $y = 120$. Now you know the lengths of the two legs of the triangle on the right, so apply the Pythagorean theorem again: $120^2 + 160^2 = x^2$, which means that $14,400 + 25,600 = x^2$. Thus, $40,000 = x^2$, and $x$ is therefore 200. (If you realize that both triangles are 3-4-5 triangles, your work will be easier.)

**45. a.** Complementary angles add up to 90°, so $j + k = 90°$, and $k = 90° - 72° = 18°$.

**46. c.** A foot in height makes a difference of 60 lbs., or 5 lbs. per inch of height over 5'. A person who is 5'5" is (5)(5 lbs.) = 25 lbs. heavier than the person who is 5', so add 25 lbs. to 110 lbs. to get 135 lbs.

**47. a.** Twelve oranges at $0.40 each is 12($0.40) = $4.80. Eleven apples at $0.60 each is 11($0.60) = $6.60. $6.60 + $4.80 = $11.40. If Alena has only $10, she needs $1.40 more.

**48. b.** When $x = 34$, then $y = \frac{2}{34}$. $(3)(34)(\frac{2}{34}) = (3)(2) = 6$.

**49. b.** The difference between 105° and 99° is 6°. Application of the ice pack plus a resting period of five minutes before reapplication means that the temperature is lowered by half a degree every six minutes, or 1° every 12 minutes. Six degrees times 12 minutes per degree is 72 minutes, or 1 hour 12 minutes.

**50. b.** The lighter liquid is $\frac{6}{15}$, or $\frac{2}{5}$, of the total solution; $\frac{2}{5} = 0.4$, or 40%.

## Section 4: General Science

**1. d.** The weak nuclear force determines beta decay, which occurs when a neutron converts to a proton with the ejection of an electron.

**2. d.** Sputnik 1 was the first satellite to be put into Earth's orbit in 1957 by the Soviet Union.

**3. a.** The periodic table has rows of elements arranged by their properties, which are derived mainly from the patterns of electrons inside their atoms.

**4. a.** The valence shell either gains or loses electrons to create atomic bonds with other atoms. Valence means *strength* (think *value*).

**5. d.** The covalent bond is a shared pair of electrons, which "spend time" in both atoms, though often in one more than the other.

**6. a.** The number 6 brings the total number of oxygen atoms on the right-hand side to 18, the same as the total on the left-hand side, thereby balancing the reaction.

**7. d.** Reduction of an element in a chemical reaction occurs when its charge is numerically lowered (in this case, from +4 to –4).

**8. b.** The liquid is warmed. The heat of fusion is the amount of energy is takes to melt a solid, or to turn it into liquid at the same temperature. Because our example is already liquid, applying any heat at all only warms it up. This may or may not also evaporate the liquid; we don't know without more information.

**9. a.** Amino acids combine to form proteins. Nucleic acids combine to form DNA and RNA.

**10. b.** Only quartz contains no carbon, a necessary condition for an organic molecule. Therefore, quartz is an inorganic molecule.

**11. a.** Wegener first proposed the idea of continental drift. Bohr gave us the Bohr model of the atom; Schrodinger developed wave mechanics to help explain the structure of atoms, and Watson studied the structure of DNA.

**12. c.** The independent variable is the one you change. The dependent variable then changes in response.

**13. a.** The breakdown of plant and animal matter over long periods of time under special conditions leads to the formation of oil.

**14. b.** Albert Einstein published the general theory of relativity in 1916. It describes gravity as a geometric property of space and time.

**15. c.** Hydrogen gas does not occur naturally; it can be made from splitting water molecules.

**16. d.** Though all forms of energy can be converted into all other forms, the efficiency varies and is sometimes very low. Heat, the most degraded form of energy, according to the law of entropy, can be made from the other forms with a conversion rate that is theoretically 100%.

**17. a.** Entropy can decrease only if the decrease is strictly local and is more than balanced by an increase on some larger scale.

**18. c.** Galileo Galilei was called the "Father of Modern Science." The Roman Inquisition investigated him and believed that his work challenged the Catholic Church. He was found guilty of heresy and ordered to live the rest of his life under house arrest.

**19. b.** Potential energy is created at the top, when the crane stops. Kinetic energy would occur were the beam dropped.

**20. c.** Chemical potential energy is released from the food we eat, when combined with oxygen in the air.

**21. c.** Entomology is the scientific study of insects. The word comes from the Greek *entomos* which means "that which is cut into pieces or segmented" (meaning insects).

**22. d.** 3,700 million years ago (equal to 3.7 billion years ago) is right between the two kinds of evidence for the origin of life, from fossils and from carbon isotopes.

**23. b.** Penicillin is derived from the fungi *Penicillium*. Penicillin antibiotics were the first drugs to cure serious bacterial infections and are still widely used today.

**24. b.** Proteins are assembled at ribosomes, from amino acids brought to the ribosomes by transfer molecules and according to the genetic code.

**25. c.** Triplets of bases—for example AAT or CGT or GAC—code for amino acids. This was discovered by, among others, English biologist Francis Crick, who, many years earlier, first discovered the double helix structure of DNA.

**26. d.** The *r* in rRNA stands for *ribosomal*. Ribosomal RNA is used to construct the universal tree of life because all organisms possess ribosomes.

**27. d.** Liposomes are hollow spheres of lipid molecules, which are similar to (though simpler than) cell membranes. Liposomes might have played a role in the origin of life and the evolution of cells.

**28. b.** Perhaps, strangely, it is modern-day pigeons that descended from ancestral birds, which descended directly from bipedal dinosaurs.

**29. c.** Eukaryotic cells have organelles; prokaryotic cells do not. The other answers are not types of cells.

**30. a.** Osteology is the study of bones, including skeletal elements, disease, pathology, teeth, the structure of bones, and any other details that help to determine age, sex, death, and development. It is a sub-discipline of anthropology and helps with the identification of human remains.

**31. b.** Sodium chloride, or NaCl, is commonly known as table salt. It is the major ingredient in edible salt, but is also responsible for the salinity of the ocean, among other things.

**32. b.** The pythons are invasive species because they have been placed in an environment in which they do not normally occur.

**33. b.** Benjamin Franklin is credited for inventing the bifocal lens and was one of the first to use them. The term "bifocal" was coined in 1824 by John Isaac Hawkins, the creator of trifocals, but the invention was credited to Franklin by Hawkins.

**34. c.** Metamorphic rocks are formed when a preexisting rock is changed through extreme heat and/or pressure. Igneous rocks are formed by the cooling and solidification of magma, and sedimentary rocks are formed by the compaction of sediments.

**35. a.** Single-celled life originated in the Archean Era.

**36. d.** Phloem is the special tube-like tissue in plants that transports food downward. Xylem conducts water and minerals up from the soil. The other choices are found in animals.

**37. a.** The evidence of a worldwide clay layer that contains unnaturally high levels of the element iridium was found first in Italy, and then in many parts of the world. Iridium at those concentrations must have come from an impactor from space.

**38. a.** Lead-acid car batteries are made up of lead and lead dioxide plates that are submerged in a solution that is 35% sulfuric acid and 65% water.

**39. c.** A seismometer (or seismograph) measures motions of the ground, including those caused by earthquakes and volcanoes. The term comes from the Greek *seismos*, meaning "shaking or quaking," and *metron*, meaning "measure."

**40. b.** An older mass extinction than the one that did away with the dinosaurs came at the end of the Permian stage of geological time, the Permian-Triassic boundary, about 250 million years ago.

**41. a.** John Glenn orbited the Earth in 1962 in *Friendship 7*. He was the first American to do so.

**42. a.** The field that studies the evolution of human behavior and the evolution of the human mind as it originated back in time is called evolutionary psychology.

**43. a.** Australopithecus, a human ancestor (or hominid), is the most recent by far.

**44. d.** The orangutan is most distantly related to us, of those on the list.

**45. b.** Alkaline is another term for basic, which is defined by a pH > 7.

**46. c.** Amphibians evolved first, then reptiles, and then mammals.

**47. b.** Electricity is the movement of electrons.

**48. a.** Voltage drives electrical current. It is the difference in electrical potential between two objects.

**49. c.** Velocity is distance per unit time, or $v = \frac{d}{t}$.

**50. b.** Spectra shifted toward the red have longer wavelengths.

## Section 5: Biology

**1. b.** Autotrophs generate energy from sunlight rather than consuming other sources of energy. Chloroplasts contain the photosynthetic machinery necessary for harvesting solar energy.

**2. d.** Xylem tissue conducts water and minerals from the roots to the rest of the plant, while phloem tissue carries sugars from the leaves down to other parts of the plant. Sieve tubes are components of phloem. Stomata are minute openings in leaves that allow air to enter.

**3. d.** Aneuploidy describes extra individual chromosomes, while polyploidy describes extra sets of homologous chromosomes.

**4. c.** Pollen released by the stamen is captured by the stigma and reaches the carpels, where the ovum cells are located.

**5. a.** Platelets are cell fragments (with no nucleus) that release serotonin and other chemicals, thus instigating the blood-clotting process.

**6. c.** Edema, also known as *dropsy*, is the interstitial collection of watery fluid.

**7. c.** Alcohol fermentation occurs during anaerobic respiration and produces ethanol and carbon dioxide.

**8. b.** Remember that the prefix *auto-* means *self*. Autogamy is a common method of fertilization used in plants. Syngamy is the union of male and female gametes also known as fertilization, and allogamy is cross-fertilization.

**9. c.** A single fertilized egg cell divides and becomes multicellular during cleavage. The other answers are all stages that a cell passes through during the four-staged cell cycle: $G_2$ phase, M phase (mitosis and cytokinesis), $G_1$ phase, and S phase.

**10. c.** Nitric oxide, NO, is an important molecule in biological systems. $O_2$ and $N_2$ are common gases and $N_2O$ is not diatomic (it contains 3 atoms).

**11. a.** Natural selection occurs through genetic traits passed on to offspring that are beneficial to survival, like adapting to harsh climates or living with limited resources. Traits learned by parents are not passed on to future generations of offspring.

**12. b.** Active transport requires energy to transport a substance through the membrane. Diffusion and osmosis rely on concentration differences, and filtration relies on pressure differences.

**13. d.** Meiosis results in four haploid gametes with half the number of chromosomes as their parent. This is unlike mitosis, which results in two daughter cells with the same number of chromosomes.

**14. d.** Essential amino acids cannot be synthesized by the body and must be ingested. The complete list of essential amino acids contains Phe, Val, Thr, Trp, Ile, Met, Leu, Lys, and His.

**15. a.** Membranes are not rigid and do not provide support like cells walls do. The cell membrane is responsible for transporting substances and forming structures to contain cytoplasm and DNA.

**16. b.** Every person's body contains an average of 4.5 to 5 liters of blood.

**17. d.** Oxygen-rich blood collects into venules and finally into a pulmonary vein from each lung. Veins return blood to the heart, while arteries carry blood away from the heart.

**18. b.** Phenylketonuria (PKU) is a hereditary disease that results in loss of function of the enzyme that converts phenylalanine to tyrosine. Build-up of phenylalanine can cause many deleterious effects, and so only limited amounts may be safely consumed for those with PKU.

**19. c.** If incorrect blood types are transfused (for example, if type B blood is injected into a person with type A blood), red cells will clump together. This process is called agglutination.

**20. c.** Threonine does not contain any aromatic rings. It contains a hydroxyl group.

**21. a.** The homozygous dominant parent has a genotype of QQ and will always give Q to its offspring. The homozygous recessive parent has a genotype of qq and will always give q to its offspring. Therefore, all the offspring will have the genotype Qq, and the chance of offspring expressing the recessive trait is 0%.

**22. b.** Bacteriophages are viruses that infect bacteria.

**23. d.** The gene appears to be sex-linked, but without more information about the genotype of an individual's parents or offspring it is not possible to determine to which chromosome the gene is linked.

**24. d.** Genetic code is broken down into codons of three base-pairs. It is helpful to separate the codons as follows: UAU UUC GCU GCA.

**25. b.** Secondary consumers eat primary consumers for energy. This transfer of energy is represented by trophic levels.

**26. b.** The cerebellum coordinates impulses sent out from the cerebrum. Its main function is to coordinate skeletal movements.

**27. d.** The myelin sheath is the outer layer that encloses the axons of many neurons.

**28. d.** tRNA is responsible for delivering amino acids to the ribosome according to the sequence on mRNA. If the mutation affected tRNA, its anticodons may not be able to read the sequence of codons, or it may not be able to attach to the appropriate amino acid.

**29. d.** The sweat glands form part of the exocrine system. The other glands form part of the endocrine system.

**30. a.** Triglycerides are the major constituent in dietary fat. To a lesser extent, phospholipids and cholesterol are also present in dietary fat. Lipase is an enzyme in vertebrates that catalyzes the breakdown of fats into fatty acids and glycerol.

**31. b.** The diastole phase of a heartbeat occurs between two contractions of the heart, during which the heart muscles relax and the ventricles fill up with blood.

**32. d.** The Malpighian layer—synonymous with *stratum basale*—is the only layer of the skin in which mitosis occurs.

**33. a.** Ribosomes, located on the endoplasmic reticulum (ER) and in the cytoplasm, are where protein synthesis occurs.

**34. a.** Hypertension is the medical term for increased blood pressure.

**35. a.** The placenta is the organ in viviparous animals which connects the embryo to its mother's uterus.

**36. c.** Draw a Punnett square diagram. Blue eye color (b) is a recessive trait, and brown (B) is dominant. Your mother must be homozygous recessive to have blue eyes (bb), and your father is heterozygous (Bb). Therefore, your chances of having blue eyes is 50%.

**37. a.** Setae (singular *seta*) are the bristle-like projections on some invertebrates. Hair only occurs on mammals, and whiskers are a type of hair.

**38. a.** Hematocrit describes the percentage of blood volume occupied by red blood cells. Anemia is a condition characterized by too few healthy red blood cells.

**39. d.** The alveoli, where carbon dioxide and oxygen are exchanged, are located at the ends of pulmonary tubes called bronchioles.

**40. c.** Light is produced without heat in bioluminscent animals when luciferin is oxidized.

**41. d.** Dentin is the thick, bony layer underneath the calcium phosphate deposit that makes up the enamel of teeth.

**42. c.** The macula is a spot near the center of the retina in the eye. Macular degeneration results in loss of central vision.

**43. d.** Prokaryotes include only unicellular organisms: bacteria and archaea. All of the other characteristics listed are seen only in eukaryotic cells.

**44. b.** Digestive organs called accessory organs contribute to the digestive process, but food does not pass through them. Choice **b**, the liver, is an example. The other choices are part of the alimentary canal or gastrointestinal tract, which is the tube through which food passes as it is digested.

**45. a.** Acquired characteristics are features that develop within the lifetime of an individual organism, as do large muscles in a weight lifter. The large ears of rabbits and nocturnal vision of owls have developed over generations to help these animals survive. The human appendix is a vestigial organ.

**46. c.** Fermentation is an anaerobic process that uses glucose for energy without oxygen. Choice **a** uses light energy to make glucose. Choice **d** uses glucose for energy when oxygen is used.

**47. c.** Individual 1 definitely has two recessive alleles, say rr. Therefore, each of his offspring will receive an "r" from him, making all of the offspring carriers of the recessive trait.

**48. a.** Fungi and plants evolved from protists. Some protists are autotrophs and contain chloroplasts like plants. Fungi are not autotrophic. Protists do not have specialized tissue.

**49. d.** Codons are three-letter codes of either DNA or mRNA that code for a specific amino acid that is added during translation.

**50. b.** The first parent showing the recessive trait has genotype nn and will always give its offspring n. The second parent not showing the recessive trait has at least one N (the possible genotypes are Nn and NN). If the offspring do not show the recessive trait, then they received N from the second parent and the first parent gave n, making the genotype Nn.

## Section 6: Chemistry

1. **c.** Sulfuric acid ($H_2SO_4$) is a strong acid. The other acid given, $HNO_2$, is a weak acid. The other choices are bases.

2. **c.** Copper oxide, a metal oxide, forms copper sulphate, a salt, and water when combined with sulphuric acid.

3. **b.** There is 1 mole of $H_2O$ in 18.0 g of water. Each mole of water contains 2 moles of hydrogen.

4. **d.** In this reaction, the iron is reduced from Fe (III) to Fe (0), and the aluminum is oxidized from Al (0) to Al (III).

5. **d.** This is the only balanced option.

6. **c.** Aldehydes consist of a central carbon atom bonded to a lone hydrogen atom and a carbon chain, and double bonded to an oxygen. Thus, choice **c** is correct.

7. **c.** Phosphate has a charge of –3, and cobalt (II) has a charge of +2. To balance the charges, they must be combined into $Co_3(PO_4)_2$.

8. **c.** Phospholipids, the major components of cell membranes, are made up of one molecule of glycerol bonded to two fatty acids and one phosphate group. Choice **a** describes a peptide bond, and choice **b** describes a fat.

9. **b.** Choice **b** is the definition of osmotic pressure. Osmotic potential, mentioned in choice **d**, is inversely proportional to osmotic pressure and is the Gibbs free energy value for the osmosis reaction.

10. **d.** An aldehyde is a molecule containing a carbonyl group, C=O, a hydrogen atom, and an alkyl group. The only choice that fits this definition is choice **d**.

11. **a.** α decay is the decay process where a helium nucleus is released.

12. **b.** Bismuth (III) has an oxidation number of +3, and the hydroxide ion has an oxidation number of –1. Therefore, three hydroxide ions must bond to each bismuth atom to form an uncharged compound.

13. **b.** When an alkali metal such as sodium reacts with water, an explosive reaction takes place, and the result is a metal hydroxide and hydrogen gas.

14. **b.** When an atom loses electrons, it is said to be oxidized; and when an atom gains electrons, it is said to be reduced. In this reaction, Br goes from negatively charged to neutral, thus losing an electron and being oxidized. Mn goes from a charge of +7 to a charge of +2, gaining electrons in the process and becoming reduced.

15. **b.** Atoms decrease in radius across rows of the periodic table to the right. For any row, the outermost orbital of electrons is the same for all elements in the row, and each added electron fills that orbital. However, each atom gains a proton as well, which increases the attraction between the nucleus and electrons, thus reducing the atomic radius. Atoms increase in radius going down a column because each successive atom adds an orbital of electrons. Since Li, N, and F are in the same row, and Li is the leftmost atom, it is the largest of the three. However, Cs is below Li and is therefore the largest.

16. **d.** Carbonic acid, $H_2CO_3$, has a pKa of 6.35, making it the weakest acid of the choices.

17. **c.** The mass of the empirical compound $CH_2O$ = (1C × 12 g) + (2H × 1 g) + (1O × 16 g) = 30 g. Since the molar mass of the compound is 90 g, the multiplier is $\frac{90}{30} = 3$, yielding a molecular formula of $C_3H_6O_3$.

18. **b.** As a general rule, atomic radius increases as you go down and to the left in the periodic table. Rb is the farthest down and to the left.

**19. c.** Gases move more freely compared with solids and liquids.

**20. a.** In redox reactions, atoms that lose electrons are being oxidized. The half reaction $Zn_{(s)} \rightarrow Zn^{2+}_{(aq)} + 2e^-$ shows that $Zn_{(s)}$ is losing two electrons in this reaction.

**21. d.** Both KOH and $NH_4^+$ are basic, leaving only $H_3PO_4$ and $H_2PO_4^-$. Because acidic compounds are generally $H^+$ donors, and $H_2PO_4^-$ has already lost one $H^+$, $H_3PO_4$ is the more acidic.

**22. b.** Because there are already either $Ag^{2+}$ or $CO_3^{2-}$ ions in the solutions in choices **a**, **c**, and **d**, $AgCO_3$ will be apt to form some solid. However, neither of these ions exist in the solution of KCl, allowing $AgCO_3$ to dissolve.

**23. b.** β decay results in the conversion of a neutron into a proton and an electron, with expulsion of the electron from the nucleus.

**24. c.** Trans fats are fatty acids with at least one trans C–C double bond. These fats are found in partially hydrogenated oils and have been associated with many negative health effects.

**25. d.** Combustion reactions produce $CO_2$ and $H_2O$.

**26. b.** A liquid will change shape according to the container it is in, whereas a gas will spread out to fill its container, and a liquid will sit at the bottom of its container, retaining the same volume. A solid always retains the same shape and volume.

**27. d.** The coefficients in the balanced reaction show that for every four P molecules reacted, there are two $P_2O_5$ molecules produced—a ratio of 2:1, as shown by the coefficients. If three moles of $P_2O_5$ are to be produced by this reaction, twice as many moles of P are required: six moles. Using Avogadro's number to calculate the number of molecules, this means: $6.02 \times 10^{23}$ molecules/mole $\times$ 6 moles of $P = 3.61 \times 10^{24}$ molecules P required.

**28. b.** The first comparison finds that the given amount of LiBr is 0.836 moles:

$$72.6\text{g LiBr} \times \frac{(1 \text{ mol LiBr})}{(86.841\text{g LiBr})} = 0.836 \text{ mol LiBr}$$

The molar ratio for LiBr and LiOH is 1:1, so if 0.836 mol LiBr is a reactant, then 0.836 mol LiOH is the product. The next step converts 0.836 mol LiOH to grams LiOH in order to calculate the mass necessary: 20.01g.

$$0.836 \text{ mol LiOH} \times \frac{(23.941\text{g LiOH})}{(1 \text{ mol LiOH})} = 20.01\text{g LiOH}$$

**29. b.** Transition metals are those with partially filled d orbitals. Iron is the only element on the list that fits that criterion.

**30. c.** Sulfur is in group VI, so it has six valence electrons.

**31. d.** Ca has two valence electrons, which occur in the 4s shell.

**32. d.** Choices **a** and **c** are not polar bonds. Fluorine will always form more polar bonds than chlorine in covalent compounds.

**33. a.** The $SO_3^{2-}$ anion is named sulfite; Li is lithium.

**34. a.** The oxidation numbers of $NO_3^-$ and $I^-$ are generally both −1; to make the net charge zero, the oxidation number for Na must be +1.

**35. b.** Choice **b** is the only one involving a beta particle.

**36. c.** It will take one half-life to decay from 40 g to 20 g; it will take another half-life to decay from 20 g to 10 g. This will take a total of $2.4 \times 10^9$ years.

**37. a.** Uranium is an actinide. Actinides are elements with partially filled 5f orbitals (elements 89–103).

**38. a.** The number of protons is the atomic number, or the lower number; the upper number is the sum of the protons and neutrons, or the atomic mass number.

**39. b.** A ketone features a carbonyl group (C=O) with 2 carbons bound to either side of it.

**40. c.** The only effect of the addition of a catalyst is to increase the rate of reaction. There is no change in the reaction's composition.

**41. a.** Allotropes are two different formats of an element. Ozone and $O_2$ are two different formats for the element oxygen.

**42. c.** For an ideal gas in a fixed volume, temperature and pressure are directly proportional. The temperature must be converted to Kelvin (27°C = 300 K and 117°C = 390 K). The temperature increased by $\frac{390}{300} = 1.3$, and so the new pressure must be 1 atm × 1.3 = 1.3 atm.

**43. a.** Oxyacids of halogens are named by the number of oxygens attached. HClO is hypochlorous acid, $HClO_2$ is chlorous acid, $HClO_3$ is chloric acid, and $HClO_4$ is perchloric acid.

**44. c.** A decomposition reaction involves a single molecule breaking down into two separate molecules.

**45. a.** The electron configuration for Cl is $[Ne]3s^2 3p^5$.

**46. d.** Amines are organic molecules with an $NR_3$ (R = alkyl or hydrogen) group.

**47. a.** $4.12 \times 10^{-3} + 9.54 \times (10^{-3} \times 10^{-2}) = (4.12 + 9.54 \times 10^{-2}) \times 10^{-3} = 4.22 \times 10^{-3}$ (two decimal places as in 4.12 and 9.54)

**48. b.** The weak base thallium (III) hydroxide has a formula of $Tl(OH)_3$, which only changes to $Tl^{3+}$ in a very strong acid.

**49. a.** The conjugate acid, or proton donor, in the system shown here is $H_2PO_4^-$.

**50. a.** This is the only balanced option.

## Scoring

After you take your nursing school entrance exam, a complicated formula will be used to convert your raw score on each section of the test into a percentile. The raw score is simply the number you get right on each section; wrong answers don't count against you. A percentile is a way of comparing your score with that of other test takers; this number indicates what percent of other test takers scored lower than you did on this section.

First, count the number of questions you got right in each section, and record them in the following blanks:

**Section 1:** _____ of 50 questions right
**Section 2:** _____ of 45 questions right
**Section 3:** _____ of 50 questions right
**Section 4:** _____ of 50 questions right
**Section 5:** _____ of 50 questions right
**Section 6:** _____ of 50 questions right

Next, convert your raw score into a *percentage* for each section of the exam. (Remember that this percentage is not the same as a *percentile*.) By now, your quantitative ability should be good enough to tell you how to arrive at a percentage, but if you've forgotten, refer back to the Scoring instructions in Chapter 3.

Now, you can compare your scores on this test with those on the first practice exam. Chances are, your scores went up. If they didn't, it's probably because you took the first practice exam without having to worry about time, whereas in this exam, you had some fairly tight time limits to meet.

So if your scores went *down* between the first practice exam and this one, the problem is not so much the limits of your knowledge as your ability to work quickly without sacrificing accuracy. In that case, reread Chapter 2, "LearningExpress Test Prep System," for tips on how to improve your time management during the exam. Then, practice your time management skills on the sample exam in the next chapter. Before you begin each section, figure out the average amount of time allotted for each question by dividing the number of minutes allowed by the number of questions. Then, as you work through the section, keep yourself moving according to the schedule you've worked out. Remember to rack up the easy points by answering the easiest questions first, leaving the harder questions for last.

On the other hand, if your scores went up, you're probably wondering if they went up enough and, if not, what you should do about it. First of all, remember that no one is expected to score 100% on a section, so don't be too hard on yourself. Here's what you should do, based on your percentage scores on this practice exam:

- **For sections on which you scored less than 50%,** you need some concentrated work in those areas. (If you scored under 50% on all five sections, you might have to postpone taking the exam while you work on your skills.) If biology and chemistry were your problem areas, more work with your textbooks and other materials might be enough, especially if you weren't very conscientious about reviewing before you took this practice exam. For other areas, and for biology and chemistry if you did review your textbooks, an extra college course is your best bet. If you don't have time or money for a complete course, find a tutor who will work with you individually. Most colleges have free or low-cost peer tutorial programs, or you may be able to get help from a professional teacher for a reasonable hourly fee.

- **For sections on which you scored 50–70%,** more review and practice is in order. Find a tutor, or form a study group with other students who are preparing for the nursing school entrance exam. Go to the library or bookstore for other books that review the relevant areas; if those books also contain practice test questions, all the better. When you've done a fair amount of review, go back to the appropriate chapters of this book to review the practice questions and strategies.

- **For sections on which you scored 70–80%,** you're on your way to a score that will look good to the admissions department of your chosen program, but a little more work wouldn't hurt. Start by reviewing the appropriate chapters in this book. If you feel at all shaky about the material, use other resources: additional books, a friend who's good at the appropriate subject, a study group, or a peer tutor.

- **For sections on which you scored more than 80%,** you're in pretty good shape. But you should keep studying and practicing up to the day before the test, so you'll know that you're as prepared as possible to score as well as you can. Keep reviewing Chapters 4–9 of this book right up until test day, and use additional resources whenever you can.

One of the biggest keys to your success on the exam is your self-confidence. The more comfortable you are with your ability to perform, the more likely you are to do well on the exam. You know what to expect, you know your strengths and weaknesses, and you can work to turn those weaknesses into strengths before the actual exam. Your preparedness should give you the confidence that you'll need to do well on exam day.

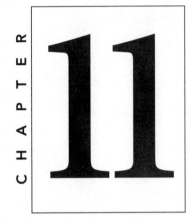

# PRACTICE EXAM III

## CHAPTER SUMMARY

How ready are you? This is the last of the three practice exams presented in this book. Use this test for extra practice and to determine the areas where you should concentrate your attention in the time leading up to exam day.

This practice test will give you additional preparation and help you focus your study in the final days before the exam. As with the two earlier practice exams, this multiple-choice test is designed to reflect the topics and format of the entrance exams used by nursing programs. The four test areas include Verbal Ability, Reading Comprehension, Math, and Science. Although this practice test is general enough to prepare you for any nursing school entrance exam, be sure to investigate the specifics of the test you will be taking. The more you know, the better prepared you will be.

Before you take this third exam, find a quiet place where you can work undisturbed for three hours. Set a timer, stopwatch, or alarm clock to time yourself according to the directions in each section. Work as quickly as you can to meet the time limits, but do not sacrifice accuracy. Stop working when you run out of time, even if you have not answered all of the questions. Allow yourself a five-minute break between each section, and a 15-minute break after Section 3.

Using a number 2 pencil, mark your answers on the answer sheet on page 341. The answer key is located on page 380—refer to this only once you have completed the test. A section about how to score your exam follows the answer key.

# Section 1: Verbal Ability

| 1. | ⓐ | ⓑ | ⓒ | ⓓ | | 18. | ⓐ | ⓑ | ⓒ | ⓓ | | 35. | ⓐ | ⓑ | ⓒ | ⓓ |
|----|---|---|---|---|---|-----|---|---|---|---|---|-----|---|---|---|---|
| 2. | ⓐ | ⓑ | ⓒ | ⓓ | | 19. | ⓐ | ⓑ | ⓒ | ⓓ | | 36. | ⓐ | ⓑ | ⓒ | ⓓ |
| 3. | ⓐ | ⓑ | ⓒ | ⓓ | | 20. | ⓐ | ⓑ | ⓒ | ⓓ | | 37. | ⓐ | ⓑ | ⓒ | ⓓ |
| 4. | ⓐ | ⓑ | ⓒ | ⓓ | | 21. | ⓐ | ⓑ | ⓒ | ⓓ | | 38. | ⓐ | ⓑ | ⓒ | ⓓ |
| 5. | ⓐ | ⓑ | ⓒ | ⓓ | | 22. | ⓐ | ⓑ | ⓒ | ⓓ | | 39. | ⓐ | ⓑ | ⓒ | ⓓ |
| 6. | ⓐ | ⓑ | ⓒ | ⓓ | | 23. | ⓐ | ⓑ | ⓒ | ⓓ | | 40. | ⓐ | ⓑ | ⓒ | ⓓ |
| 7. | ⓐ | ⓑ | ⓒ | ⓓ | | 24. | ⓐ | ⓑ | ⓒ | ⓓ | | 41. | ⓐ | ⓑ | ⓒ | ⓓ |
| 8. | ⓐ | ⓑ | ⓒ | ⓓ | | 25. | ⓐ | ⓑ | ⓒ | ⓓ | | 42. | ⓐ | ⓑ | ⓒ | ⓓ |
| 9. | ⓐ | ⓑ | ⓒ | ⓓ | | 26. | ⓐ | ⓑ | ⓒ | ⓓ | | 43. | ⓐ | ⓑ | ⓒ | ⓓ |
| 10. | ⓐ | ⓑ | ⓒ | ⓓ | | 27. | ⓐ | ⓑ | ⓒ | ⓓ | | 44. | ⓐ | ⓑ | ⓒ | ⓓ |
| 11. | ⓐ | ⓑ | ⓒ | ⓓ | | 28. | ⓐ | ⓑ | ⓒ | ⓓ | | 45. | ⓐ | ⓑ | ⓒ | ⓓ |
| 12. | ⓐ | ⓑ | ⓒ | ⓓ | | 29. | ⓐ | ⓑ | ⓒ | ⓓ | | 46. | ⓐ | ⓑ | ⓒ | ⓓ |
| 13. | ⓐ | ⓑ | ⓒ | ⓓ | | 30. | ⓐ | ⓑ | ⓒ | ⓓ | | 47. | ⓐ | ⓑ | ⓒ | ⓓ |
| 14. | ⓐ | ⓑ | ⓒ | ⓓ | | 31. | ⓐ | ⓑ | ⓒ | ⓓ | | 48. | ⓐ | ⓑ | ⓒ | ⓓ |
| 15. | ⓐ | ⓑ | ⓒ | ⓓ | | 32. | ⓐ | ⓑ | ⓒ | ⓓ | | 49. | ⓐ | ⓑ | ⓒ | ⓓ |
| 16. | ⓐ | ⓑ | ⓒ | ⓓ | | 33. | ⓐ | ⓑ | ⓒ | ⓓ | | 50. | ⓐ | ⓑ | ⓒ | ⓓ |
| 17. | ⓐ | ⓑ | ⓒ | ⓓ | | 34. | ⓐ | ⓑ | ⓒ | ⓓ | | | | | | |

# Section 2: Reading Comprehension

| 1. | ⓐ | ⓑ | ⓒ | ⓓ | | 16. | ⓐ | ⓑ | ⓒ | ⓓ | | 31. | ⓐ | ⓑ | ⓒ | ⓓ |
|----|---|---|---|---|---|-----|---|---|---|---|---|-----|---|---|---|---|
| 2. | ⓐ | ⓑ | ⓒ | ⓓ | | 17. | ⓐ | ⓑ | ⓒ | ⓓ | | 32. | ⓐ | ⓑ | ⓒ | ⓓ |
| 3. | ⓐ | ⓑ | ⓒ | ⓓ | | 18. | ⓐ | ⓑ | ⓒ | ⓓ | | 33. | ⓐ | ⓑ | ⓒ | ⓓ |
| 4. | ⓐ | ⓑ | ⓒ | ⓓ | | 19. | ⓐ | ⓑ | ⓒ | ⓓ | | 34. | ⓐ | ⓑ | ⓒ | ⓓ |
| 5. | ⓐ | ⓑ | ⓒ | ⓓ | | 20. | ⓐ | ⓑ | ⓒ | ⓓ | | 35. | ⓐ | ⓑ | ⓒ | ⓓ |
| 6. | ⓐ | ⓑ | ⓒ | ⓓ | | 21. | ⓐ | ⓑ | ⓒ | ⓓ | | 36. | ⓐ | ⓑ | ⓒ | ⓓ |
| 7. | ⓐ | ⓑ | ⓒ | ⓓ | | 22. | ⓐ | ⓑ | ⓒ | ⓓ | | 37. | ⓐ | ⓑ | ⓒ | ⓓ |
| 8. | ⓐ | ⓑ | ⓒ | ⓓ | | 23. | ⓐ | ⓑ | ⓒ | ⓓ | | 38. | ⓐ | ⓑ | ⓒ | ⓓ |
| 9. | ⓐ | ⓑ | ⓒ | ⓓ | | 24. | ⓐ | ⓑ | ⓒ | ⓓ | | 39. | ⓐ | ⓑ | ⓒ | ⓓ |
| 10. | ⓐ | ⓑ | ⓒ | ⓓ | | 25. | ⓐ | ⓑ | ⓒ | ⓓ | | 40. | ⓐ | ⓑ | ⓒ | ⓓ |
| 11. | ⓐ | ⓑ | ⓒ | ⓓ | | 26. | ⓐ | ⓑ | ⓒ | ⓓ | | 41. | ⓐ | ⓑ | ⓒ | ⓓ |
| 12. | ⓐ | ⓑ | ⓒ | ⓓ | | 27. | ⓐ | ⓑ | ⓒ | ⓓ | | 42. | ⓐ | ⓑ | ⓒ | ⓓ |
| 13. | ⓐ | ⓑ | ⓒ | ⓓ | | 28. | ⓐ | ⓑ | ⓒ | ⓓ | | 43. | ⓐ | ⓑ | ⓒ | ⓓ |
| 14. | ⓐ | ⓑ | ⓒ | ⓓ | | 29. | ⓐ | ⓑ | ⓒ | ⓓ | | 44. | ⓐ | ⓑ | ⓒ | ⓓ |
| 15. | ⓐ | ⓑ | ⓒ | ⓓ | | 30. | ⓐ | ⓑ | ⓒ | ⓓ | | 45. | ⓐ | ⓑ | ⓒ | ⓓ |

## Section 3: Quantitative Ability

| | | | | | | | | | | | | | | |
|---|---|---|---|---|---|---|---|---|---|---|---|---|---|---|
| 1. | ⓐ | ⓑ | ⓒ | ⓓ | 18. | ⓐ | ⓑ | ⓒ | ⓓ | 35. | ⓐ | ⓑ | ⓒ | ⓓ |
| 2. | ⓐ | ⓑ | ⓒ | ⓓ | 19. | ⓐ | ⓑ | ⓒ | ⓓ | 36. | ⓐ | ⓑ | ⓒ | ⓓ |
| 3. | ⓐ | ⓑ | ⓒ | ⓓ | 20. | ⓐ | ⓑ | ⓒ | ⓓ | 37. | ⓐ | ⓑ | ⓒ | ⓓ |
| 4. | ⓐ | ⓑ | ⓒ | ⓓ | 21. | ⓐ | ⓑ | ⓒ | ⓓ | 38. | ⓐ | ⓑ | ⓒ | ⓓ |
| 5. | ⓐ | ⓑ | ⓒ | ⓓ | 22. | ⓐ | ⓑ | ⓒ | ⓓ | 39. | ⓐ | ⓑ | ⓒ | ⓓ |
| 6. | ⓐ | ⓑ | ⓒ | ⓓ | 23. | ⓐ | ⓑ | ⓒ | ⓓ | 40. | ⓐ | ⓑ | ⓒ | ⓓ |
| 7. | ⓐ | ⓑ | ⓒ | ⓓ | 24. | ⓐ | ⓑ | ⓒ | ⓓ | 41. | ⓐ | ⓑ | ⓒ | ⓓ |
| 8. | ⓐ | ⓑ | ⓒ | ⓓ | 25. | ⓐ | ⓑ | ⓒ | ⓓ | 42. | ⓐ | ⓑ | ⓒ | ⓓ |
| 9. | ⓐ | ⓑ | ⓒ | ⓓ | 26. | ⓐ | ⓑ | ⓒ | ⓓ | 43. | ⓐ | ⓑ | ⓒ | ⓓ |
| 10. | ⓐ | ⓑ | ⓒ | ⓓ | 27. | ⓐ | ⓑ | ⓒ | ⓓ | 44. | ⓐ | ⓑ | ⓒ | ⓓ |
| 11. | ⓐ | ⓑ | ⓒ | ⓓ | 28. | ⓐ | ⓑ | ⓒ | ⓓ | 45. | ⓐ | ⓑ | ⓒ | ⓓ |
| 12. | ⓐ | ⓑ | ⓒ | ⓓ | 29. | ⓐ | ⓑ | ⓒ | ⓓ | 46. | ⓐ | ⓑ | ⓒ | ⓓ |
| 13. | ⓐ | ⓑ | ⓒ | ⓓ | 30. | ⓐ | ⓑ | ⓒ | ⓓ | 47. | ⓐ | ⓑ | ⓒ | ⓓ |
| 14. | ⓐ | ⓑ | ⓒ | ⓓ | 31. | ⓐ | ⓑ | ⓒ | ⓓ | 48. | ⓐ | ⓑ | ⓒ | ⓓ |
| 15. | ⓐ | ⓑ | ⓒ | ⓓ | 32. | ⓐ | ⓑ | ⓒ | ⓓ | 49. | ⓐ | ⓑ | ⓒ | ⓓ |
| 16. | ⓐ | ⓑ | ⓒ | ⓓ | 33. | ⓐ | ⓑ | ⓒ | ⓓ | 50. | ⓐ | ⓑ | ⓒ | ⓓ |
| 17. | ⓐ | ⓑ | ⓒ | ⓓ | 34. | ⓐ | ⓑ | ⓒ | ⓓ | | | | | |

## Section 4: General Science

| | | | | | | | | | | | | | | |
|---|---|---|---|---|---|---|---|---|---|---|---|---|---|---|
| 1. | ⓐ | ⓑ | ⓒ | ⓓ | 18. | ⓐ | ⓑ | ⓒ | ⓓ | 35. | ⓐ | ⓑ | ⓒ | ⓓ |
| 2. | ⓐ | ⓑ | ⓒ | ⓓ | 19. | ⓐ | ⓑ | ⓒ | ⓓ | 36. | ⓐ | ⓑ | ⓒ | ⓓ |
| 3. | ⓐ | ⓑ | ⓒ | ⓓ | 20. | ⓐ | ⓑ | ⓒ | ⓓ | 37. | ⓐ | ⓑ | ⓒ | ⓓ |
| 4. | ⓐ | ⓑ | ⓒ | ⓓ | 21. | ⓐ | ⓑ | ⓒ | ⓓ | 38. | ⓐ | ⓑ | ⓒ | ⓓ |
| 5. | ⓐ | ⓑ | ⓒ | ⓓ | 22. | ⓐ | ⓑ | ⓒ | ⓓ | 39. | ⓐ | ⓑ | ⓒ | ⓓ |
| 6. | ⓐ | ⓑ | ⓒ | ⓓ | 23. | ⓐ | ⓑ | ⓒ | ⓓ | 40. | ⓐ | ⓑ | ⓒ | ⓓ |
| 7. | ⓐ | ⓑ | ⓒ | ⓓ | 24. | ⓐ | ⓑ | ⓒ | ⓓ | 41. | ⓐ | ⓑ | ⓒ | ⓓ |
| 8. | ⓐ | ⓑ | ⓒ | ⓓ | 25. | ⓐ | ⓑ | ⓒ | ⓓ | 42. | ⓐ | ⓑ | ⓒ | ⓓ |
| 9. | ⓐ | ⓑ | ⓒ | ⓓ | 26. | ⓐ | ⓑ | ⓒ | ⓓ | 43. | ⓐ | ⓑ | ⓒ | ⓓ |
| 10. | ⓐ | ⓑ | ⓒ | ⓓ | 27. | ⓐ | ⓑ | ⓒ | ⓓ | 44. | ⓐ | ⓑ | ⓒ | ⓓ |
| 11. | ⓐ | ⓑ | ⓒ | ⓓ | 28. | ⓐ | ⓑ | ⓒ | ⓓ | 45. | ⓐ | ⓑ | ⓒ | ⓓ |
| 12. | ⓐ | ⓑ | ⓒ | ⓓ | 29. | ⓐ | ⓑ | ⓒ | ⓓ | 46. | ⓐ | ⓑ | ⓒ | ⓓ |
| 13. | ⓐ | ⓑ | ⓒ | ⓓ | 30. | ⓐ | ⓑ | ⓒ | ⓓ | 47. | ⓐ | ⓑ | ⓒ | ⓓ |
| 14. | ⓐ | ⓑ | ⓒ | ⓓ | 31. | ⓐ | ⓑ | ⓒ | ⓓ | 48. | ⓐ | ⓑ | ⓒ | ⓓ |
| 15. | ⓐ | ⓑ | ⓒ | ⓓ | 32. | ⓐ | ⓑ | ⓒ | ⓓ | 49. | ⓐ | ⓑ | ⓒ | ⓓ |
| 16. | ⓐ | ⓑ | ⓒ | ⓓ | 33. | ⓐ | ⓑ | ⓒ | ⓓ | 50. | ⓐ | ⓑ | ⓒ | ⓓ |
| 17. | ⓐ | ⓑ | ⓒ | ⓓ | 34. | ⓐ | ⓑ | ⓒ | ⓓ | | | | | |

## Section 5: Biology

| | | | |
|---|---|---|---|
| 1. | (a) | (b) | (c) | (d) |
| 2. | (a) | (b) | (c) | (d) |
| 3. | (a) | (b) | (c) | (d) |
| 4. | (a) | (b) | (c) | (d) |
| 5. | (a) | (b) | (c) | (d) |
| 6. | (a) | (b) | (c) | (d) |
| 7. | (a) | (b) | (c) | (d) |
| 8. | (a) | (b) | (c) | (d) |
| 9. | (a) | (b) | (c) | (d) |
| 10. | (a) | (b) | (c) | (d) |
| 11. | (a) | (b) | (c) | (d) |
| 12. | (a) | (b) | (c) | (d) |
| 13. | (a) | (b) | (c) | (d) |
| 14. | (a) | (b) | (c) | (d) |
| 15. | (a) | (b) | (c) | (d) |
| 16. | (a) | (b) | (c) | (d) |
| 17. | (a) | (b) | (c) | (d) |
| 18. | (a) | (b) | (c) | (d) |
| 19. | (a) | (b) | (c) | (d) |
| 20. | (a) | (b) | (c) | (d) |
| 21. | (a) | (b) | (c) | (d) |
| 22. | (a) | (b) | (c) | (d) |
| 23. | (a) | (b) | (c) | (d) |
| 24. | (a) | (b) | (c) | (d) |
| 25. | (a) | (b) | (c) | (d) |
| 26. | (a) | (b) | (c) | (d) |
| 27. | (a) | (b) | (c) | (d) |
| 28. | (a) | (b) | (c) | (d) |
| 29. | (a) | (b) | (c) | (d) |
| 30. | (a) | (b) | (c) | (d) |
| 31. | (a) | (b) | (c) | (d) |
| 32. | (a) | (b) | (c) | (d) |
| 33. | (a) | (b) | (c) | (d) |
| 34. | (a) | (b) | (c) | (d) |
| 35. | (a) | (b) | (c) | (d) |
| 36. | (a) | (b) | (c) | (d) |
| 37. | (a) | (b) | (c) | (d) |
| 38. | (a) | (b) | (c) | (d) |
| 39. | (a) | (b) | (c) | (d) |
| 40. | (a) | (b) | (c) | (d) |
| 41. | (a) | (b) | (c) | (d) |
| 42. | (a) | (b) | (c) | (d) |
| 43. | (a) | (b) | (c) | (d) |
| 44. | (a) | (b) | (c) | (d) |
| 45. | (a) | (b) | (c) | (d) |
| 46. | (a) | (b) | (c) | (d) |
| 47. | (a) | (b) | (c) | (d) |
| 48. | (a) | (b) | (c) | (d) |
| 49. | (a) | (b) | (c) | (d) |
| 50. | (a) | (b) | (c) | (d) |

## Section 6: Chemistry

| | | | |
|---|---|---|---|
| 1. | (a) | (b) | (c) | (d) |
| 2. | (a) | (b) | (c) | (d) |
| 3. | (a) | (b) | (c) | (d) |
| 4. | (a) | (b) | (c) | (d) |
| 5. | (a) | (b) | (c) | (d) |
| 6. | (a) | (b) | (c) | (d) |
| 7. | (a) | (b) | (c) | (d) |
| 8. | (a) | (b) | (c) | (d) |
| 9. | (a) | (b) | (c) | (d) |
| 10. | (a) | (b) | (c) | (d) |
| 11. | (a) | (b) | (c) | (d) |
| 12. | (a) | (b) | (c) | (d) |
| 13. | (a) | (b) | (c) | (d) |
| 14. | (a) | (b) | (c) | (d) |
| 15. | (a) | (b) | (c) | (d) |
| 16. | (a) | (b) | (c) | (d) |
| 17. | (a) | (b) | (c) | (d) |
| 18. | (a) | (b) | (c) | (d) |
| 19. | (a) | (b) | (c) | (d) |
| 20. | (a) | (b) | (c) | (d) |
| 21. | (a) | (b) | (c) | (d) |
| 22. | (a) | (b) | (c) | (d) |
| 23. | (a) | (b) | (c) | (d) |
| 24. | (a) | (b) | (c) | (d) |
| 25. | (a) | (b) | (c) | (d) |
| 26. | (a) | (b) | (c) | (d) |
| 27. | (a) | (b) | (c) | (d) |
| 28. | (a) | (b) | (c) | (d) |
| 29. | (a) | (b) | (c) | (d) |
| 30. | (a) | (b) | (c) | (d) |
| 31. | (a) | (b) | (c) | (d) |
| 32. | (a) | (b) | (c) | (d) |
| 33. | (a) | (b) | (c) | (d) |
| 34. | (a) | (b) | (c) | (d) |
| 35. | (a) | (b) | (c) | (d) |
| 36. | (a) | (b) | (c) | (d) |
| 37. | (a) | (b) | (c) | (d) |
| 38. | (a) | (b) | (c) | (d) |
| 39. | (a) | (b) | (c) | (d) |
| 40. | (a) | (b) | (c) | (d) |
| 41. | (a) | (b) | (c) | (d) |
| 42. | (a) | (b) | (c) | (d) |
| 43. | (a) | (b) | (c) | (d) |
| 44. | (a) | (b) | (c) | (d) |
| 45. | (a) | (b) | (c) | (d) |
| 46. | (a) | (b) | (c) | (d) |
| 47. | (a) | (b) | (c) | (d) |
| 48. | (a) | (b) | (c) | (d) |
| 49. | (a) | (b) | (c) | (d) |
| 50. | (a) | (b) | (c) | (d) |

## Section 1: Verbal Ability

Find the correctly spelled word in the following questions. You have 15 minutes to complete 50 questions.

1. a. compete
   b. compeet
   c. compeete
   d. compet

2. a. audable
   b. audible
   c. audiable
   d. auddable

3. a. entirity
   b. entirrety
   c. entirety
   d. intirety

4. a. gradually
   b. gradualy
   c. gradualely
   d. gradualey

5. a. preambel
   b. preamble
   c. priambel
   d. priamble

6. a. stomacheache
   b. stomacache
   c. stomachache
   d. stomackache

7. a. madness
   b. maddness
   c. maddnes
   d. madnesse

8. a. porcelain
   b. porcelin
   c. porcilin
   d. porcilain

9. a. delirious
   b. delerious
   c. delireous
   d. dilerious

10. a. pleed
    b. plede
    c. plead
    d. plaed

11. a. inundated
    b. innundated
    c. inondatted
    d. inundatid

12. a. funnyer
    b. funier
    c. funyer
    d. funnier

13. a. obediant
    b. obeddient
    c. obedient
    d. obedeint

14. a. prosecuted
    b. prossecuted
    c. prosecutted
    d. prosecuited

15. a. counterfiet
    b. counterfit
    c. countirfit
    d. counterfeit

**16. a.** symetricaly
**b.** symetrically
**c.** symmetricully
**d.** symmetrically

**17. a.** dalaying
**b.** delaing
**c.** deleying
**d.** delaying

**18. a.** vacuum
**b.** vaccuum
**c.** vacum
**d.** vacume

**19. a.** acomodate
**b.** acommodate
**c.** acommedate
**d.** accommodate

**20. a.** incredulus
**b.** incredulous
**c.** increduluos
**d.** incredulis

**21. a.** trauma
**b.** trouma
**c.** troma
**d.** trama

**22. a.** marrigeable
**b.** marrageable
**c.** marriageable
**d.** mariageable

**23. a.** ilegible
**b.** illegible
**c.** ilegable
**d.** illegable

**24. a.** penicillen
**b.** penicillin
**c.** penicillen
**d.** penicilin

**25. a.** adolescense
**b.** adolessents
**c.** adolescence
**d.** adolscence

Find the misspelled word in the following questions.

**26. a.** eloquent
**b.** eased
**c.** cheesey
**d.** no mistakes

**27. a.** potatoes
**b.** sopranoes
**c.** albinos
**d.** no mistakes

**28. a.** aggitate
**b.** pigment
**c.** vault
**d.** no mistakes

**29. a.** trophy
**b.** replenish
**c.** simultaneus
**d.** no mistakes

**30. a.** coughing
**b.** oasis
**c.** laughable
**d.** no mistakes

**31. a.** encapsulate
**b.** thesisis
**c.** braided
**d.** no mistakes

**32. a.** debateable
   **b.** enviable
   **c.** despicable
   **d.** no mistakes

**33. a.** flys
   **b.** business
   **c.** acquisition
   **d.** no mistakes

**34. a.** border
   **b.** bullitin
   **c.** magazine
   **d.** no mistakes

**35. a.** recoyle
   **b.** perspiration
   **c.** fumble
   **d.** no mistakes

**36. a.** marginal
   **b.** syllable
   **c.** fraudelent
   **d.** no mistakes

**37. a.** problematic
   **b.** questionniare
   **c.** controversial
   **d.** no mistakes

**38. a.** pungaent
   **b.** aromatic
   **c.** spicy
   **d.** no mistakes

**39. a.** hybrid
   **b.** hypnosis
   **c.** hygeinic
   **d.** no mistakes

**40. a.** judge
   **b.** ilegal
   **c.** magistrate
   **d.** no mistakes

**41. a.** correspondent
   **b.** corrosivness
   **c.** coronation
   **d.** no mistakes

**42. a.** acrobat
   **b.** somersault
   **c.** gymnist
   **d.** no mistakes

**43. a.** tenacious
   **b.** consequence
   **c.** glorify
   **d.** no mistakes

**44. a.** inept
   **b.** plentiful
   **c.** shawl
   **d.** no mistakes

**45. a.** panicy
   **b.** jittery
   **c.** nervous
   **d.** no mistakes

**46. a.** spiteful
   **b.** hungrier
   **c.** crazyness
   **d.** no mistakes

**47. a.** yellowish
   **b.** spoiled
   **c.** returnable
   **d.** no mistakes

**48. a.** chiase
 **b.** lounge
 **c.** seat
 **d.** no mistakes

**49. a.** extremly
 **b.** abundance
 **c.** dancing
 **d.** no mistakes

**50. a.** spiteful
 **b.** freindly
 **c.** laughing
 **d.** no mistakes

# Section 2:
# Reading Comprehension

Read each passage and answer the accompanying questions based only on the information found in the passage. You have 45 minutes to complete this section.

It is well known that the early months and years of life are critical for brain development. But the question remains: Just how do early influences act on the brain to promote or challenge the developmental process? Research has suggested that both positive and negative experiences, chronic stressors, and various other environmental factors may affect a young child's developing brain. And now, studies involving animals are revealing in greater detail how this may occur.

One important line of research has focused on brain systems that control stress hormones—cortisol, for example. Cortisol and other stress hormones play an important role in emergencies: they help our bodies make energy available to enable effective responses, temporarily suppress the immune response, and sharpen attention. However, a number of studies conducted in people with depression

indicate that excess cortisol released over a long span of time may have many negative health consequences. Excess cortisol may cause shrinking of the hippocampus, a brain structure required for the formation of certain types of memory.

In experiments with animals, scientists have shown that a well-defined period of early postnatal development may be an important determinant of the capacity to handle stress throughout life. In one set of studies, rat pups were removed from their mothers each day for a period as brief as 15 minutes and then returned. The natural maternal response of instinctively licking and grooming the returned pup was shown to alter the brain chemistry of the pup in a positive way, making the animal less reactive to stressful stimuli. While these pups are able to mount an appropriate stress response in the face of threat, their response does not become excessive or inappropriate. Rat mothers who spontaneously lick and groom their pups with the same intensity even without human handling of the pups also produce pups that have a similarly stable reaction, including an appropriate stress hormone response.

Striking differences were seen in rat pups that were removed from their mothers for periods of three hours a day, a model of maternal neglect, when compared to pups that were not separated. After three hours, the mother rats tended to ignore the pups, at least initially, upon their return. In sharp contrast to those pups that were greeted attentively by their mothers after a short absence, the "neglected" pups were shown to have a more profound and excessive stress response in subsequent tests. This response appeared to last into adulthood.

It is far too early to draw firm conclusions from these animal studies about the extent to which early life experience produces a long-lived or permanent set point for stress responses or influences the development of the cerebral cortex in humans. However, animal models that show the interactive effect of stress and brain development deserve serious consideration and continued study.

1. As used in paragraph five, what does the word *draw* mean?
   a. attract
   b. sketch
   c. make
   d. tie

2. Which of the following is true of rat pups that were removed from their mothers for periods of three hours a day in the study?
   a. They helped to prove the validity of the study.
   b. They displayed relatively normal stress response levels.
   c. They received little attention when first returned to their mothers.
   d. They developed physical problems that lasted into adulthood.

3. What was the overall point of the study discussed in the passage?
   a. to show that rats facing stressful experiences when young remained distressed as they aged
   b. to study how the parenting skills of rats differ from the parenting skills of humans
   c. to prove that parental neglect can occur in animals as much as it can in humans
   d. to measure the amount of separation time between parent and child that will lead to distress

4. What is the main idea of this passage?
   a. to prove via a clinical study that parental neglect leads to significant turmoil and stress as an adult
   b. to introduce the concept that significant stress when young can permanently alter brain functions
   c. to show via animals that parents should not leave a child alone for more than 15 minutes
   d. to prove that good parenting will lead to children who do not easily get stressed

5. Which of the following is true, according to paragraphs 3 and 4?
   a. The animals removed from their parents for only 15 minutes did not show signs of stress.
   b. Scientists found that the pups removed for three hours had heightened levels of cortisol compared with those removed for 15 minutes.
   c. Rat pups are used to being licked and groomed by their mothers.
   d. The goal of the experiment was to eliminate stress levels from the pups in order to apply their findings to humans.

6. What is the best definition of the word *promote* in paragraph 1?
   a. endorse
   b. advance
   c. affect
   d. hinder

**7.** According to the passage, which of the following is NOT true about stress?

**a.** Parents should avoid exposing their children to any stress at the critical early ages.

**b.** Stress helps drive the body during an emergency situation.

**c.** Stress can help delay physical response to stimuli during a crisis.

**d.** Excessive stress as a toddler may permanently alter the brain.

A very low-calorie diet (VLCD) is a doctor-supervised diet that typically uses commercially prepared formulas to promote rapid weight loss in patients who are obese. These formulas, usually liquid shakes or bars, replace all food intake for several weeks or months. VLCD formulas need to contain appropriate levels of vitamins and micronutrients to ensure that patients meet their nutritional requirements. Some physicians also prescribe VLCDs made up almost entirely of lean protein foods, such as fish and chicken. People on a VLCD consume about 800 calories per day or less. VLCD formulas are not the same as the meal replacements you can find at grocery stores or pharmacies, which are meant to replace one or two meals a day. Over-the-counter meal replacements, such as bars, entrees, or shakes, should account for only part of one's daily calories.

When used under proper medical supervision, VLCDs may produce significant short-term weight loss in patients who are moderately to extremely obese. VLCDs should be part of comprehensive weight-loss treatment programs that include behavioral therapy, nutrition counseling, physical activity, and/or drug treatment.

VLCDs are designed to produce rapid weight loss at the start of a weight-loss program in patients with a body mass index (BMI) greater than 30 and significant co-morbidities.

BMI correlates significantly with total body fat content. It is calculated by dividing a person's weight in pounds by height in inches squared and multiplied by 703. Use of VLCDs in patients with a BMI of 27 to 30 should be reserved for those who have medical conditions due to being overweight, such as high blood pressure. In fact, all candidates for VLCDs undergo a thorough examination by their healthcare provider to make sure the diet will not worsen preexisting medical conditions. These diets are not appropriate for children or adolescents, except in specialized treatment programs.

Very little information exists regarding the use of VLCDs in older adults. Because adults over age 50 already experience depletion of lean body mass, use of a VLCD may not be warranted. Also, people over 50 may not tolerate the side effects associated with VLCDs because of preexisting medical conditions or the need for other medicines. Doctors must evaluate on a case-by-case basis the potential risks and benefits of rapid weight loss in older adults, as well as in patients who have significant medical problems or are on medications. Furthermore, doctors must monitor all VLCD patients regularly—ideally every two weeks in the initial period of rapid weight loss—to be sure they are not experiencing serious side effects.

A VLCD may allow a patient who is moderately to extremely obese to lose about three to five pounds per week for an average total weight loss of 44 pounds over 12 weeks. Such a weight loss can rapidly improve obesity-related medical conditions, including diabetes, high blood pressure, and high cholesterol. The rapid weight loss experienced by most people on a VLCD can be very motivating. Patients who participate in a VLCD program that includes lifestyle treatment typically lose about 15% to 25% of their initial weight during the first three to six months. They may maintain a 5% weight loss after four years if they adopt a healthy eating plan and physical activity habits.

Many patients on a VLCD for four to 16 weeks report minor side effects, such as fatigue, constipation, nausea, or diarrhea. These conditions usually improve within a few weeks and rarely prevent patients from completing the program. The most common serious side effect is gallstone formation. Gallstones, which often develop in people, especially women, who are obese, are even more common during rapid weight loss. Research indicates that rapid weight loss may increase cholesterol levels in the gallbladder and decrease its ability to contract and expel bile. Some medicines can prevent gallstone formation during rapid weight loss. A healthcare provider can determine if these treatments are appropriate.

8. What is a good title for this passage?
   a. VLCDs: An Easy Path to Weight-Loss Success
   b. The Risks of a VLCD Diet
   c. An Option for Combating Obesity in Adults
   d. What Your BMI Says about Your Health

9. According to the passage, which of the following is often related to obesity?
   a. nausea
   b. diabetes
   c. body mass depletion
   d. diarrhea

10. A person of which age would likely have the least lean body mass?
    a. 11
    b. 21
    c. 41
    d. 61

11. According to the passage, which of the following is true about people on a VLCD?
    a. They may eventually start feeling excessively weary.
    b. They always suffer permanent negative side effects.
    c. They will not see results until six months after starting the diet.
    d. They enjoy health benefits such as a decrease of gallstones

12. According to the passage, what is true of a person's BMI level?
    a. A person who is 200 pounds and 6 feet tall will have a lower BMI than a person who is 200 pounds and 5.5 feet tall.
    b. BMI takes your age into account.
    c. A person with obese parents will have a higher BMI than a person with parents of a normal weight.
    d. You should start a VLCD if your BMI level is over 30.

13. What can be inferred from the passage about the specifics of a VLCD?
    a. Maintaining a successful VLCD is a simple matter of exact calories.
    b. Patients on VLCDs eat only about two times a day.
    c. VLCDs work best if they are comprised only of liquid shakes that contain all the appropriate nutrients.
    d. VLCDs must be rich in vitamins in order to work to their full potential.

A government report addressing concerns about the many implications of genetic testing outlined policy guidelines and legislative recommendations intended to avoid involuntary and ineffective testing and protect confidentiality.

The report identified urgent concerns, such as quality control measures (including federal oversight for testing laboratories) and better genetics training for medical practitioners. It recommended voluntary screening, urged couples in high-risk populations to consider carrier screening, and advised caution in using and interpreting presymptomatic or predictive tests, as certain information could easily be misused or misinterpreted.

About three in every 100 children are born with a severe disorder presumed to be genetic or partially genetic in origin. Genes, often in concert with environmental factors, are being linked to the causes of many common adult diseases, such as coronary artery disease, hypertension, various cancers, diabetes, and Alzheimer's disease. Tests to determine predisposition to a variety of conditions are under study, and some are beginning to be applied.

The report recommended that all screening, including screening of newborns, be voluntary. Citing results of two different voluntary newborn screening programs, the report said that these programs can achieve compliance rates equal to or better than those of mandatory programs. State health departments could eventually mandate the offering of tests for diagnosing treatable conditions in newborns; however, careful pilot studies for conditions diagnosable at birth need to be conducted first.

Although the report asserted that it would prefer all screening to be voluntary, it did note that if a state requires newborn screening for a particular condition, the state should do so only if there is strong evidence that a newborn would benefit from effective treatment at the earliest possible age. Newborn screening is the most common type of genetic screening today. More than four million newborns are tested annually so that effective treatment can be started in a few hundred affected infants.

Prenatal testing can pose the most difficult issues. The ability to diagnose genetic disorders in the fetus far exceeds any ability to treat or cure them. Parents must be fully informed about risks and benefits of testing procedures, the nature and variability of the disorders they would disclose, and the options available if test results are positive. Obtaining informed consent—a process that would include educating participants, not just processing documents—would enhance voluntary participation. When offered testing, parents should receive comprehensive counseling, which should be nondirective. Relevant medical advice, however, is recommended for treatable or preventable conditions.

Genetics also can predict whether certain diseases might develop later in life. For single-gene diseases, population screening should only be considered for treatable or preventable conditions of relatively high frequency. Children should be tested only for disorders for which effective treatments or preventive measures could be applied early in life.

14. Based on how it is used in the passage, the word *prenatal* most nearly means
   a. newborn.
   b. genetic disorder.
   c. before birth.
   d. undisclosed.

15. Out of 300 children, about how many are likely to be born with severe genetic disorders?
   a. 3
   b. 9
   c. 30
   d. 100

**16.** How many infants are treated for genetic disorders as a result of newborn screening?
a. dozens
b. hundreds
c. thousands
d. millions

**17.** One intention of the policy guidelines was to
a. implement compulsory testing.
b. minimize concerns about quality control.
c. endorse the expansion of screening programs.
d. preserve privacy in testing.

**18.** According to the report, states should implement mandatory infant screening only
a. if the compliance rate for voluntary screening is low.
b. for mothers who are at high risk for genetic disease.
c. after meticulous research is undertaken.
d. to avoid the abuse of sensitive information.

**19.** The most prevalent form of genetic testing is conducted on
a. high-risk populations.
b. adults.
c. fetuses prior to birth.
d. infants shortly after birth.

Scientists have developed an innovative procedure that reveals details of tissues and organs that are difficult to see by conventional magnetic resonance imaging (MRI). By using "hyperpolarized" gases, scientists have taken the first clear MRI pictures of human lungs and airways. Researchers hope the new technique will aid the diagnosis and treatment of lung disorders and perhaps lead to improved visualization of blood flow.

The air spaces of the lungs have been notoriously difficult for clinicians to visualize. Chest X-rays can detect tumors or inflamed regions in the lungs but provide poor soft-tissue contrast and no clear view of air passages. Computed tomography, a cross sectional X-ray scan, can provide high-resolution images of the walls of the lungs and its airways but gives no measure of function. Conventional MRI, because it images water protons, provides poor images of the lungs, which are filled with air, not water.

The new MRI technique detects not water, but inert gases whose nuclei have been strongly aligned, or hyperpolarized, by laser light. Initially, this technique seemed to have no practical application, but exhaustive research has proven its potential. Scientists plan to further refine this technology with animal and human studies, in part because they have yet to produce a viable 3-D image of human lungs (as of this editing).

By 1995, researchers had produced the first 3-D MRI pictures of a living animal's lungs. In the first human test, a member of the research team inhaled hyperpolarized helium-3. His lungs were then imaged using a standard MRI scanner that had been adjusted to detect helium. The results were impressive, considering that the system had yet to be optimized and there was only a relatively small volume of gas with which to work.

When a standard MRI is taken, the patient enters a large magnet. Many of the body's hydrogen atoms (primarily the hydrogen atoms in water) align with the magnetic field like tiny bar magnets, and the nucleus at the center of each atom spins constantly about its north-south axis. Inside the MRI scanner, a radio pulse temporarily knocks the spinning nuclei out of position, and as their axes gradually realign within the magnetic field, they emit faint radio signals. Computers convert these faint signals into an image.

The new gas-based MRI is built around similar principles. But circularly polarized light, rather than a magnet, is used to align spinning nuclei, and the inert gases helium-3 or xenon-129 (rather than hydrogen) provide the nuclei that emit the image-producing signals. The laser light polarizes the gases through a technique known as *spin exchange*. Helium-3 and xenon-129 are ideal for gas-based MRI because they take hours to lose their polarization. Most other gases readily lose their alignment. The clarity of an MRI picture depends in part on the volume of aligned nuclei.

**20.** The MRI innovation is different from the standard MRI in that it
  **a.** distinguishes gases rather than water.
  **b.** uses magnets rather than light.
  **c.** has a range of useful applications.
  **d.** provides better images of blood circulation.

**21.** The inability to generate satisfactory images of air routes is a deficiency of
  **a.** computed tomography.
  **b.** the spin exchange process.
  **c.** 3-D pictures.
  **d.** chest X-rays.

**22.** Which of the following is a flaw of conventional MRI?
  **a.** It cannot detect water.
  **b.** It provides poor images of the lungs.
  **c.** It only visualizes blood flow.
  **d.** It polarizes gases.

**23.** The word that can best be interchanged with *hyperpolarization* in the passage is
  **a.** visualization.
  **b.** alignment.
  **c.** emission.
  **d.** tomography.

**24.** Use of which of the following is substituted for use of a magnet in one of the MRI techniques?
  **a.** light
  **b.** hydrogen
  **c.** helium-3
  **d.** X-rays

**25.** An image lacking in clarity is likely to be the result of
  **a.** a high number of aligned nuclei.
  **b.** hydrogen being replaced with xenon.
  **c.** an abbreviated period of alignment.
  **d.** nuclei regaining their aligned position.

Once people wore garlic around their necks to ward off disease. Today, most Americans would scoff at the idea of wearing a necklace of garlic cloves to enhance their well-being. However, you might find a number of Americans willing to ingest capsules of pulverized garlic or other herbal supplements in the name of health.

Complementary and alternative medicine (CAM), which includes a range of practices outside of conventional medicine, such as herbs, homeopathy, massage, yoga, and acupuncture, holds increasing appeal for Americans. In fact, according to one estimate, 42% of Americans have used alternative therapies. A Harvard Medical School survey found that adults born between 1965 and 1979 are the most likely to use alternative treatments, whereas people born before 1945 are the least likely to use these therapies. Nonetheless, in all age groups, the use of unconventional healthcare practices has steadily increased since the 1950s, and the trend is likely to continue.

CAM has become a big business as Americans dip into their wallets to pay for alternative treatments. A 1997 American Medical Association study estimated that the public spent $21.2 billion for alternative medicine therapies in that year, more than half of which were "out-of-pocket" expenditures, meaning they were not covered by health insurance. Indeed, Americans made more out-of-pocket expenditures for alternative services than they did for out-of-pocket payments for hospital stays in 1997. In addition, the number of total visits to alternative medicine providers (about 629 million) exceeded the number of visits to primary care physicians (386 million) in that year.

However, the public has not abandoned conventional medicine for alternative healthcare. Most Americans seek out alternative therapies as a complement to their conventional healthcare, whereas only a small percentage of Americans rely primarily on alternative care. Why have so many patients turned to alternative therapies? Frustrated by the time constraints of managed care and alienated by conventional medicine's focus on technology, some feel that a holistic approach to healthcare better reflects their beliefs and values. Others seek therapies that will relieve symptoms associated with chronic disease, symptoms that mainstream medicine cannot treat.

Some alternative therapies have crossed the line into mainstream medicine as scientific investigation has confirmed their safety and efficacy. For example, today physicians may prescribe acupuncture for pain management or to control the nausea associated with chemotherapy. Most U.S. medical schools teach courses in alternative therapies, and many health insurance companies offer some alternative medicine benefits. Yet, despite their gaining acceptance, the majority of alternative therapies have not been researched in controlled studies. New research efforts aim at testing alternative methods and providing the public with information about which ones are safe and effective and which ones are a waste of money or possibly dangerous.

So what about those who swear by the health benefits of the "smelly rose," garlic?

Observational studies that track disease incidence in different populations suggest that garlic use in the diet may act as a cancer-fighting agent, particularly for prostate and stomach cancer. However, these findings have not been confirmed in clinical studies. And, yes, reported side effects include garlic odor.

26. The author describes wearing garlic as an example of
    a. an arcane practice considered odd and superstitious today.
    b. the ludicrous nature of complementary and alternative medicine.
    c. a scientifically tested medical practice.
    d. a socially unacceptable style of jewelry.

27. As it is used in the second paragraph, the word *practices* most nearly means
    a. businesses.
    b. routines.
    c. usages.
    d. studies.

28. The author most likely uses the Harvard survey results in the second paragraph to imply that
    a. as people age, they always become more conservative.
    b. people born before 1945 view alternative therapies with disdain.
    c. the survey did not question baby boomers (those born between 1945 and 1965) on the topic.
    d. many younger adults are open-minded to alternative therapies.

**29.** The statistic in the third paragraph comparing total visits to alternative medicine practitioners with those to primary care physicians is used to illustrate the
  a. popularity of alternative medicine.
  b. public's distrust of conventional healthcare.
  c. accessibility of alternative medicine.
  d. affordability of alternative therapies.

**30.** In paragraph four, *complement* most nearly means
  a. tribute.
  b. commendation.
  c. replacement.
  d. addition.

**31.** The information in the fourth paragraph indicates that Americans believe that conventional healthcare
  a. offers the best relief from the effects of chronic diseases.
  b. should not use technology in treating illness.
  c. combines caring for the body with caring for the spirit.
  d. falls short of their expectations in some aspects.

In space flight, there are the obvious hazards of meteors, debris, and radiation; however, astronauts must also deal with two vexing physiological foes—muscle atrophy and bone loss. Space shuttle astronauts undergo minimal wasting of bone and muscle because they spend only about a week in space. But when longer stays in microgravity or zero gravity are contemplated, as in the space station or a two-year round-trip voyage to Mars, these problems are of particular concern because they could become acute.

Some studies show that muscle atrophy can be kept largely at bay with appropriate exercise, but bone loss caused by reduced gravity cannot. Scientists can measure certain flight-related hormonal changes and obtain animal bone biopsies immediately after flights, but they do not completely understand how gravity affects the bones or what happens at the cellular level.

Even pounding the bones or wearing a suspender-like pressure device does nothing to avert loss of calcium from bones. Researchers say that after a three-month or longer stay in space, much of the profound bone loss may be irreversible. Some argue that protracted missions should be curtailed. They are conducting a search for the molecular mechanisms behind bone loss, and they hope these studies will help develop a prevention strategy to control tissue loss associated not only with weightlessness but also with prolonged bed rest.

Doctors simulate bone-depleting microgravity conditions by putting volunteers to bed for long time periods. The bed support of the supine body decreases the load on it significantly, thus simulating reduced gravity. One study involves administering either alendronate, a drug that blocks the breakdown of bone, or a placebo, a look-alike substance without medical effects, to volunteers for two weeks prior to and then during a three-week bed rest.

Prior to bed rest, alendronate-treated volunteers excreted only about one-third as much calcium as did the persons receiving the placebo. Bed rest increased urinary calcium excretion in both groups, but in alendronate-treated persons, the urinary calcium levels were even lower than those in the placebo group before bed rest. Blood levels of parathyroid hormone and vitamin D, which are involved in regulation of bone metabolism, were also significantly elevated in drug recipients.

Although these results suggest that alendronate inhibits bone loss and averts high urinary calcium concentrations that can cause kidney stones, they do not point to the precise molecular mechanisms at work.

**32.** Astronauts who exercise regularly can
   **a.** expect bone loss to be temporary.
   **b.** greatly reduce the amount of muscle atrophy.
   **c.** use special implements that maintain calcium levels.
   **d.** minimize the percentage of bone loss.

**33.** Compared to volunteers who received a placebo, volunteers who received alendronate experienced
   **a.** lower levels of parathyroid hormone.
   **b.** lower levels of hormonal changes.
   **c.** more elevated levels of vitamin D.
   **d.** higher levels of calcium excretion.

**34.** Specialized equipment for astronauts in weightless conditions
   **a.** reduces the amount of calcium in their bones.
   **b.** makes lengthy space flights more feasible.
   **c.** enables scientists to better comprehend molecular mechanisms.
   **d.** has a negligible impact on bone loss.

**35.** The passage suggests that the bone-loss studies may yield information that could aid the treatment of
   **a.** kidney stones.
   **b.** muscular atrophy.
   **c.** thyroid disease.
   **d.** urinary infections.

**36.** What is the minimum amount of time someone would have to be in space in order to lose an amount of bone that may never be regained?
   **a.** about 15 days
   **b.** about 30 days
   **c.** about 60 days
   **d.** about 90 days

About three million Americans have open-angle glaucoma, the most common form of glaucoma in the United States. For unknown reasons, small changes within the eye gradually interfere with the normal flow of fluids that feed tissues in the front of the eye. If these fluids do not drain properly, the resulting higher pressure inside the eye can damage the optic nerve and narrow the field of vision. This change happens so slowly that many people are not diagnosed with glaucoma until they have significant loss of vision.

Laser therapy is a safe and effective alternative to eye drops as a first-line treatment for patients with newly diagnosed primary open-angle glaucoma. This finding comes from a follow-up study undertaken to learn if early laser treatment is safe and whether it offers any medical advantages over eye drops for newly diagnosed open-angle glaucoma. A total of 271 patients were enrolled in the initial study. Each patient had laser treatment in one eye and medication in the other eye. Over two hundred patients were followed for an average of seven years after treatment.

Post-study analysis revealed that all measures used to evaluate the two treatments showed that the "laser-first" eyes and the "medication-first" eyes had a similar status on all measures used to evaluate the two treatments. Researchers assessed changes in the patient's visual field, visual acuity, intraocular pressure, and optic nerve. The results suggested that initial treatment with laser surgery is at least as effective as initial treatment with eye drops. However, researchers cautioned that neither treatment method is a "magic bullet" for long-term control of glaucoma. They noted that two years after the start of treatment, 56% of "laser-first" eyes and 70% of "medication-first" eyes needed new or extra medications to control pressure inside the eye.

Researchers noted that both treatments caused side effects. However, the side effects of laser treatment were temporary or made no apparent difference in the long run, whereas the side effects of eye drops were troublesome for some patients for as long as the drops were used. Eye drops used for glaucoma treatment can cause discomfort in the eye, blurry vision, headaches, and fast or slow heartbeat.

In 34% of "laser-first" eyes, the laser treatment caused a temporary jump in intraocular pressure for the first few days after treatment. Also, about 30% of the "laser-first" eyes developed *peripheral anterior synechiae*—adhesions that form when the iris sticks to part of the cornea.

**37.** Over half the patients in the study discussed in the passage required supplemental treatment for
   **a.** optic nerve damage.
   **b.** intraocular pressure.
   **c.** visual field weakness.
   **d.** lack of visual acuity.

**38.** The primary purpose of the passage is to
   **a.** advocate the use of glaucoma medication.
   **b.** define the needs of glaucoma patients.
   **c.** defend the safety of laser treatment for glaucoma.
   **d.** weigh the effects of glaucoma treatments.

**39.** Greater pressure within the eye results from
   **a.** a disruption of fluid concentration.
   **b.** the rapid accumulation of fluids.
   **c.** a gradual broadening of the field of vision.
   **d.** initial treatment with eye drops.

**40.** The study concluded that, compared with medication, laser therapy is
   **a.** slightly more effective.
   **b.** significantly more effective.
   **c.** just as effective.
   **d.** less effective.

**41.** The study was conducted on patients who were
   **a.** in the initial stages of open-angle glaucoma.
   **b.** experiencing a rare form of glaucoma.
   **c.** given eye drop medication in both eyes.
   **d.** in the late stages of open-angle glaucoma.

Almost 50% of American teens are not vigorously active on a regular basis, contributing to a trend of sluggishness among Americans of all ages, according the U.S. Centers for Disease Control (CDC). Adolescent female students are particularly inactive—29% are inactive compared with 15% of male students. Unfortunately, the sedentary habits of young "couch potatoes" often continue into adulthood. According to the Surgeon General's 1996 Report on Physical Activity and Health, Americans become increasingly less active with each year of age. Inactivity can be a serious health risk factor, setting the stage for obesity and associated chronic illnesses like heart disease or diabetes. The benefits of exercise include building bone, muscle, and joints; controlling weight; and preventing the development of high blood pressure.

Some studies suggest that physical activity may have other benefits as well. One CDC study found that high school students who take part in team sports or are physically active outside of school are less likely to engage in risky behaviors, such as using drugs or smoking. Physical activity does not need to be strenuous to be beneficial. The CDC recommends moderate, daily physical activity for people of all ages, such as brisk walking for 30 minutes or 15 to 20 minutes of more intense exercise. A survey conducted by the National Association for Sport and Physical Education questioned teens about their attitudes toward exercise and what it would take to get them moving. Teens chose friends (56%) as their most likely motivators for becoming more active, followed by parents (18%) and professional athletes (11%).

**42.** The first paragraph of the passage serves all of the following purposes EXCEPT
   **a.** to provide statistical information to support the claim that teenagers do not exercise enough.
   **b.** to list long-term health risks associated with lack of exercise.
   **c.** to express skepticism that teenagers can change their exercise habits.
   **d.** to show a correlation between inactive teenagers and inactive adults.

**43.** In the first paragraph, *sedentary* most nearly means
   **a.** slothful.
   **b.** apathetic.
   **c.** stationary.
   **d.** stabilized.

**44.** Which of the following techniques is used in the last sentence of the passage?
   **a.** explanation of terms
   **b.** comparison of different arguments
   **c.** contrast of opposing views
   **d.** illustration by example

**45.** The primary purpose of the passage is to
   **a.** refute an argument.
   **b.** make a prediction.
   **c.** praise an outcome.
   **d.** promote a change.

## Section 3: Quantitative Ability

Choose the correct answer for each problem. You have 45 minutes to complete this section.

**1.** How many inches are there in $3\frac{1}{3}$ yards?
   **a.** 120
   **b.** 126
   **c.** 160
   **d.** 168

**2.** $\frac{3}{4} + \frac{5}{7}$ is equal to
   **a.** $\frac{8}{11}$
   **b.** $1\frac{6}{7}$
   **c.** $1\frac{1}{4}$
   **d.** $1\frac{13}{28}$

**3.** 0.97 is equal to
   **a.** 97%
   **b.** 9.7%
   **c.** 0.97%
   **d.** 0.097%

**4.** In triangle *ABC*, angle *A* is 70° and angle *B* is 30°. What is the measure of angle *C*?
   **a.** 90°
   **b.** 70°
   **c.** 80°
   **d.** 100°

**5.** Rectangle *QRST* is divided into two congruent triangles by line segment *QS*. What is the area of triangle *QRS*?

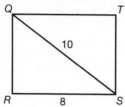

a. 24 units$^2$

b. 40 units$^2$

c. 48 units$^2$

d. 80 units$^2$

**6.** With Ace Insurance, the co-payment for a visit to Dr. Patel's office is $20. If the co-payment is $13\frac{1}{3}$% of the full price, how much does Dr. Patel charge for an office visit, rounded to the nearest dollar?

a. $133

b. $150

c. $200

d. $267

**7.** The nursing assistants give baths to the patients every morning at 7:00. NA Garcia gives Ms. Rogers her bath in 20 minutes. NA West gives Mr. Taft his bath in 17 minutes, and NA Owens gives Ms. Johnson her bath in 14 minutes. What is the average time for the three baths?

a. 20 minutes

b. 17 minutes

c. 14 minutes

d. 12 minutes

**8.** In Lake City, the average time it takes a fire engine to travel from the firehouse to the scene of a fire is 6 minutes. If the fire engine travels at a speed of 58 miles per hour, what is the average distance of a fire from the firehouse?

a. 5.8 miles

b. 6.0 miles

c. 9.7 miles

d. 10.3 miles

**9.** A hospital waiting room is 8 feet wide and 10 feet long. What is the area of the waiting room?

a. 18 square feet

b. 40 square feet

c. 60 square feet

d. 80 square feet

**10.** Mr. Beard's temperature is 98°F. What is his temperature in degrees Celsius?

$C = \frac{5}{9}(F - 32)$

a. 35.8°

b. 36.7°

c. 37.6°

d. 31.1°

**11.** $\frac{2}{5} \times \frac{3}{7}$ is equal to

a. $\frac{6}{35}$

b. $\frac{14}{15}$

c. $\frac{5}{12}$

d. $\frac{29}{35}$

**12.** $12 + (14 \times 7)$ is equal to

a. 98

b. 266

c. 110

d. 100

**13.** Which of the following is 14% of 232?
   **a.** 3.248
   **b.** 32.48
   **c.** 16.57
   **d.** 165.7

**14.** One side of a square bandage is 4 inches long. What is the perimeter of the bandage?
   **a.** 4 inches
   **b.** 8 inches
   **c.** 12 inches
   **d.** 16 inches

**15.** What is the value of $x$ if $38 = x^2 - 11$?
   **a.** $3\sqrt{3}$
   **b.** 7
   **c.** 27
   **d.** 49

**16.** If Marisol orders her textbooks at least two weeks before the semester starts, she will save 15% on her order. Unfortunately, she does not have a chance to order her textbooks until a week after the semester starts and spends $385. How much money would she have saved if she had been able to order her textbooks two weeks before the semester started?
   **a.** $25.67
   **b.** $57.75
   **c.** $327.25
   **d.** $370.00

**17.** $945.6 \div 24$ is equal to
   **a.** 3,940
   **b.** 394
   **c.** 39.4
   **d.** 3.946

**18.** At a local clinic, there are twice as many nurses as doctors on staff. There are also three fewer medical technicians than nurses. If the total number of staff equals 37, how many doctors are there?
   **a.** 8
   **b.** 19
   **c.** 25
   **d.** 34

**19.** The radius of a circle is 13. What is the approximate area of the circle?
   **a.** 81.64
   **b.** 1,666.27
   **c.** 530.66
   **d.** 169

**20.** $\frac{7}{8} - \frac{3}{5}$ is equal to
   **a.** $\frac{11}{40}$
   **b.** $1\frac{1}{3}$
   **c.** $\frac{1}{10}$
   **d.** $1\frac{19}{40}$

**21.** How many hours are in $4\frac{1}{6}$ days?
   **a.** 86
   **b.** 96
   **c.** 100
   **d.** 102

**22.** 0.15% of what number is equal to 0.5?
   **a.** $6\frac{2}{3}$
   **b.** $13\frac{1}{3}$
   **c.** $333\frac{1}{3}$
   **d.** $1,333\frac{1}{3}$

**23.** What is the value of $5x + 3y + 6xy$ when $x = 2$ and $y = 3$?
   **a.** 31
   **b.** 55
   **c.** 57
   **d.** 60

**24.** What is the diameter of a circle with an area of $121\pi$?
 a. 11
 b. 12
 c. 21
 d. 22

**25.** There are three different-colored candies in a bag. If $\frac{1}{3}$ of the candies are red and $\frac{1}{4}$ of the candies are blue, what fraction of the candies is green?
 a. $\frac{5}{12}$
 b. $\frac{1}{2}$
 c. $\frac{7}{12}$
 d. $\frac{6}{7}$

**26.** If Tyrone can type 62 words per minute, how many words can he type in $1\frac{1}{8}$ hours?
 a. $67\frac{1}{2}$
 b. $69\frac{3}{4}$
 c. 3,720
 d. 4,185

**27.** What percentage of 18,000 is 234?
 a. 1,300%
 b. 130%
 c. 13%
 d. 1.3%

**28.** How many minutes are in $7\frac{1}{6}$ hours?
 a. 430 minutes
 b. 2,580 minutes
 c. 4,300 minutes
 d. 258 minutes

**29.** 72.687 + 145.29 is equal to
 a. 87.216
 b. 217.977
 c. 217.877
 d. 882.16

**30.** $12(84 - 5) - (3 \times 54)$ is equal to
 a. 54,000
 b. 841
 c. 796
 d. 786

**31.** $43 + (-5) - 12 - (-2) + 12$ is equal to
 a. 36
 b. 40
 c. 46
 d. 50

**32.** After four books were put on a shelf, there were three times as many books on the shelf as before. How many books were on the shelf before the addition?
 a. one
 b. two
 c. three
 d. four

**33.** The value of $2x + 1$ is how much greater than the value of $x - 2$?
 a. $x - 1$
 b. $x - 3$
 c. $x + 3$
 d. $2x - 1$

**34.** When Gary left the house on his way to work, he saw that the mileage gauge on his car registered $10,593\frac{4}{5}$ miles. When he arrived at work, he noted that the gauge registered $10,610\frac{1}{5}$ miles. How far does Gary live from work?
 a. $16\frac{2}{5}$ miles
 b. 17 miles
 c. $17\frac{2}{5}$ miles
 d. 18 miles

**35.** $2\frac{3}{4} \div \frac{3}{8}$ is equal to
   **a.** $1\frac{1}{32}$
   **b.** 6
   **c.** $7\frac{1}{3}$
   **d.** 16

**36.** $4\frac{1}{5} + 1\frac{2}{5} + 3\frac{3}{10}$ is equal to
   **a.** $9\frac{1}{10}$
   **b.** $8\frac{9}{10}$
   **c.** $8\frac{4}{5}$
   **d.** $8\frac{6}{15}$

**37.** What is the reciprocal of $8\frac{8}{7}$?
   **a.** $\frac{64}{7}$
   **b.** $7\frac{7}{8}$
   **c.** $\frac{7}{64}$
   **d.** $\frac{56}{8}$

**38.** $\frac{14}{25}$ is equal to
   **a.** 0.056
   **b.** 0.56
   **c.** 5.6
   **d.** 56.0

**39.** 5.9 − 4.166 is equal to
   **a.** 1.844
   **b.** 1.843
   **c.** 1.744
   **d.** 1.734

**40.** A truck is 16 feet 2 inches long and a car is 13 feet 6 inches long. How much longer is the truck?
   **a.** 2 feet 6 inches
   **b.** 2 feet 8 inches
   **c.** 3 feet 4 inches
   **d.** 3 feet 8 inches

**41.** 172 × 0.56 is equal to
   **a.** 9.632
   **b.** 96.32
   **c.** 963.2
   **d.** 0.9632

**42.** There are 16 patients in the waiting room. After an hour, the number of waiting patients is reduced by 62.5%. After another hour, the number of patients is reduced by $66\frac{2}{3}$%. How many patients are left in the waiting room after 2 hours?
   **a.** 2
   **b.** 4
   **c.** 6
   **d.** 7

**43.** A nurse administering medication to the patients on her floor spends 30 seconds traveling from one patient to the next and 1 minute with each patient while they take their medication. If there are 22 patients on the floor, how long does it take the nurse to administer medication to all the patients on the floor?
   **a.** 22 minutes 30 seconds
   **b.** 32 minutes
   **c.** 32 minutes 30 seconds
   **d.** 33 minutes

**44.** 35% of what number is equal to 14?
   **a.** 4
   **b.** 40
   **c.** 49
   **d.** 400

**45.** A piece of gauze 3 feet 4 inches long was divided into five equal parts. How long was each part?
   **a.** 1 foot 2 inches
   **b.** 10 inches
   **c.** 8 inches
   **d.** 6 inches

**46.** There were three robberies in Glenville this month, down 25% from the previous month. How many robberies were there in Glenville last month?
   **a.** 4
   **b.** 5
   **c.** 6
   **d.** 7

**47.** Myrna's Beauty Salon is open from 8:45 A.M. to 7:30 P.M. and is closed from 12:15 P.M. to 1:00 P.M. for lunch. How many total hours is the salon in business?
   **a.** 9 hours 15 minutes
   **b.** 10 hours
   **c.** 10 hours 30 minutes
   **d.** 10 hours 45 minutes

**48.** If $4x + 8 = 40$, then what is $3x - 4$?
   **a.** 2
   **b.** 8
   **c.** 12
   **d.** 20

**49.** A certain faucet can fill a 255-gallon tank in 15 minutes. At this rate, how many more minutes would it take to drain a full 340-gallon tank?
   **a.** 5
   **b.** $5\frac{2}{3}$
   **c.** $7\frac{2}{3}$
   **d.** 20

**50.** A gymnast earned the following scores from the judges: 8.7, 8.9, 9.1, 9.0, 8.7. What was her average score?
   **a.** 8.70
   **b.** 8.88
   **c.** 8.95
   **d.** 11.10

# Section 4: General Science

There are 50 questions in this section. You have 45 minutes to complete this section.

**1.** The Earth's core is
   **a.** divided into two parts.
   **b.** also called the mantle.
   **c.** largely composed of lead.
   **d.** located 400 miles beneath the surface.

**2.** When did Earth form?
   **a.** 4.6 billion years ago
   **b.** 3.5 billion years ago
   **c.** 4.6 hundred million years ago
   **d.** 3.5 hundred million years ago

**3.** The lithosphere is
   **a.** relatively light and deep.
   **b.** relatively light and uppermost.
   **c.** relatively heavy and deep.
   **d.** relatively heavy and uppermost.

**4.** Most weather phenomena occur in the
   **a.** lithosphere.
   **b.** troposphere.
   **c.** thermosphere.
   **d.** stratosphere.

**5.** The average depth of the ocean is about
   **a.** 0.5 km.
   **b.** 10 km.
   **c.** 2 km.
   **d.** 4 km.

**6.** Earth's mantle
   **a.** is between the crust and the core.
   **b.** is under the core and the crust.
   **c.** is heavier than the core.
   **d.** contains both crust and core.

**7.** Most of the rock at the Earth's surface is
   **a.** sedimentary.
   **b.** metamorphic.
   **c.** igneous.
   **d.** bedrock.

**8.** 49% of natural diamonds originate from
   **a.** North America.
   **b.** Central and Southern Africa.
   **c.** Australia.
   **d.** Russia.

**9.** The four planets in the Solar System known as the gas giants are Jupiter, Saturn, Neptune, and
   **a.** Mars.
   **b.** Uranus.
   **c.** Mercury.
   **d.** Venus.

**10.** What kind of rock is obsidian?
   **a.** sedimentary
   **b.** igneous
   **c.** metamorphic
   **d.** mantle

**11.** In which century did the world see the biggest population increase?
   **a.** 13th
   **b.** 20th
   **c.** 19th
   **d.** 17th

**12.** How long does it take the global atmosphere to circulate?
   **a.** one day
   **b.** one year
   **c.** one decade
   **d.** one century

**13.** What ultimately drives the circulation of the atmosphere and ocean?
   **a.** the biosphere
   **b.** the sun
   **c.** volcanism
   **d.** the lithosphere

**14.** The atmospheres of Venus and Mars, unlike that of Earth, are mainly composed of what gas?
   **a.** carbon dioxide
   **b.** oxygen
   **c.** nitrogen
   **d.** argon

**15.** The timescale for the entire ocean to mix is about
   **a.** one year.
   **b.** one decade.
   **c.** one thousand years.
   **d.** one hundred thousand years.

**16.** If you have $10^6$ grams of a metal, how many grams do you have?
   **a.** 1,000 (one thousand)
   **b.** 100,000 (one hundred thousand)
   **c.** 1,000,000 (one million)
   **d.** 1,000,000,000 (one billion)

**17.** Which type of chemical reaction is responsible for the radiation emitted by stars?
   **a.** nuclear fission
   **b.** nuclear fusion
   **c.** oxidation-reduction
   **d.** acid-base

**18.** Which trait best describes the nucleus of an atom?
   **a.** contains the electrons of the atom
   **b.** has an overall positive charge
   **c.** has no mass
   **d.** cannot be altered

**19.** Which of the following contributes to acid rain?
a. deforestation
b. burning fossil fuels
c. invasive species
d. carbon sequestration

**20.** After cigarette smoking, what is the second leading cause of lung cancer?
a. carbon monoxide
b. acid rain
c. ozone
d. radon gas

**21.** In which biome are the solar collecting organs of the net primary producers particularly tough due to large amounts of the chemical called lignin?
a. tundra
b. tropical dry forest
c. deciduous forest
d. boreal forest

**22.** Which of the following is true in biological classification?
a. Family is equal to genus.
b. A genus has many families.
c. Genus is equal to species.
d. A genus has many species.

**23.** Uranus and Neptune are composed mainly of
a. rocks.
b. metals.
c. various ices.
d. hydrogen.

**24.** High-temperature magma behaves much like
a. running water.
b. rubber.
c. thick oil.
d. a sponge.

**25.** The special type of cell division that creates gametes (cells with half the number of chromosomes) from an individual male or female in a sexual species is called
a. mitosis.
b. symbiosis.
c. parthenogenesis.
d. meiosis.

**26.** Carbon monoxide is a primary air pollutant that is derived from
a. incomplete combustion of fossil fuels.
b. deforestation.
c. burning hydrogen gas.
d. photochemical smog.

**27.** The upper part of the ocean that receives light is the
a. benthos.
b. heterotrophic zone.
c. hyphae.
d. pelagic zone.

**28.** Which of the following biomes is characterized by short growing seasons and small plants that reproduce quickly?
a. boreal forest
b. deciduous forest
c. deserts
d. tundra

**29.** Which of the following levels of classification is most inclusive?
a. class
b. kingdom
c. order
d. family

30. Dolly the sheep was involved in what scientific achievement?
    a. the first genetically modified animal
    b. the first animal-to-human organ transplant
    c. the first cloned mammal
    d. the first animal-human hybrid

31. The limit to a population of a species in a community, determined by environmental conditions or species interactions, is called the
    a. ultimate yield.
    b. maximum sustainable yield.
    c. carrying capacity.
    d. deadlock number.

32. A source of marine protein that is increasing in supply is
    a. aquaculture.
    b. upwelling zones.
    c. pelagic fishing.
    d. benthic fishing.

33. In addition to performing photosynthesis, plants also perform respiration for an internal function. They do this when
    a. animals eat them.
    b. capturing sunlight.
    c. creating photosynthesized molecules.
    d. building other molecules from simple sugars.

34. Two gases that contain carbon and are released by bacteria are
    a. sulfuric acid and methane.
    b. carbon dioxide and methane.
    c. sulfuric acid and water.
    d. water and carbon dioxide.

35. Bacteria that live in nodules attached to the roots of certain plants perform the chemical transformation called
    a. denitrification.
    b. ammonification.
    c. nitrification.
    d. nitrogen fixation.

36. Negative population growth in some countries is due to
    a. sub-replacement fertility rates.
    b. overpopulation.
    c. high fertility rates.
    d. medical technology.

37. The main supply of phosphorus to the ocean (and thus to marine life in the ocean) is carried as phosphate ions via
    a. wind.
    b. undersea volcanoes.
    c. rain.
    d. rivers.

38. From most to least, in terms of mass, the four most abundant elements in the human body are
    a. H, C, Fe, P.
    b. H, C, P, Fe.
    c. C, H, P, Fe.
    d. C, P, Fe, H.

39. Which is NOT a macronutrient?
    a. copper
    b. magnesium
    c. nitrogen
    d. sulfur

**40.** During the hunting and gathering period of human history, prior to agriculture, the global population was about
   **a.** ten thousand.
   **b.** ten billion.
   **c.** one hundred thousand.
   **d.** ten million.

**41.** How does the seafloor change as you move outward from the mid-ocean ridge?
   **a.** It gets older.
   **b.** It gets younger.
   **c.** It gets rockier.
   **d.** It gets thinner.

**42.** Toxicology is the study of
   **a.** viruses.
   **b.** transportation.
   **c.** poisons.
   **d.** cancers.

**43.** The Cambrian Explosion refers to a time when
   **a.** Earth became populated with many new forms of life.
   **b.** the universe began expanding outward.
   **c.** Earth's tectonic plates began splitting apart.
   **d.** the seafloor began spreading.

**44.** Which of the following parts of a cell convert food nutrients into high-energy molecules?
   **a.** chloroplasts
   **b.** microtubes
   **c.** lipids
   **d.** mitochondria

**45.** What is removed from water in the process of desalination?
   **a.** salt
   **b.** lead
   **c.** electrolytes
   **d.** pollution

**46.** The burning of a fossil fuel does not create
   **a.** greenhouse gases.
   **b.** stratospheric ozone.
   **c.** carbon dioxide.
   **d.** acid rain.

**47.** Methane in Earth's atmosphere is a greenhouse gas, as is $CO_2$. A greenhouse gas
   **a.** absorbs shortwave radiation and is transparent to longwave radiation.
   **b.** absorbs shortwave radiation and reflects longwave radiation.
   **c.** absorbs longwave radiation and is transparent to shortwave radiation.
   **d.** absorbs longwave radiation and reflects shortwave radiation.

**48.** The chemical formula for ozone is
   **a.** $O$.
   **b.** $O_2$.
   **c.** $O_3$.
   **d.** $O_4$.

**49.** Nitrates and sulfates in Earth's atmosphere create
   **a.** polar melting.
   **b.** acid rain.
   **c.** the greenhouse effect.
   **d.** equilibrium clouds.

**50.** The most poisoning deaths annually occur due to
   **a.** carbon monoxide poisoning.
   **b.** carbon trioxide poisoning.
   **c.** ozone poisoning.
   **d.** hydroxide poisoning.

# Section 5: Biology

There are 50 questions in this section. You have 45 minutes to complete this section.

1. Which of the following vitamins prevents scurvy, aids in the production of collagen, and may boost the immune system?
   a. vitamin K
   b. vitamin C
   c. vitamin A
   d. vitamin D

2. What is another term for the meat preservatives that contain the $NO_2^-$ ion?
   a. nitrites
   b. nitrates
   c. sodium chloride
   d. sodium hydrochloride

3. Which of the following actions is controlled by smooth muscles?
   a. running
   b. heartbeat
   c. peristalsis
   d. movement of bones and joints

4. The resting potential of a neuron is
   a. −70 mV.
   b. +70 mV.
   c. −50 mV.
   d. 0 mV.

5. An important function of a plant's root system is to
   a. produce glucose through photosysnthesis.
   b. break down organic compounds.
   c. release carbon dioxide.
   d. absorb minerals and water from the soil.

6. A defect in an organism's alveoli would affect which function of what organ system?
   a. constant blood pressure by the circulatory system
   b. air exchange by the respiratory system
   c. nutrient absorption by the digestion system
   d. enzyme secretion by the endocrine system

7. Organisms with greater diversity and more adaptations typically utilize
   a. asexual reproduction.
   b. meiosis.
   c. natural selection.
   d. mitosis.

8. The resulting single cell from an egg fertilized by a sperm is called a(n)
   a. monomer.
   b. embryo.
   c. fetus.
   d. zygote.

9. A flowering plant relies on fruit for all of the following EXCEPT
   a. protection of the embryo.
   b. pollination.
   c. seed dispersal.
   d. propagation.

10. Instead of providing nutrients to the embryo in the form of an egg, mammalian mothers provide nutrients to the developing embryo through the
    a. fallopian tubes.
    b. uterus.
    c. placenta.
    d. ovaries.

**11.** Which of the following groups of organisms produces flowers?
a. angiosperms
b. mosses
c. gymnosperms
d. fungi

**12.** Which of the following is NOT an effect of the hormone adrenaline?
a. enhancement of the effects of sympathetic nerves
b. decrease in blood sugar
c. increase in heart rate
d. inhibition of the movement of smooth muscles in the stomach and intestines

**13.** A disease related to the thyroid gland is
a. diabetes mellitus.
b. Addison's disease.
c. rickets.
d. goiter.

**14.** To which specialist would a patient with a suspected tumor most likely be referred?
a. an oncologist
b. a urologist
c. a podiatrist
d. a cardiologist

**15.** All of the following bones are found in the human leg EXCEPT the
a. fibula.
b. ulna.
c. patella.
d. femur.

**16.** Which of the following parts of the brain controls breathing rates?
a. the medulla oblongata
b. the cerebellum
c. the thalamus
d. the temporal lobe

**17.** For the DNA segment 5′ AAT-GAC-TGG 3′, what mRNA segment will be generated by transcription?
a. 5′ TTA-CTG-ACC 3′
b. 5′ UUA-CUG-ACC 3′
c. 5′ CCA-GUC-AUU 3′
d. 5′ CCA-GTC-ATT 3′

**18.** In what organelle does most protein synthesis occur?
a. the nucleus
b. the ribosome
c. the cytoplasm
d. the lysosome

**19.** Which of the following best defines an antigen?
a. a chemical that prevents blood clotting
b. a chemical extracted from a living microbe
c. an antibody that attaches itself to a toxin and renders the toxin harmless
d. a substance that stimulates the production of antibodies

**20.** Cell membranes generally have which of the following structures?
a. phospholipid bilayer
b. amino acid monolayer
c. amino peptide bilayer
d. phosphopeptide monolayer

**21.** Which of the following is a vertebrate?
a. a sponge
b. a starfish
c. an octopus
d. a snake

**22.** In genetics, what kind of diagram indicates all of the possible genotypes in the offspring generation of a Mendelian cross?
a. Punnett square
b. flow chart
c. periodic table
d. test square

**23.** Which of the following is the function of a ligament?
  **a.** to connect bones
  **b.** to connect muscles
  **c.** to attach muscle to bone
  **d.** to serve as a cushion between vertebrae

**24.** Which of the following plants lacks a vascular system?
  **a.** a moss
  **b.** a fern
  **c.** a fir tree
  **d.** a peanut plant

**25.** An energy-rich molecule found in cells is
  **a.** adrenaline.
  **b.** adenosine triphosphate.
  **c.** acetylcholine.
  **d.** amino acids.

**26.** Processes that have encouraged genetic diversity include all of the following EXCEPT
  **a.** sexual reproduction.
  **b.** cross linking.
  **c.** mitosis.
  **d.** genetic recombination.

**27.** Mutations are favored when they lead to adaptations. However, which of the following does NOT cause a beneficial mutation?
  **a.** a toxin
  **b.** a carcinogen
  **c.** gene linkage
  **d.** codons

**28.** Which of the following is an example of an exocrine gland?
  **a.** pineal
  **b.** pituitary
  **c.** salivary
  **d.** adrenal

**29.** A plant expresses yellow flowers (Y) over white flowers (y) and tall stalks (T) are dominant over short (t). Two of these plants are crossed and the results recorded in the table below. What must the genotypes of the parents be?

| | |
|---|---|
| Yellow/Tall | 30 |
| Yellow/Short | 25 |
| White/Tall | 27 |
| White/Short | 20 |

  **a.** YYTT × yytt
  **b.** YyTt × YyTt
  **c.** YyTt × yytt
  **d.** yytt × yytt

**30.** Blood type is determined by the three alleles A, B, and i. Type AB blood results from having both the A and B alleles. What will the genotype be for type O blood?
  **a.** ii
  **b.** AB
  **c.** Ai
  **d.** Bi

**31.** What molecule is the terminal source of electrons during photosynthesis?
  **a.** $H_2O$
  **b.** $O_2$
  **c.** $CO_2$
  **d.** $C_6H_{12}O_6$

**32.** Which of the following structures prevents the rupture of the tympanic membrane when a person changes altitude?
  **a.** the cochlea
  **b.** the ossicles
  **c.** the Eustachian tube
  **d.** the pinna

**33.** An osteocyte is a
a. muscle cell.
b. blood cell.
c. nerve cell.
d. bone cell.

**34.** Bat wings and bird wings are an example of
a. homologous structures.
b. vestigial structures.
c. analogous structures.
d. divergent structures.

**35.** In the scientific name for the emperor penguin, *Aptenodytes forsteri*, the word *Aptenodytes* indicates the
a. phylum.
b. genus.
c. species.
d. order.

**36.** Which of the following substances is NOT an enzyme?
a. lactase
b. lactose
c. sucrase
d. amylase

**37.** The human appendix and the coccyx are examples of
a. homologous structures.
b. vestigial structures.
c. analogous structures.
d. convergent structures.

**38.** A chemical signal emitted by one animal to stimulate a specific response in another animal of the same species is called a(n)
a. hormone.
b. pheromone.
c. antigen.
d. receptor.

**39.** In messenger RNA, a codon contains how many nucleotides?
a. one
b. two
c. three
d. four

**40.** Which of the following is another word for the digits in the hands and feet of vertebrates?
a. carpals
b. tarsals
c. phalanges
d. metacarpals

**41.** Fungi eating the nutrients of a dead plant is an example of
a. mutualism.
b. commensalism.
c. parasitism.
d. decomposition.

**42.** Which of the following is an example of a predator-prey relationship?
a. a goat grazing grass
b. a tick feeding off of a deer
c. a scorpion eating a spider
d. a caterpillar eating leaves

**43.** All of the following are forms of connective tissue EXCEPT
a. tendons.
b. adipose tissue.
c. blood.
d. nerves.

**44.** The specialized organ system that is responsible for filtering out impurities from the blood and excreting them is the
a. respiratory system.
b. renal system.
c. circulatory system
d. endocrine system

45. Sickle-cell anemia is a recessive genetic disorder that decreases the amount of oxygen carried by red blood cells. Individuals have painful attacks, and their life expectancy is shortened. Which of the following statements is true?
    a. Both parents must pass the defective allele to offspring with the disease.
    b. The allele should disappear from the gene pool in the future.
    c. One parent must show symptoms of the disorder.
    d. The mutation is not useful at all.

46. Which of the following is the region between two nerve cells across which electrical and chemical signals are transmitted?
    a. neuron
    b. myelin sheath
    c. synapse
    d. axon

47. When egg cells are created and grow in an animal ovary, the process is called
    a. oogenesis.
    b. oocyte.
    c. oogonia.
    d. ova.

48. A genetic disorder caused by a mutation on the X chromosome
    a. will only affect men.
    b. will only affect women.
    c. is more likely to affect men.
    d. is more likely to affect women.

49. In humans, the ossicles, utricle, and cochlea are all part of which organ?
    a. the stomach
    b. the heart
    c. the ear
    d. the brain

50. Which of the following drugs is NOT a stimulant?
    a. cocaine
    b. nicotine
    c. alcohol
    d. amphetamines

## Section 6: Chemistry

There are 50 questions in this section. Use the periodic table on this page when necessary to help you answer the questions. You have 45 minutes to complete this section.

1. Which of the following has the greatest mass?
   a. 0.5 moles of uranium (U)
   b. 5 moles of electrons
   c. 10 molecules of $C_6H_{12}O_6$
   d. 20 molecules of protons

2. Iodine-123, which is used in tumor scans, has a half-life of 13 hours. If the hospital currently has 110 grams of iodine-123, how long will it be before the sample decays to less than 12 grams?
   a. about 6.5 hours
   b. about 13 hours
   c. about 22 hours
   d. about 44 hours

3. What is the formula for the compound copper (II) oxide?
   a. CuO
   b. $Cu_2O$
   c. $CuO_2$
   d. $Cu_2O_2$

| IA | | | | | | | | | | | | | | | | | VIIA | VIIIA |
|---|---|---|---|---|---|---|---|---|---|---|---|---|---|---|---|---|---|---|
| 1 **H** 1.00794 | IIA | | | | | | | | | | | | | | | | 1 **H** 1.00794 | 2 **He** 4.002602 |
| 3 **Li** 6.941 | 4 **Be** 9.012182 | | | | | | | | | | | IIIA | IVA | VA | VIA | | | |
| | | | | | | | | | | | | 5 **B** 10.811 | 6 **C** 12.0107 | 7 **N** 14.00674 | 8 **O** 15.9994 | 9 **F** 18.9984032 | 10 **Ne** 20.1797 | |
| 11 **Na** 22.989770 | 12 **Mg** 24.3050 | IIIB | IVB | VB | VIB | VIIB | | VIIIB | | | IB | IIB | 13 **Al** 26.981538 | 14 **Si** 28.0855 | 15 **P** 30.973761 | 16 **S** 32.066 | 17 **Cl** 35.4527 | 18 **Ar** 39.948 |
| 19 **K** 39.0983 | 20 **Ca** 40.078 | 21 **Sc** 44.955910 | 22 **Ti** 47.867 | 23 **V** 50.9415 | 24 **Cr** 51.9961 | 25 **Mn** 54.938049 | 26 **Fe** 55.845 | 27 **Co** 58.933200 | 28 **Ni** 58.6934 | 29 **Cu** 63.546 | 30 **Zn** 65.39 | 31 **Ga** 69.723 | 32 **Ge** 72.61 | 33 **As** 74.92160 | 34 **Se** 78.96 | 35 **Br** 79.904 | 36 **Kr** 83.80 |
| 37 **Rb** 85.4678 | 38 **Sr** 87.62 | 39 **Y** 88.90585 | 40 **Zr** 91.224 | 41 **Nb** 92.90638 | 42 **Mo** 95.94 | 43 **Tc** (98) | 44 **Ru** 101.07 | 45 **Rh** 102.90550 | 46 **Pd** 106.42 | 47 **Ag** 107.8682 | 48 **Cd** 112.411 | 49 **In** 114.818 | 50 **Sn** 118.710 | 51 **Sb** 121.760 | 52 **Te** 127.60 | 53 **I** 126.90447 | 54 **Xe** 131.29 |
| 55 **Cs** 132.90545 | 56 **Ba** 137.327 | 57 **La*** 138.9055 | 72 **Hf** 178.49 | 73 **Ta** 180.9479 | 74 **W** 183.84 | 75 **Re** 186.207 | 76 **Os** 190.23 | 77 **Ir** 192.217 | 78 **Pt** 195.078 | 79 **Au** 196.96655 | 80 **Hg** 200.59 | 81 **Tl** 204.3833 | 82 **Pb** 207.2 | 83 **Bi** 208.98038 | 84 **Po** (209) | 85 **At** (210) | 86 **Rn** (222) |
| 87 **Fr** (223) | 88 **Ra** (226) | 89 **Ac**** (227) | 104 **Rf** (261) | 105 **Db** (262) | 106 **Sg** (263) | 107 **Bh** (262) | 108 **Hs** (265) | 109 **Mt** (266) | 110 **Ds** (269) | 111 **Rg** (281) | 112 **Cn** (285) | 113 **Uut** (286) | 114 **Uuq** (289) | 115 **Uup** (289) | 116 **Uuh** (289) | 117 **Uus** (294) | 118 **Uuo** (293) |

| * Lanthanide series | 58 **Ce** 140.116 | 59 **Pr** 140.90765 | 60 **Nd** 144.24 | 61 **Pm** (145) | 62 **Sm** 150.36 | 63 **Eu** 151.964 | 64 **Gd** 157.25 | 65 **Tb** 158.92534 | 66 **Dy** 162.50 | 67 **Ho** 164.93032 | 68 **Er** 167.26 | 69 **Tm** 168.93421 | 70 **Yb** 173.04 | 71 **Lu** 174.967 |
|---|---|---|---|---|---|---|---|---|---|---|---|---|---|---|
| ** Actinide series | 90 **Th** 232.0381 | 91 **Pa** 231.03588 | 92 **U** 238.0289 | 93 **Np** (237) | 94 **Pu** (244) | 95 **Am** (243) | 96 **Cm** (247) | 97 **Bk** (247) | 98 **Cf** (251) | 99 **Es** (252) | 100 **Fm** (257) | 101 **Md** (258) | 102 **No** (259) | 103 **Lr** (262) |

**4.** $2Al_{(s)} + Fe_2O_{3(s)} \overset{\rightarrow}{\leftarrow} Al_2O_{3(s)} + 2Fe_{(l)}$
If a reaction produces 1.2 moles of Fe, how much $Fe_2O_3$ was consumed in the reaction?

a. 0.6 moles

b. 0.6 grams

c. 1.2 moles

d. 1.2 grams

**5.**

Capsaicin, the molecule shown above, is responsible for the spicy taste of chilies. It possesses all of the following functional groups except

a. amide.

b. alcohol.

c. ether.

d. carboxylic acid

**6.** What is the product when an acid and a base combine?

a. water and a salt

b. hydrogen and a salt

c. an oxidant and a reductant

d. no reaction occurs

**7.** Identify the oxidizing agent and the reducing agent in the following reaction:
$8H^+_{(aq)} + 6Cl^-_{(aq)} + Sn_{(s)} + 4NO^-_{3(aq)} \rightarrow$
$SnCl^{2-}_{6(aq)} + 4NO_{2(g)} + 4H_2O_{(l)}$

a. oxidizing agent: $8H^+_{(aq)}$, reducing agent: $Sn_{(s)}$

b. oxidizing agent: $4NO^-_{3(aq)}$, reducing agent: $Sn_{(s)}$

c. oxidizing agent: $4NO^-_{3(aq)}$, reducing agent: $4NO_{2(g)}$

d. oxidizing agent: $4NO^-_{3(aq)}$, reducing agent: $8H^+_{(aq)}$

**8.** Balance the following redox reaction:
$Mg_{(s)} + H_2O_{(g)} \rightarrow Mg(OH)_{2(s)} + H_{2(g)}$

a. $Mg_{(s)} + H_2O_{(g)} \rightarrow Mg(OH)_{2(s)} + H_{2(g)}$

b. $Mg_{(s)} + 4H_2O_{(g)} \rightarrow Mg(OH)_{2(s)} + H_{2(g)}$

c. $Mg_{(s)} + 2H_2O_{(g)} \rightarrow Mg(OH)_{2(s)} + H_{2(g)}$

d. $Mg_{(s)} + H_2O_{(g)} \rightarrow Mg(OH)_{2(s)} + \frac{1}{2}H_{2(g)}$

**9.** Classify the following reaction as a combination, decomposition, or single or double displacement reaction:
$Cr(NO_3)_{3(aq)} + Al_{(s)} \rightarrow Al(NO_3)_{3(aq)} + Cr_{(s)}$

a. combination

b. decomposition

c. single displacement

d. double displacement

**10.** Classify the following reaction as a combination, decomposition, or single or double displacement reaction:
$PF_{3(g)} + F_{2(g)} \rightarrow PF_{5(g)}$

a. decomposition

b. combination

c. single displacement

d. double displacement

**11.** Balance the following equation:
$Ba(OH)_{2(aq)} + HNO_{3(aq)} \rightarrow Ba(NO_3)_{2(aq)} + H_2O_{(l)}$

a. $Ba(OH)_{2(aq)} + 2HNO_{3(aq)} \rightarrow Ba(NO_3)_{2(aq)} + 2H_2O_{(l)}$

b. $Ba(OH)_{2(aq)} + 2HNO_{3(aq)} \rightarrow Ba(NO_3)_{2(aq)} + 4H_2O_{(l)}$

c. $Ba(OH)_{2(aq)} + 2HNO_{3(aq)} \rightarrow Ba(NO_3)_{2(aq)} + H_2O_{(l)}$

d. $Ba(OH)_{2(aq)} + HNO_{3(aq)} \rightarrow Ba(NO_3)_{2(aq)} + H_2O_{(l)}$

**12.** What is the chemical formula for the polyatomic ion nitrite?

a. $N_2O^-$

b. $NO^{2-}$

c. $NO_2^-$

d. $NO_3^-$

**13.** Which reactant is oxidized and which is reduced in the following reacton?

$$C_2H_{4(g)} + 3O_{2(g)} \rightarrow 2CO_{2(g)} + 2H_2O_{(g)}$$

a. oxidized: $C_2H_{4(g)}$, reduced: $3O_{2(g)}$

b. oxidized: $C_2H_{4(g)}$, reduced: $2H_2O_{(g)}$

c. oxidized: $C_2H_{4(g)}$, reduced: $2CO_{2(g)}$

d. oxidized: $2CO_{2(g)}$, reduced: $C_2H_{4(g)}$

**14.** Which one of the following compounds is a nonelectrolyte when dissolved in water?

a. KOH

b. $NH_3$

c. NaBr

d. $CaCl_2$

**15.** Which of the following solutions will have the highest electrical conductivity?

a. 0.1M $AlCl_3$

b. 0.15M $SrBr_2$

c. 0.2M NaBr

d. 0.25M $Mg(NO_3)_2$

**16.** A precipitate will form when an aqueous solution of $Ba(NO_3)_2$ is added to an aqueous solution of $Na_2SO_4$. How many moles of sodium sulfate are required to produce 10.0 g of the precipitate?

a. 1 mole

b. 10.0 mole

c. 0.04 mole

d. 0.4 mole

**17.** Which of the following is an element?

A) NO    B) Ca    C) Na    D) Xe

a. A, B, and C

b. B, C, and D

c. A and D

d. B and C

**18.** When vinegar (acetic acid, $CH_3COOH$) is combined with baking soda (sodium bicarbonate, $NaHCO_3$) a gas is released. What is the identity of the gas?

a. $O_2$

b. $H_2$

c. $CO_2$

d. CO

**19.** What ions form NaCl?

a. Na and Cl

b. $Na^+$ and $Cl^+$

c. $Na^+$ and $Cl^-$

d. $Na^-$ and $Cl^+$

**20.** The density of acetic acid is 1.05 g/mL. What is the volume of 275 g of acetic acid?

a. 275 mL

b. ~262 mL

c. ~100 mL

d. 22.4 L

**21.** The correct formula for converting Fahrenheit to Celsius is given by: $°C = \frac{5}{9}(°F - 32)$. Convert 72 °F into degrees Celsius.

a. 72°C

b. 40°C

c. 25°C

d. 22.2°C

**22.** Which of the following compounds is held together by ionic bonds?

a. $CaCl_2$

b. $CCl_4$

c. $SiO_4$

d. $H_2O$

**23.** Convert $4.50 \times 10^2$ nm into _____ m.

    **a.** $4.50 \times 10^2$ m

    **b.** $4.50 \times 10^{11}$ m

    **c.** $4.50 \times 10^{-7}$ m

    **d.** $4.50 \times 10^8$ m

**24.** What is the concentration of ions when 47.6 g of magnesium chloride is dissolved in 2 L of water?

    **a.** 0.250 M

    **b.** 0.500 M

    **c.** 0.750 M

    **d.** 1.50 M

**25.** Find all the enantiomeric (i.e., mirror-image) pairs among the sets of stereoisomers (a), (b), (c), (d), (e), (f), (g), (h) shown below.

    **a.** (a), (b), (c), (e), (h)

    **b.** (b), (c), (d), (h)

    **c.** (a), (c), (f)

    **d.** (d), (e), (g)

**26.** Find all the diastereomeric pairs among the sets of stereoisomers shown below.

    **a.** (b), (d), (g)

    **b.** (b), (d)

    **c.** (g)

    **d.** (h)

**27.** Write the correct answer (with the correct number of significant figures) for the following calculation: $3.33 \times 10^{-5} + 8.13 \times 10^{-7}$
 a. $3.41 \times 10^{-5}$
 b. $11.46 \times 10^{-7}$
 c. $11.46 \times 10^{-5}$
 d. $11.46 \times 10^{-12}$

**28.** Express 0.05620 in exponential notation.
 a. $0.057 \times 10^{-3}$
 b. $57 \times 10^{-3}$
 c. $563 \times 10^{-4}$
 d. $5.62 \times 10^{-2}$

**29.** How many neutrons does $^{131}$I have?
 a. 53
 b. 78
 c. 131
 d. 262

**30.** What is the atomic number of an ion with a −1 charge and the following electron configuration: $1s_2\, 2s_2\, 2p_5$?
 a. 2
 b. 5
 c. 8
 d. 9

**31.** What volume of a 0.5 M solution of NaOH is required to fully neutralize a 100 mL solution of 1 M $H_2SO_4$?
 a. 50 mL
 b. 100 mL
 c. 200 mL
 d. 400 mL

**32.** How many significant figures are there in the value 0.00250?
 a. 2
 b. 3
 c. 5
 d. 6

**33.** $AgNO_3 + NaCl \leftrightarrow AgCl + NaNO_3$
 The reaction shown here is best described as a
 a. synthesis reaction.
 b. decomposition reaction
 c. single replacement reaction.
 d. double replacement reaction.

**34.** When linoleic acid, an unsaturated fatty acid, reacts with hydrogen, it forms a saturated fatty acid.
 $C_{18}H_{32}O_2 + 2H_2 \rightarrow C_{18}H_{36}O_2$
 Is linoleic acid oxidized, reduced, or hydrogenated in the reaction?
 a. oxidized
 b. reduced
 c. hydrogenated
 d. choices b and c

**35.** When linoleic acid, an unsaturated fatty acid, reacts with hydrogen, it forms a saturated fatty acid.
 $C_{18}H_{32}O_2 + 2H_2 \rightarrow C_{18}H_{36}O_2$
 How many moles of hydrogen ($H_2$) are required to hydrogenate 5.0 g of unsaturated linoleic acid?
 a. 1 mol
 b. 10 mol
 c. $\frac{1}{5}$ mol
 d. $\frac{1}{28}$ mol

**36.** Valence electrons are those in the outermost shell of an atom. Indicate the number of valence electrons for Sc (Scandium).
 a. 1
 b. 2
 c. 4
 d. 3

**37.** What are the names of the orbitals in the 2nd atomic shell?
- **a.** $1s, 2s$
- **b.** $2s, 2p$
- **c.** $s, p, d$
- **d.** $p_x, p_y, p_z$

**38.** In an atom, how many orbitals have a principle quantum number, n, of 2?
- **a.** 1
- **b.** 2
- **c.** 3
- **d.** 4

**39.** Knowing the *group* of an element in the periodic table, how would you find the number of *valence electrons* for an atom of that element?
- **a.** The group number is equal to the number of valence electrons for that element.
- **b.** The group number is equal to the number of bonds an atom of that element can form.
- **c.** The group number indicates the number of orbitals for an element.
- **d.** The group number is equal to the number of shells in an atom of that element.

**40.** Knowing the *period* of an element in the periodic table, what could you say about the number of *electron shells* of an atom of that element?
- **a.** The period number indicates the number of bonds an atom of that element can form.
- **b.** The period number is equal to the number of valence electrons for that element.
- **c.** The period number is equal to the number of electron shells in an atom of that element.
- **d.** The period number changes from left to right of the periodic table.

**41.** When a chemical reaction occurs between two atoms, their valence electrons are reorganized so that an attractive force, called a *chemical bond*, occurs between the atoms. Name the type of bond that is formed when electrons are transferred from one atom to another.
- **a.** molecular bond
- **b.** covalent bond
- **c.** ionic bond
- **d.** transfer bond

**42.** When $CO_2$ is processed by plants during photosynthesis, what happens to the carbon?
- **a.** It is oxidized.
- **b.** It is reduced.
- **c.** It undergoes $\alpha$-decay.
- **d.** It is expelled as waste.

**43.** In bonding, what would happen between the electrons of K and Br?
- **a.** transfer
- **b.** sharing
- **c.** neither of the above
- **d.** both transfer and sharing

**44.** From the periodic table, which is larger, K or Br?
- **a.** K is larger.
- **b.** Br is larger.
- **c.** They are the same size.
- **d.** We cannot know which one is larger.

**45.** Give the number of valence electrons for boron (B).
- **a.** 5
- **b.** 3
- **c.** 2
- **d.** 13

**46.** What is the maximum number of electrons in an atom that can be described by a principal quantum number of 3 and an orbital quantum number of 2?
a. 1
b. 2
c. 5
d. 10

**47.** What is the formula for lead (II) hydroxide?
a. $PbOH$
b. $Pb(OH)_2$
c. $Pb_2OH$
d. $Pb_2(OH)_2$

**48.** Which of these bonds involves the sharing of electrons?
a. ionic
b. proton
c. covalent
d. hydrogen

**49.** Unlike most compounds, water is at its densest when it is
a. solid.
b. liquid.
c. gas.
d. changing from a liquid to a gas.

**50.** A group of students learning to use a triple-beam balance measures a child who weighs 13.0 kg. Which of these groups of measurements shows the greatest precision?
a. 12.9, 13.5, 14.2, 14.0
b. 12.9, 13.6, 13.0, 13.4
c. 14.5, 13.0, 13.6, 15.8
d. 15.2, 15.0, 15.1, 15.2

## Answers

### Section 1: Verbal Ability
1. **a.** compete
2. **b.** audible
3. **c.** entirety
4. **a.** gradually
5. **b.** preamble
6. **c.** stomachache
7. **a.** madness
8. **a.** porcelain
9. **a.** delirious
10. **c.** plead
11. **a.** inundated
12. **d.** funnier
13. **c.** obedient
14. **a.** prosecuted
15. **d.** counterfeit
16. **d.** symmetrically
17. **d.** delaying
18. **a.** vacuum
19. **d.** accommodate
20. **b.** incredulous
21. **a.** trauma
22. **c.** marriageable
23. **b.** illegible
24. **b.** penicillin
25. **c.** adolescence
26. **c.** The correct spelling is cheesy.
27. **b.** The correct spelling is sopranos.
28. **a.** The correct spelling is agitate.
29. **c.** The correct spelling is simultaneous.
30. **d.** no mistakes
31. **b.** The correct spelling is thesis.
32. **a.** The correct spelling is debatable.
33. **a.** The correct spelling is flies.
34. **b.** The correct spelling is bulletin.
35. **a.** The correct spelling is recoil.
36. **c.** The correct spelling is fraudulent.
37. **b.** The correct spelling is questionnaire.
38. **a.** The correct spelling is pungent.
39. **c.** The correct spelling is hygienic.

**40. b.** The correct spelling is illegal.

**41. b.** The correct spelling is corrosiveness.

**42. c.** The correct spelling is gymnast.

**43. d.** no mistakes

**44. d.** no mistakes

**45. a.** The correct spelling is panicky.

**46. c.** The correct spelling is craziness.

**47. d.** no mistakes

**48. a.** The correct spelling is chaise.

**49. a.** The correct spelling is extremely.

**50. b.** The correct spelling is friendly.

## Section 2: Reading Comprehension

**1. c.** It is too early to make, or *draw*, conclusions about early life experiences based on the animal studies described in the passage.

**2. c.** According to paragraph four, the mothers of the rat pups that were separated for three hours *tended to ignore the pups, at least initially, upon their return.*

**3. a.** The author introduced the study to show a clinical example of the long-term effects of stress on the young, as recreated in a lab setting.

**4. b.** The passage presents the idea that excessive distress on a young child can have permanent effects on his or her brain function as the child ages. The author later backs up this notion with a clinical example.

**5. c.** Paragraph three states that *the natural maternal response of instinctively licking and grooming the returned pup was shown to alter the brain chemistry of the pup in a positive way.* Later, paragraph four explains the negative effects on the rat pup when licking and grooming did not occur.

**6. b.** The author wants to know how early influences either *promote* or challenge developmental processes. The two words are opposites, so an opposite to "challenge" is *advance.*

**7. a.** Paragraph two explains that stress is as much a good thing as it is a bad one—*cortisol and other stress hormones play an important role in emergencies: they help our bodies make energy available to enable effective responses, temporarily suppress the immune response, and sharpen attention.*

**8. c.** The passage goes into detail discussing the pros and cons of VLCDs, one option for very obese individuals. It doesn't necessarily say that it's *an easy path* (choice **a**).

**9. b.** Paragraph five states, *such a weight loss can rapidly improve obesity-related medical conditions, including* diabetes, *high blood pressure, and high cholesterol.*

**10. d.** According to paragraph four, *adults over age 50 already experience depletion of lean body mass.*

**11. a.** According to the first sentence of the final paragraph, *many patients on a VLCD for four to 16 weeks report minor side effects such as fatigue,* which means excessive weariness.

**12. a.** Paragraph three states that BMI is calculated by dividing a person's weight by height and then multiplying by a constant. If two people are the same weight and one is taller, then the shorter person will have the larger BMI.

**13. d.** The passages states from the very beginning that *VLCD formulas need to contain appropriate levels of vitamins and micronutrients to ensure that patients meet their nutritional requirements.* Since there are many physical side effects, nutrients are key to keeping the body healthy during a VLCD.

**14. c.** According to paragraph six, prenatal testing is performed on fetuses, which are developing mammals still in the womb.

**15. b.** According to paragraph three, *about three in every 100 children are born with a severe disorder presumed to be genetic.* 300 is 100 multiplied by three, and nine is three multiplied by three.

**16. b.** See the last sentence of the fifth paragraph, which states that *effective treatment can be started in a few hundred infants.*

**17. d.** The first paragraph says that the report addressed concerns about *protecting confidentiality.*

**18. c.** The last sentence of the fourth paragraph states that *careful pilot studies . . . need to be conducted first.*

**19. d.** See the fifth paragraph: *Newborn screening is the most common type of genetic screening today.*

**20. a.** According to the first sentence of the third paragraph, the new MRI *detects not water, but inert gases.*

**21. d.** See the second sentence of the second paragraph, which states that X-rays cannot provide a clear view of air passages.

**22. b.** The last sentence of paragraph two states that *conventional MRI, because it images water protons, provides poor images of the lungs, which are filled with air, not water.*

**23. b.** The first sentence of the third paragraph states the equivalency: nuclei are *aligned, or hyperpolarized.*

**24. a.** The last paragraph says that light, rather than a magnet, is used to align nuclei, suggesting that the two serve equivalent purposes in the two MRI processes.

**25. c.** See the last sentence of the passage. Since lesser gases lose their alignment more quickly, a shorter period of alignment would lead to poorer clarity. A higher number of aligned nuclei would theoretically lead to a better image.

**26. a.** The author contrasts the public's dismissal of the arcane practice of wearing garlic with its increasing acceptance of herbal remedies.

**27. a.** In this context, *practices* refer to unconventional healthcare businesses.

**28. d.** Choice **a** is overly general, and choice **b** is too negative to be inferred from the survey's findings. Choice **c** is incorrect—the author does not mention the "baby boom" age group, but that does not imply that the survey does not include it.

**29. a.** The statistic illustrates the popularity of alternative therapies without giving any specific information as to why.

**30. d.** The author states that Americans are not replacing conventional healthcare but are adding to or supplementing it with alternative care.

**31. d.** The shortcomings of conventional healthcare mentioned in paragraph four are the time constraints of managed care, focus on technology, and inability to relieve the symptoms associated with chronic disease.

**32. b.** The second paragraph states that *muscle atrophy can be kept largely at bay with appropriate exercise.*

**33. c.** According to the fifth paragraph, levels of vitamin D were elevated in drug recipients.

**34. d.** According to information in the third paragraph, a pressure device *does nothing to avert loss of calcium from bones.*

**35. a.** The last paragraph states that high urinary calcium concentrations can cause kidney stones. Treatment that inhibits urinary discharge of calcium, such as use of alendronate, could therefore help the treatment of kidney stones.

**36. d.** According to paragraph three, after a three-month or longer stay in space, much of the profound bone loss may be irreversible. Since three months is about 90 days, choice **d** is correct.

**37. b.** The last sentence of the third paragraph states that 56% of "laser-first" and 70% of "medication-first" patients needed *new or extra medications to control pressure inside the eye.*

**38. d.** The passage focuses primarily on the effects of both laser and medication treatments. It does not advocate either method.

**39. a.** See the second and third sentences of the first paragraph.

**40. c.** The third sentence of the third paragraph states that *initial treatment with laser surgery is at least as effective as initial treatment with eye drops.*

**41. a.** The second paragraph says that the patients were *newly diagnosed.*

**42. c.** Nowhere in the passage does the author speculate about whether teenagers can change their exercise habits.

**43. c.** One meaning of *sedentary* is settled; another meaning is doing or requiring much sitting. *Stationary,* defined as fixed in a course or mode, is closest in meaning.

**44. d.** The last sentence illustrates factors that motivate teenagers to exercise by using the results of a national survey to provide specific examples.

**45. d.** The passage promotes change in teenagers' exercise habits by emphasizing the benefits of exercise, the moderate amount of exercise needed to achieve benefits, and some factors that may encourage teenagers to exercise.

## Section 3: Quantitative Ability

**1. a.** To solve this problem, you must first convert yards to inches. There are 36 inches in a yard. $36 \times 3\frac{1}{3} = 120$ inches.

**2. d.** The least common denominator is 28. When the fractions are converted, the problem becomes $\frac{21}{28} + \frac{20}{28} = \frac{41}{28}$. When the answer is reduced, it is $1\frac{13}{28}$.

**3. a.** 0.97 multiplied by 100 is 97; therefore, the correct answer is 97%.

**4. c.** The sum of the measures of the angles in a triangle is 180°; $70° + 30° = 100°$; $180° - 100° = 80°$. Therefore, angle $C$ is 80°.

**5. a.** Since quadrilateral $QRST$ is a rectangle, we know that angle $R$ is a right angle and triangle $QRS$ is a right triangle. The area of a triangle is $\frac{1}{2}$ (*base* $\times$ *height*) but we are only given the base of triangle $QRS$. Since this is a right triangle, we can find the height $h$ using the Pythagorean theorem. $h^2 + 8^2 = 10^2$; $h^2 + 64 = 100$; $h^2 = 36$; $h = 6$. The area of triangle $QRS$ is $\frac{1}{2}(6)(8) = \frac{1}{2}(48) = 24$ units$^2$.

**6. b.** First, convert $13\frac{1}{3}\%$ to a decimal: $13\frac{1}{3}\% \approx 0.1333$. If $p$ is the full price of an office visit, then $0.1333p = \$20$. Divide both sides by 0.1333 and round to the nearest dollar to get the answer: $p = \frac{\$20}{0.1333} = \$150.04 \approx \$150$.

**7. b.** To find the average time for the three baths, you must add the times for all the baths and divide by the number of baths: $20 + 17 + 14 = 51$; $51 \div 3 = 17$ minutes.

**8. a.** The formula to use to solve this problem is *distance = rate × time*. Rate and time must be in the same units to get the correct answer, so first convert the time to hours: $6 \text{ min} \times \frac{1 \text{ hr}}{60 \text{ min}} = 0.1$ hr. Then multiply to get the answer: *distance* $= (0.1 \text{ hr})(58 \text{ miles/hr}) = 5.8$ miles.

**9. d.** The area of a rectangular space is the width times the length—in this case, $10 \times 8$, or 80 square feet.

**10. b.** Use the formula beginning with the operation in parentheses: $98 - 32 = 66$. After that, multiply 66 by $\frac{5}{9}$, first multiplying 66 by 5 to get 330; 330 divded by 9 is 36.6, which is rounded up to 36.7.

**11. a.** To multiply fractions, you must multiply the numerators to reach the numerator of the answer ($2 \times 3 = 6$) and multiply the denominitors to reach the denominator of the answer ($5 \times 7 = 35$), so the answer is $\frac{6}{35}$.

**12. c.** Perform the operation in parentheses first: $14 \times 7 = 98$, and then add 12 to get 110.

**13. b.** Convert the percentage to a decimal and multiply: $232 \times 0.14 = 32.48$.

**14. d.** The perimeter is the total length of all sides. In a square, all four sides are of equal length, so the perimeter is $4 + 4 + 4 + 4$, or 16.

**15. b.** First, add 11 to both sides to isolate $x$: $x^2 = 38 + 11 = 49$. Then, find the square root of both sides to solve for $x$: $\sqrt{x^2} = \sqrt{49}$; $x = 7$.

**16. b.** Read the question carefully: it asks how much she would have *saved*, not how much she would have *spent*, if she had ordered her books early. The amount she would have saved is the discount amount: 15%. So, she would have saved $(0.15)(\$385) = \$57.75$.

**17. c.** It is important to keep the decimal values straight. Divide as usual, and then bring the decimal point straight up into the answer in order to get 39.4.

**18. a.** Let $n$ equal the number of nurses, $d$ equal the number of doctors, and $t$ equal the number of technicians. There are twice as many nurses as doctors, so $2d = n$, or $d = \frac{n}{2}$. There are three fewer medical technicians than nurses, so $t = n - 3$. The total number of staff is 37, so $n + \frac{n}{2} + (n - 3) = 37$. Collect like terms to get $\frac{5n}{2} = 40$; $5n = 80$; $n = 16$. To solve for $d$, divide $n$ by 2, so $d = \frac{16}{2} = 8$.

**19. c.** The formula for finding the area of a circle is $A = \pi r^2$. First, square the radius: $13 \times 13 = 169$. Then, multiply by the approximate value of $\pi$, 3.14, to get 530.66.

**20. a.** In order to subtract fractions, you must first find the least common denominator, in this case, 40. The problem is then $\frac{35}{40} - \frac{24}{40}$, or $\frac{11}{40}$.

**21. c.** There are 24 hours in a day: $24 \times 4\frac{1}{6} = 24 \times \frac{25}{6} = 4 \times 25 = 100$ hours.

**22. c.** Use the formula: $\frac{x}{100} = \frac{is}{of}$
$$\frac{0.15}{100} = \frac{0.5}{x}$$
$$\frac{0.5 \times 100}{0.15} = x$$
$$x = 333.33 \text{ or } 333\frac{1}{3}$$

**23. b.** Carefully plug in the given values. $5x + 3y + 6xy = 5(2) + 3(3) + 6(2)(3) = 10 + 9 + 36 = 55$.

**24. d.** The question is asking you to find the diameter. In order to find the diameter, you will first have to find the radius. The formula for the area of a circle is $A = \pi r^2$. Plug in the given values: $121\pi = \pi r^2$; $121 = r^2$; $r = 11$. Don't stop there! $d = 2(r)$; $d = 2(11)$; $d = 22$.

**25. a.** The fractions of red, blue, and green candies must add up to 1, so the number of green candies equals $1 - \left(\frac{1}{3} + \frac{1}{4}\right) = \frac{12}{12} - \frac{4}{12} - \frac{3}{12} = \frac{5}{12}$.

**26. d.** Note that Tyrone's typing speed is given in words per *minute*, but the question is asking for words typed in $1\frac{1}{8}$ *hours*. First convert the number of hours to minutes: $1\frac{1}{8} \text{ hr} \times \frac{60 \text{ min}}{1 \text{ hr}} = \frac{9}{8} \times 60 = 67\frac{1}{2} \text{ min}$. Then multiply by the typing speed to get the answer: $67\frac{1}{2} \text{ min} \times 62 \frac{\text{words}}{\text{min}} = \frac{135}{2} \times 62 = 135 \times 31 = 4{,}185$ words.

**27. d.** A percentage is a portion of 100, or $\frac{x}{100}$. The equation here is $\frac{x}{100} = \frac{234}{18{,}000}$, or $234 \times 100 = 18{,}000x$; $23{,}400 \div 18{,}000 = 1.3$.

**28. a.** There are 60 minutes in an hour. Multiply $60 \times 7\frac{1}{6}$ by multiplying $60 \times 7 = 420$ and $60 \times \frac{1}{6} = 10$. Then add $420 + 10$ to get 430 minutes.

**29. b.** Think of 145.29 as 145.290, and then line up the decimal points and add the numbers to get the correct answer, 217.977.

**30. d.** Perform the operations in parentheses first, left to right: $84 - 5 = 79$. Next, do the other parenthetical operation: $3 \times 54 = 162$. Now, multiply $12(79) = 948$. Now, do the final operation: $948 - 162 = 786$.

**31. b.** Take the time to make sure you are performing the correct operations: $43 + (-5) = 43 - 5 = 38$; $38 - 12 = 26$; $26 - (-2) = 26 + 2 = 28$; $28 + 12 = 40$.

**32. b.** Use the answers provided and work backward. Start with choice **c**. If three books were on the shelf and four are added, there are now seven books on the shelf. 3(3) does NOT equal 7, so choice **c** is incorrect. Try choice **b**. If two books were on the shelf and four are added, there are now six books. 2(3) = 6. Choice **b** is correct.

**33. c.** Subtract the equations as you would any other normal values: $2x + 1 - (x - 2) = 2x + 1 - x + 2 = x + 3$.

**34. a.** One way to solve is to change the fractions into decimals: $10,593\frac{4}{5} = 10,593.80$; $10,610\frac{1}{5} = 10,610.20$.

$$\begin{array}{r} 10,610.20 \\ -10,593.80 \\ \hline 16.40 \end{array}$$

$16.40 = 16\frac{2}{5}$

**35. c.** Change the first fraction into an improper fraction so it is easier to work with: $2\frac{3}{4} = \frac{11}{4}$. To divide, multiply by the reciprocal: $\frac{11}{4} \div \frac{3}{8} = \frac{11}{4} \times \frac{8}{3} = 11 \times \frac{2}{3} = \frac{22}{3} = 7\frac{1}{3}$.

**36. b.** The correct answer is $8\frac{9}{10}$. Incorrect answers include adding both the numerator and the denominator and not converting fifths to tenths properly.

**37. c.** First convert $8\frac{8}{7}$ into an improper fraction: $\frac{64}{7}$. The reciprocal of this fraction is $\frac{7}{64}$.

**38. b.** You can estimate that 14 is a little more than half of 25, so the answer should be a little more than 0.5, or 0.56. You can also calculate the answer by dividing 14 by 25 and getting 0.56.

**39. d.** This is a simple subtraction problem with decimals. The correct answer is 1.734.

**40. b.** To subtract the length of the car from the truck, you have to "borrow" 12 inches from the feet of the truck and add them to the inches, since 6 is greater than 2. This gives you (16 − 1) feet (2 + 12) inches, or 15 feet 14 inches for the truck. Subtract to get the answer: 15 feet 14 inches − 13 feet 6 inches = 2 feet 8 inches.

**41. b.** The correct answer has only two decimal places: 96.32.

**42. a.** First, figure out how many patients are left after the first hour: $16 - 16(0.625) = 16 - 10 = 6$. Then calculate how many patients are left after the second hour: $6 - 6(0.66\frac{2}{3}) = 6 - 4 = 2$.

**43. c.** The nurse will spend 1 minute with each patient while he or she take his or her medication, so she will spend $22 \times 1$ min = 22 min total giving medication to patients. She will also need to travel from the first patient to the second patient, from the second to the third, and so on, but will not have to travel from the last patient to another. That means she will be making the 30-second trip from one patient to another $22 - 1 = 21$ times. So, she will spend $21 \times 30$ sec = 630 sec or $\frac{630 \text{ sec}}{60 \text{ sec/min}} = 10.5$ min = 10 min 30 sec traveling between patients. Add the time spent with patients with the time spent traveling to get 32 minutes 30 seconds.

**44. b.** To find the answer, divide 14 by 0.35 to get 40.

**45. c.** Three feet 4 inches equals 40 inches; 40 inches divided by 5 is 8 inches.

**46. a.** To save time, use the given answers here and work backward. Start with choice **b**. If there were five robberies last month, a 25% decrease would mean .25(5) = 1.25 fewer robberies this month. That does not make sense, so choice **b** is incorrect. Try choice **a**. If there were four robberies last month, a 25% decrease would mean 0.25(4) = 1 fewer this month. $4 - 3 = 1$, so this choice is correct.

**47. b.** Calculate the total time in chunks. The total time from opening at 8:45 A.M. to noon is 3 hours 15 minutes. The time from noon to lunch is 15 minutes. The time from 1:00 P.M. to closing is 6 hours 30 minutes. 3 hours 15 minutes + 15 minutes + 6 hours 30 minutes = 10 hours.

**48. d.** Solve for $x$ and then plug your answer into the second equation. First, subtract eight from both sides to get $4x = 32$. Divide both sides by 4 to get $x = 8$. Don't stop there! $3(8) - 4 = 24 - 4 = 20$.

**49. a.** Remember the formula *total = rate × time*. $225 = r(15)$, so the rate = 17 gallons per minute. Now, plug this rate into a new formula using the new total. $340 = 17t$, so $t = 20$. Don't stop there; you need to find how many more minutes the second tank will take: $20 - 15 = 5$ more minutes.

**50. b.** To find the average, add all of the scores and divide by the total number of scores: $8.7 + 8.9 + 9.1 + 9.0 + 8.7 = 44.4$; $\frac{44.4}{5} = 8.88$.

## Section 4: General Science

**1. a.** The Earth's core is divided into two parts – the solid inner core and the liquid outer core.

**2. a.** The Earth formed 4.6 billion years ago, which we know from radioactive dating of meteorites.

**3. b.** The lithosphere has a light density and "floats" on the more dense layers of Earth that are below.

**4. b.** The troposphere is the lowest portion of the Earth's atmosphere, where most weather phenomena takes place. The word comes from the Greek *tropos*, meaning "turning or mixing," since the troposphere's structure and behavior are caused by mixing.

**5. d.** The deepest parts of the ocean are remarkably uniform in depth, from 3 to 5 km deep, for an average of 4 km, or about 2.5 miles.

**6. a.** The mantle is the thick zone beneath Earth's crust but not as deep as the inner core.

**7. a.** Most of Earth's surface is sedimentary rock, or recycled rock. Bedrock is simply surface rock as a definition, so that answer contains no content and makes no sense.

**8. b.** Central and Southern Africa are home to 49% of all natural diamonds. Natural diamonds have caused controversy in this part of the world due to African paramilitary groups selling "blood diamonds," or diamonds mined in war zones and sold to fund a warlord's activities.

**9. b.** Uranus is the fourth planet in the Solar System known as a gas giant—a large planet not composed primarily of rock or solid matter.

**10. b.** Obsidian is igneous rock, formed by lava that has cooled rapidly.

**11. b.** The 20th century had the world's largest population increase. This is due to medical advances and improved agricultural technology.

**12. b.** In about one year, the entire atmosphere mixes, even between Northern and Southern Hemispheres.

**13. b.** The energy of the sun that falls upon the land and ocean creates differences in temperature that drive the circulation of the atmosphere and ocean.

**14. a.** Earth's atmosphere has only a tiny amount of the greenhouse gas carbon dioxide. In the atmospheres of Mars and Venus, carbon dioxide is the dominant gas.

**15. c.** The mixing time for the entire ocean is about one thousand years.

**16. c.** $10^6$ is equal to one million in scientific notation.

**17. b.** Nuclear fusion is the process responsible for the energy emitted by stars. In this type of reaction, light nuclei fuse together into heavier ones.

**18. b.** The nucleus contains protons and neutrons. Since protons are positive and neutrons are neutral, the nucleus has an overall positive charge.

**19. b.** Burning fossil fuels contributes to acid rain because such burning emits the acid-forming elements sulfur and nitrogen into the atmosphere.

**20. d.** Radon gas is the second leading cause of lung cancer and occurs naturally in some areas.

**21. d.** Boreal forests, with their evergreens of fir and pine, sport tough needles with lots of lignin to give them strength to endure the winds and freezing of winter in very high latitudes.

**22. d.** A genus consists of many species (in rare cases, a genus might have only one living species, but it would have had more in the past). A family consists of many genera.

**23. c.** Uranus and Neptune are mostly composed of ammonia, water, and methane molten ices, and are often referred to as "ice giants."

**24. c.** Magma is a high-temperature fluid substance that behaves like thick oil.

**25. d.** Meiosis is the process in which parent cells from males and females create four gametes (eggs or sperm in the case of animals) with half the genes and chromosomes of the parents. (Note that it's not a simple process of splitting in half.)

**26. a.** Carbon monoxide is derived from the incomplete combustion of fossil fuels. Carbon dioxide, on the other hand, comes from complete combustion.

**27. d.** The upper part of the ocean that receives light is the pelagic zone. The benthos is the deeper layer.

**28. d.** The tundra has a short growing season and small plants that reproduce quickly. They reproduce quickly because the climate is so severe for most of the year.

**29. b.** The kingdom level is the most inclusive.

**30. c.** In 1996, Dolly became the first mammal to be cloned using a process called nuclear transfer.

**31. c.** The carrying capacity is the limit asked for in the question. Terms with "yield" usually refer to the human harvesting of creatures, such as fish.

**32. a.** The only supply of marine protein that is growing is aquaculture, or "farms" of fish and other aquatic organisms.

**33. d.** Photosynthesis creates simple sugars, but to create more complex molecules needed for their tissues, plants must also perform respiration.

**34. b.** Various types of bacteria release carbon dioxide and methane as wastes from their metabolisms.

**35. d.** Bacteria in root nodules are nitrogen fixers.

**36. a.** Negative population growth in some countries is due to sub-replacement fertility rates (less than 2.1 children per woman in developed countries).

**37. d.** Rivers carry the most phosphorus to the sea. There is some phosphorus in the dust carried by wind, which is less than the phosphorus in rivers. Regardless, the phosphorus in dust is not in the dissolved ion form, which is what the question asked for.

**38. c.** Although you wouldn't be expected to memorize numbers, it should be noted that carbon is the most abundant, and that iron is a micronutrient. In between these two, hydrogen is in all organic molecules, while phosphorus has specialized uses in cells. Therefore, it is logical that carbon is first, followed by hydrogen, then phosphorus, then iron.

**39. a.** Copper is needed by cells in only trace amounts; it is therefore not a macronutrient, but a micronutrient.

**40. d.** Estimates place the preagricultural worldwide population at about ten million. The other answers are either definitely too small or too big.

**41. a.** The seafloor gets older as you move outward from the mid-ocean ridge. This is evidence of seafloor spreading and continental drift.

**42. c.** Toxicology is the study of poisons and the adverse effects of chemicals on living organisms. It comes from the Greek *toxicos*, which means "poisonous."

**43. a.** The Cambrian Explosion refers to a time in Earth's history when many new forms of life appeared in the fossil record.

**44. d.** Mitochondria convert food nutrients into energy.

**45. a.** Desalination is the process of removing salt from water. It is done to convert salt water into fresh water that is suitable for human use.

**46. b.** The burning of fossil fuels creates all of those items except stratospheric ozone. Natural processes high in the Earth's atmosphere create that type of ozone.

**47. c.** A greenhouse gas traps heat because it absorbs outgoing longwave radiation and is transparent to incoming shortwave radiation.

**48. c.** Ozone has three oxygen atoms in a single molecule.

**49. b.** Acid rain occurs when nitrates and sulfates in clouds fall to Earth as nitric and sulfuric acids in rainwater.

**50. a.** Carbon monoxide, an odorless gas that is lethal in very small quantities, is the number one cause of poisoning deaths annually.

## Section 5: Biology

**1. b.** Vitamin K is important in the clotting of blood, vitamin A is important in vision, and vitamin D is important in the formation of bone.

**2. a.** Any salts or esters with the $NO_2^-$ ion are called nitrites and can be found in such cured meat products as bacon and hot dogs.

**3. c.** The other actions are controlled by skeletal muscles (choices **a** and **d**) or cardiac muscles (choice **b**).

**4. a.** The resting potential of a neuron is $-70$ millivolts (mV).

**5. d.** Glucose production (glycolysis) is done primarily in the leaf chloroplasts, and breakdown of organic compounds is primarily done in the mitochondria. Roots do not release carbon dioxide.

**6. b.** Alveoli are found in the lungs and are the site of oxygen and carbon dioxide exchange by the respiratory system.

**7. b.** Meiosis results in daughter cells that are genetically different than their parent cells. This leads to greater diversity when compared to reproduction through mitosis or asexual reproduction.

**8. d.** After sexual reproduction leads to fertilization, the first stage of development is a single-celled zygote. Choices **b** and **c** are later stages in development; the zygote becomes an embryo, which then becomes a fetus.

**9. b.** Fruits serve the functions of choices **a**, **c**, and **d**, but are formed after pollination.

**10. c.** The placenta is specialized tissue that provides nutrients to the developing embryo in the mother's uterus.

**11. a.** Gymnosperms produce pine cones with seeds, not flowers; mosses are not vascular plants and do not produce flowers; fungi are not plants and produce spores from fruiting bodies, not flowers.

**12. b.** Adrenaline causes an increase in blood sugar by releasing stored carbohydrates. Choice **d** is incorrect because adrenaline does inhibit these muscles, even though it stimulates muscles in the spleen, hair follicles, and eyes.

**13. d.** Goiter is an enlargement of the thyroid gland.

**14. a.** Oncology is the study and treatment of cancer and tumors.

**15. b.** The ulna is a bone in the lower arm.

**16. a.** The medulla oblongata controls many involuntary responses, including heart and breathing rates.

**17. c.** DNA is transcribed into mRNA by pairing A→U, T→A, G→C, and C→G. The 5′ end of DNA aligns with the 3′ end of mRNA, so the DNA is read in reverse when starting at the 5′ end.

**18. b.** The ribosomes are the sites of protein synthesis within the cell. The nucleus houses the genetic material, the lysosomes manage waste, and the cytoplasm is the fluid inside the cell membrane.

**19. d.** Antigens are chemicals that are recognized as foreign by the immune system, thus stimulating the production of antibodies. Viruses and bacteria are typically antigenic because of their structure.

**20. a.** Cell membranes are generally composed of phospholipids—molecules arranged in two layers, with the phosphate ends pointing in toward the cell's center in one layer and to the outside environment in the other layer. The lipid ends of the molecules are sandwiched in the middle of the membrane.

**21. d.** The snake is the only vertebrate listed—it is the only one of the four animals that has a backbone.

**22. a.** The Punnett square is a grid that represents all of the possible genotypic combinations in the offspring generation produced by a male (gametes listed horizontally) and a female (gametes listed vertically).

**23. a.** Ligaments are the dense parallel bundles of collagen fibers that hold bones together at a joint.

**24. a.** Mosses are bryophytes, which are characterized by their lack of a vascular system.

**25. b.** Adrenaline is a hormone, acetylcholine is a neurotransmitter, and amino acids are the building block molecules of proteins.

**26. c.** Mitosis results in daughter cells with genes identical to their parent cell. This is used by the simplest living organisms, as well as advanced life forms, but it does not result in genetic diversity.

**27. b.** Carcinogens cause mutations that lead to cancerous growth, which is unhealthy in most cases.

**28. c.** The salivary glands have ducts and are called exocrine glands. The others are endocrine glands, which are ductless and pour their secretions directly into the blood.

**29. c.** The proportions of offspring are relatively equal. Choice **a** is eliminated, because since the recessive traits showed up in the offspring, then the offspring must have received recessive alleles from both parents. Choice **d** is eliminated because dominant traits were also present. Of the remaining possibilities, choice **c** would produce equal numbers of offspring. One parent will always give yt, and the other has equal chances of providing YT, Yt, yT, and yt.

**30. a.** Type O results from the recessive genotype, without alleles for type A or type B. Types A and B are codominant, so they can be expressed together.

**31. a.** Photosynthesis oxidizes water into $O_2$ and protons ($H^+$). These electrons and protons are ultimately used in the Calvin Cycle to reduce $CO_2$ into more complex molecules.

**32. c.** The Eustachian tube allows the air pressure in the middle ear to remain equal to that on the outside of the tympanic membrane.

**33. d.** Osteocytes are living cells within the minerals of bone. *Osteo* is the combining form meaning *bone*.

**34. c.** Analogous structures describe traits that independently evolved in two unrelated species. The closest common ancestor of birds and bats did not have wings, yet each group evolved them.

**35. b.** In binomial nomenclature, the genus name (*Aptenodytes*) precedes the species name (*forsteri*).

**36. b.** The correct answer is lactose. Most enzymes are named according to the substance that they act on plus the suffix *-ase*. For example, choice **c** is incorrect because suc*rase* is an enzyme that degrades sucrose.

**37. b.** Vestigial structures are structures within an organism that have lost their original function through evolution. The appendix was part of the digestive system of a human ancestor, and the coccyx is the remnant of a tail.

**38. b.** Pheromones are chemical signals that may be released either in a secretion or as an odor.

**39. c.** A codon is a triplet of nucleotides that usually represents a genetic code for an amino acid added during protein synthesis.

**40. c.** Vertebrate digits are also referred to as phalanges.

**41. d.** Fungi are decomposers that return nutrients into the soil by breaking them down from decaying organic matter. Fungi rely on dead organisms, like the dead plant in the question, for nutrients, but this is not a form of symbiosis, which is considered a relationship between living organisms. Choices **a** through **c** are examples of symbiosis.

**42. c.** This is the only example of a true predator-prey dynamic. The other choices are all examples of consumption, but choice **c** is an interaction that results in the death of the prey organism, which is a requirement of the act of predation.

**43. d.** Nerves are composed of nervous tissue, not connective tissue.

**44. b.** The renal system, also called the excretory system, consists of the kidneys and excretory accessory organs.

**45. a.** Because the trait is recessive, an individual must be homozygous recessive for the disease to present the disorder. Even with a shortened life expectancy, the gene is not expected to leave the gene pool, eliminating choice **b**. Choice **c** is not true because a parent carrying one recessive gene is a carrier and will not show symptoms. Choice **d** is not true because carriers are resistant to malaria, which is extremely useful in parts of the world where malaria is a risk.

**46. c.** The junction of two nerve cells is called a synapse.

**47. a.** Oogenesis is the name of the process in which the ova (egg cells) are produced and grow in the ovary. Special ovarian cells called oogonia divide repeatedly to make large numbers of prospective eggs called oocytes.

**48. c.** Men are more likely to be affected by an X-linked disorder as they possess only one copy of the gene, whereas women possess two. X-linked recessive disorders are often inherited through the mother when she is a carrier and shows no symptoms because she also has a second, functional allele.

**49. c.** The ossicles, utricle, and cochlea are all components of the human ear.

**50. c.** Alcohol acts as a depressant, not as a stimulant.

## Section 6: Chemistry

**1. a.** Protons and $C_6H_{12}O_6$ have mass, but not enough to matter in such small quantities as 20 molecules. Electrons have almost no mass regardless of how much you have, so the greatest mass is 0.5 moles of uranium (U).

**2. d.** Three half-lives, or 39 hours, leave $\frac{1}{8}$ of the iodine-123 undecayed: 13.75 grams. A few more hours, a total of about 44, leaves less than 12 grams.

**3. a.** The correct formula for copper (II) oxide is CuO.

**4. a.** The molar ratio of $Fe_2O_3$ to Fe is 1:2, so the number of moles of Fe produced is twice the number of moles of $Fe_2O_3$ used.

**5. d.** Capsaicin is not a carboxylic acid. Carboxylic acids contain a –COOH group.

**6. a.** Acids and bases neutralize each other, creating water and a salt. ($HA + BOH \rightarrow H_2O + AB$).

**7. b.** Oxidation: increase of the oxidation # of Sn from Sn [0] to $SnCl_6^{2-}$ [+4]. Oxidizing agent: $4NO_{3(aq)}^-$, while $Sn_{(s)}$ is the reducing agent (because it is oxidized).

**8. c.** Balance Mg first [1 in $Mg_{(s)}$ for 1 in $Mg(OH)_2$], then O [2 in $2H_2O$ for 2 in $Mg(OH)_2$], and finally H [4 in $2H_2O$ for 2 in $Mg(OH)_2$ and 2 in $H_2$].

**9. c.** Cr in $Cr(NO_3)_3$ is displaced by Al.

**10. b.** Combination of $PF_{3(g)}$ and $F_{2(g)}$.

**11. a.** $Ba(OH)_{2(aq)} + 2HNO_{3(aq)} \rightarrow$ $Ba(NO_3)_{2(aq)} + 2H_2O(l)$
The number of each atom on the left side of the equation must equal the number on the right side of the equation:
1 Ba [in $Ba(OH)_2$] for 1 Ba [in $Ba(NO_3)_2$],
2 N [in $2HNO_3$] for 2 N [in $Ba(NO_3)_2$],
8 O [2 in $Ba(OH)_2$ and 6 in $2HNO_3$] for 8 O [6 in $Ba(NO_3)_2$ and 2 in $2H_2O$]
4 H [2 in $Ba(OH)_2$ and 2 in $2HNO_3$] for 4 H [4 in $2H_2O$]

**12. c.** The chemical formula for nitrite is $NO_2^-$.

**13. a.** $C_2H_{4(g)} + 3O_{2(g)} \rightarrow 2CO_{2(g)} + 2H_2O_{(g)}$
Oxidation: increase of the oxidation # of C from [–2] in $C_2H_{4(g)}$ to [+4] in $CO_{2(g)}$.
Reduction: decrease of the oxidation # of O from [0] in $O_{2(g)}$ to [–4] in $CO_{2(g)}$.

**14. b.** Only $NH_3$ is not ionic and cannot be broken into ions.

**15. d.** 3 ions: 2 $NO_3^-$ and 1 $Mg^{2+}$: $3 \times 0.25M = 0.75M$, which is greater than 0.4M ($Al^{3+}$ and 3 $Cl^-$), 0.45M ($Sr^{2+}$ and 2 $Br^-$), 0.4M ($Na^+$ and $Br^-$).

**16. c.** In the equation $Ba(NO_3)_2 + Na_2SO_4 \rightarrow BaSO_4$ (sol) + $2NaNO_3$, 1 mole of sodium sulfate produces 1 mole of the precipitate barium sulfate [137.3 (Ba) + 32 (S) + [$4 \times 16$ (4O)] = 233.3 g]. So, to produce 10.0 g of barium sulfate, only ($\frac{10.0}{233.3}$) $\times$ 1 mol= 0.04 mol of sodium sulfate is needed.

**17. b.** Only NO is not an element.

**18. c.** $CH_3COOH + NaHCO_3 \rightarrow NaCH_3COO + H_2CO_3$ is an acid-base reaction. Carbonic acid decomposes to $H_2O$ and $CO_2$ which is released as a gas.

**19. c.** $Na^+$ and $Cl^-$ combine to form NaCl.

**20. b.** $d = \frac{m}{v}$ implies that $v = \frac{m}{d} = \frac{275 \text{ g}}{1.05 \text{ g/mL}} \sim$ 262 mL.

**21. d.** $\frac{5}{9}(72 - 32) = \frac{5}{9} \times 40 = 22.2°C$

**22. a.** Ionic compounds are formed from combinations of metals and nonmetals held together by ionic bonds. All other choices contain only nonmetals, which form covalent bonds with each other.

**23. c.** $4.50 \times 10^2 \times 10^{-9}$ m $= 4.50 \times 10^{-7}$ m

**24. c.** 47.6 g $MgCl_2$ is equivalent to 0.500 mol. 0.500 mol/2.00 L = 0.250 M $MgCl_2$. In solution, $MgCl_2$ dissociates into 3 ions (1 $Mg^{2+}$ and 2 $Cl^-$), so the total concentration of ions is 0.750 M.

**25. b.** Mirror-images are two structures that are not superposable (upon rotation/flipping of the structure or not). In (a), (e), (f), we have the same structure: On rotating the *second* structure (in plane strictly for (a) and (e) since these are Fischer projections and out of plane for (f)) by 180°, we obtain the *first* structure: (a), (e), (f) are not constituted by pairs of enantiomers or mirror-images. Set (g) is labeled (R),(S) for one and (R),(R) for the other structure, and cannot therefore constitute a set of enantiomers (in which absolute configuration shouldn't be the same for the same chiral carbon of the structures). (b), (c), (d), (h) are sets of enantiomers or mirror-images by the same procedure, (h) showing (R),(R) and (S),(S) that is characteristic of enantiomeric pairs.

**26. c.** Since (g) is labeled (R),(S) for one structure and (R),(R) for the other and cannot therefore constitute a set of enantiomers, it's a set of diastereomers.

**27. a.** $3.33 \times 10^{-5} + 8.13 \times (10^{-5} \times 10^{-2}) = (3.33 + 8.13 \times 10^{-2}) \times 10^{-5} = 3.41 \times 10^{-5}$ (2 decimal digits as in 3.33 and 8.13).

**28. d.** $0.05620 = 0.5620 \times 10^{-1} = 5.620 \times 10^{-2}$.

**29. b.** The number of neutrons can be found by subtracting the atomic number for iodine, 53, from the mass number, 131. That number is 78.

**30. c.** If an ion has a charge of $-1$, it has 1 more electron than it has protons. The ion shown has 9 electrons so it has 8 protons.

**31. d.** The acid concentration of $H_2SO_4$ is 2 M (2 $H^+$ per $H_2SO_4$). The acid is neutralized when it has been reacted with an equimolar amount of base. Using $M_1V_1 = M_2V_2$: $(2\ M)(0.1\ L) = (0.5\ M)(x\ L) \rightarrow$ $x = 0.4\ L$ (400 m L).

**32. b.** Significant figures include all nonzero digits and trailing zeroes in a number that contains a decimal point. In the number 0.00**250**, the bolded digits are significant.

**33. d.** The reactants are both replaced, making this a double replacement reaction.

**34. c.** Hydrogen atoms have been incorporated, i.e., *hydrogenation*.

**35. d.** 2 mol of $H_2$ react with 1 mol (280 g) of linoleic acid. To hydrogenate 5.0 g of linoleic acid, the required amount of $H_2$ is $\left(\frac{5.0}{280}\right) \times 2\ \text{mol} = \frac{1}{28}\ \text{mol}$.

**36. d.** Sc has 3 valence electrons ($3d^1 4s^2$) and is therefore in group IIIB (transition metals).

**37. b.** 2nd shell: 2 for "second" ($s$ and $p$ are the types of orbitals found in the second shell).

**38. d.** For a principle quantum number of 2, there are four orbitals: 2s, $2p_x$, $2p_y$, and $2p_z$.

**39. a.** The group number of an element corresponds to the number of valence electrons for an atom of that element.

**40. c.** The period number of an element is equal to the number of electron shells in an atom of that element.

**41. c.** An ionic bond forms when electrons are transferred from one atom (now a cation) to another (which becomes an anion).

**42. b.** In $CO_2$, carbon has a +4 oxidation state. During photosynthesis, it is reduced to a lower oxidation state as it is converted into carbohydrates to be used as fuel.

**43. a.** K is transferring its valence electron (1 electron) to Br (which becomes $Br^-$ with 8 valence electrons, a complete octet).

**44. a.** The size of atoms decreases from left to right in the same period and increases from top to bottom in the same group of the periodic table.

**45. b.** Boron is in group III, so it has 3 valence electrons.

**46. d.** An orbital quantum number of 2 corresponds to a d orbital. There are 5 d orbitals, each of which can hold 2 electrons, for a total of 10 electrons that can have these quantum numbers.

**47. b.** The formula for lead (II) hydroxide is $Pb(OH)_2$.

**48. c.** The ionic bond involves the exchange of electrons, the hydrogen bond involves electrostatic attraction between polar molecules, and there is no such thing as a "proton bond." The covalent bond involves the sharing of valence electrons.

**49. b.** While most compounds become slightly denser upon solidifying, water's crystalline structure causes it to expand upon freezing, making it less dense as a solid than as a liquid.

**50. d.** Precision is the degree to which the measurements are replicated, regardless of how close those measurements are to the true value. The group of measurements closest to each other, though not necessarily to 13.0, is 15.2, 15.0, 15.1, and 15.2.

## Scoring

Your scores on the six sections of the exam and on the test as a whole will be reported both as scaled scores and as percentiles. A scaled score is a way of converting the number you got right on this test to a number that can be compared with the number other people got right on other forms of the test, which may have been harder or easier. A percentile is a comparison of your scaled score with the scaled scores of other test takers. If your percentile score is 60, you scored higher than 60% of all test takers; if your percentile score is 84, you scored higher than 84% of all test takers. By definition, a scaled score of 200 is a percentile score of 50.

There is no "passing" scale or percentile score. Individual schools set their own standards, and it's worth your while to find out what scores the schools you want to apply to will accept.

The testing agency uses complicated formulas to come up with scaled and percentile scores. A more meaningful way for you to look at your performance on this practice test is to convert your scores to percentages so that you will be able to compare how you did on the six sections of the test. A *percentage* is not the same as the *percentile* that will appear on your score report. The percentage is simply the number you would have gotten right if there had been 100 questions in the section; it will enable you to compare your scores among the various sections. The *percentile* compares your score with that of other candidates.

In order to find your percentage scores, first add up the number you got right in each section and write it in the following blanks. Questions you didn't answer or got wrong don't count; only count the ones you got right. Then add up the total number of questions you got right.

**Section 1:** _____ of 50 questions right
**Section 2:** _____ of 45 questions right
**Section 3:** _____ of 50 questions right
**Section 4:** _____ of 50 questions right
**Section 5:** _____ of 50 questions right
**Section 6:** _____ of 50 questions right

To figure the percentages for each section and for your total, divide your raw score by the number of questions, and then move the decimal point two places to the right to arrive at a percentage.

Now that you know what percentage of the questions on each section you got right, you can diagnose your strengths and weaknesses. The sections on which you got the lowest percentages are the ones you should plan on studying hardest. Sections on which you got higher percentages may not need as much of your time. However, unless you scored over 90% on a given section, you can't afford to skip studying that section altogether. After all, you want the highest score you can manage in the time left before the exam.

Having taken this practice exam is one important step toward that high score. Simply knowing what to expect is a big help in taking a standardized exam. You are now familiar with the format and content of nursing school entrance exams. Make the most of this advantage by using your scores to help you focus your additional study.

# ADDITIONAL ONLINE PRACTICE ▶

**W**hether you need help building basic skills or preparing for an exam, visit the LearningExpress Practice Center! On this site, you can access additional practice materials. Using the code below, you'll be able to log in and access a practice Nursing School Entrance Exam. This online practice will also provide you with:

**Immediate Scoring**
**Detailed answer explanations**
**Personalized recommendations for further practice and study**

Log in to the LearningExpress Practice Center by using the URL: **www.learnatest.com/practice**

This is your Access Code: **9025**

Follow the steps online to redeem your access code. After you've used your access code to register with the site, you will be prompted to create a username and password. For easy reference, record them here:

**Username:** _____ **Password:** _____

With your username and password, you can log in and access your additional practice materials. If you have any questions or problems, please contact LearningExpress customer service at 1-800-295-9556 ext. 2, or e-mail us at **customerservice@learningexpressllc.com**